Lecture Notes in Computer Science 8700

Commenced Publication in 1973
Founding and Former Series Editors:
Gerhard Goos, Juris Hartmanis, and Jan van Leeuwen

Andreas Holzinger · Carsten Röcker
Martina Ziefle (Eds.)

Smart Health

Open Problems and Future Challenges

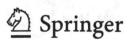 Springer

Editors
Andreas Holzinger
Research Unit HCI-KDD
Medical University of Graz
Graz
Austria

Carsten Röcker
Industrial HCI Research Lab
Fraunhofer Institute
Lemgo
Germany

Martina Ziefle
Human-Computer Interaction Center
RWTH Aachen University
Aachen
Germany

ISSN 0302-9743 ISSN 1611-3349 (electronic)
Lecture Notes in Computer Science
ISBN 978-3-319-16225-6 ISBN 978-3-319-16226-3 (eBook)
DOI 10.1007/978-3-319-16226-3

Library of Congress Control Number: 2015932653

CR Subject Classification (1998): H.2, H.3, H.4, H.5, I.2, I.7, J.3

LNCS Sublibrary: SL3 – Information Systems and Applications, incl. Internet/Web, and HCI

Springer Cham Heidelberg New York Dordrecht London

Printed on acid-free paper

Springer International Publishing AG Switzerland is part of Springer Science+Business Media (www.springer.com)

Foreword

A popular vision of future technology is to make things smart – from homes to cities and phones to cars. The current buzz is all about smart health. But what does it mean to make health smart? Ever more sensing and tracking of body data? But for what reason? From one perspective, it is about raising awareness about people's health and well-being so they can be better informed and be able to act and make intelligent decisions. From society's perspective, it is about accumulating increasing amounts of knowledge about people's health and habits in order to provide better health policies, guidance, and medical care.

While technology has been developed and used for many years to help improve healthcare in hospitals, medical centers, and in the home, we are now witnessing the dawn of a new digital health-tech revolution. Mobile apps and a diversity of sensing devices are becoming more commonplace – placed in and on our bodies to track, monitor, and detect patterns, anomalies, and deviations about how parts of us are behaving. Not only can it tell us more about our blood, urine, and sugar levels but it can also give us fresh insights into our moods, mental states, and motivations. Multiple streams of data are being collated, mined, analyzed, and visualized in new ways to provide new insights into what goes on under the skin. Not only doctors, but also the general public are starting to learn and understand more about how their fitness levels, their illnesses, and their well-being change over time.

A central question this smart health revolution raises, however, is whether it can be put to good use so that people are truly empowered to act upon the knowledge rather than become obsessively concerned about their data or frightened when discovering new patterns in it. How can we design new tools and interfaces so that individuals can be reassured about their data that is being collected, monitored, and aggregated over time and space?

Being smart about health data is not straightforward. There are many questions that need to be addressed from whether to automate or hand over more control to patients to care for themselves; whether to let people know what diseases they are genetically prone to, and so on. Smart health has the potential to enable more people to manage their own health, and in doing so become more aware and better informed. But it also raises a host of moral questions. Who owns the health data being collected? Who is willing to share their health data? Where do the new streams of health data end up? This book is all about how smart health can change society's lives for the better.

December 2014   Yvonne Rogers

About the Editors

Andreas Holzinger is head of the Research Unit HCI-KDD, Institute for Medical Informatics at the Medical University Graz, Lead at the HCI-KDD network, head of the first Austrian IBM Watson Think Group in close cooperation with the Software Group of IBM Austria, Associate Professor of Applied Informatics at the Faculty of Computer Science, Institute of Information Systems and Computer Media, and Lecturer at the Bioinformatics Group at Graz University of Technology. He serves as consultant for the Canadian, Swiss, French, and Dutch Governments, for the German Excellence Initiative, and as national expert in the European Commission (Lisbon Delegate). Andreas was Visiting Professor in Berlin, Innsbruck, Vienna, London, and Aachen. Andreas and his team are passionate on bringing together Human-Computer Interaction and Knowledge Discovery/Data Mining, with the goal of supporting human intelligence with machine learning. Andreas holds a PhD in Cognitive Science and a second PhD (Habiliation) in Computer Science. http://www.hci-kdd.org

Carsten Röcker is head of the Research Unit Usability Engineering at the Fraunhofer Application Center Industrial Automation (IOSB-INA) and professor for User Experience and Interaction Design at the Ostwestfalen-Lippe University of Applied Sciences. Prior to these appointments, he held positions at the RWTH Aachen University (Germany), University of California, San Diego (USA) as well as Fraunhofer IPSI, Darmstadt (Germany) and was guest researcher at the Nara Institute of Science and Technology, Ikoma (Japan), the Medical University Graz (Austria), and the University of Tokyo, Tokyo (Japan). He serves as a consultant for the Australian Research Council (ARC), the Academy of Finland and the Luxembourg National Research Fund (FNR). His current research interests include intelligent systems, human-computer interaction, and technology acceptance. Carsten has an interdisciplinary background with a PhD in Computer Science and a PhD in Psychology. http://www.iosb-ina.fraunhofer.de.

Martina Ziefle is professor for Communication Science at RWTH Aachen University and director of the Human-Computer Interaction Center at RWTH Aachen University. Martina Ziefle studied Psychology at the universities of Göttingen and Würzburg (Germany), where she finished her studies with honors. From the University of Fribourg, Switzerland, she received her PhD in Psychology summa cum laude. After her habilitation at RWTH, in which she examined reading processes in electronic media, Martina Ziefle took up positions as Assistant Professor at the University of Münster and, subsequently, as Full Professor at the RWTH Aachen. The research of Martina addresses human factors in different technology types and using contexts. Technology acceptance decisively depends on the extent to which user diversity is considered and implemented in technological design. A special research focus is directed to the design of medical technologies with a focus on users' specific needs. http://www.comm.rwth-aachen.de.

Preface

Health costs worldwide are rapidly increasing. Demographic structures are dramatically changing. Technological advances are tremendously increasing. The invariable need for quality remains.

Advances in Biomedical Informatics and Biomedical Engineering provide the foundations for our modern and future patient-centered medical and healthcare solutions, biomedical systems, technologies, and techniques.

The majority of computer-supported healthcare solutions of the last decades focused on the support of caregivers and medical professionals; this changed dramatically with the introduction of ubiquitous computing technologies and the enormous success of mobile computing: in particular, smart phones with multi-touch interaction along with sophisticated sensor networks. Future smart technologies using the power of grid computers and supercomputing – driven by examples including IBM Watson and Apple Siri – will enable that a new concept of smart health provides support for a more diverse end user group to enable individualized medicine, i.e., the P4-medicine (preventive, participatory, predictive, personalized).

However, all these advances produce enormous amounts of data and one of the grand challenges in our networked world are the large and high-dimensional datasets, and the massive amounts of unstructured information. To keep pace with these growing amounts of complex data, smart hospital approaches are a commandment of the future, necessitating context-aware computing along with advanced interaction paradigms in new physical-digital ecosystems. In such a smart hospital the medical doctors are supported by smart technologies. At the same time people at home can be supported by their technological health assistants to facilitate an overall healthier life, wellness and well-being – and the circle of P4-medicine is closed.

The very successful synergistic combination of methodologies and approaches from two areas offer ideal conditions toward solving the aforementioned problems: Human-Computer Interaction (HCI) and Knowledge Discovery and Data Mining (KDD). The vision is to support human intelligence with machine learning.

Consequently, the objective is to combine the best of both worlds: HCI, with the emphasis on human issues including perception, cognition, interaction, reasoning, decision making, human learning, and human intelligence; and KDD, encompassing the wide range of artificial intelligence. Whatever we do, issues of privacy, data-protection, safety, and security are mandatory in the medicine and health domains.

Volume 8700 of the Springer Lecture Notes in Computer Science is a State-of-the-Art Volume focusing on hot topics on smart health. Each paper describes the state-of-the-art and focuses on open problems and future challenges in order to provide a research agenda to stimulate further research and progress.

To acknowledge here all those who contributed toward all our efforts and stimulating discussions would be sheer impossible. Many people contributed to the development of this book, either directly or indirectly, so we will use the plural form here:

First of all we thank the members of our international advisory board (http://hci-kdd. org/phealth), for their expertise and patient reviews on the papers collected in this book – we are grateful for critical comments and discussions from members of the HCI-KDD network (http://hci-kdd.org/expert-network-hci-kdd).

We thank our institutes for the academic freedom we enjoy, the intellectual environments, and the opportunity for carrying out such crazy scientific enterprises.

We thank our families, our friends, and our colleagues for their nurturing and positive encouragement. Last but not least we thank the Springer management team and the Springer production team for their constant smooth support.

December 2014
Andreas Holzinger
Carsten Röcker
Martina Ziefle

Organization

International Scientific Committee

Additionally to the experts below we are grateful for the support and help of members of the expert group HCI-KDD, see http://hci-kdd.org/expert-network-hci-kdd/.

International Scientific Committee

Gregory D. Abowd	Georgia Tech, Atlanta, USA
Rosa Arriaga	Georgia Tech, Atlanta, USA
Juan Carlos Augusto	Middlesex University, UK
Jakob Bardram	IT University of Copenhagen, Denmark
Bert Bongers	University of Technology Sydney, Australia
Pam Briggs	Northumbria University, UK
Matt-Mouley Bouamrane	University of Glasgow, UK
Stefan Carmien	Tecnalia, Spain
John M. Carroll	Human-Computer Interaction, Pennsylvania State University, USA
Brian Caulfield	University College Dublin, Ireland
Mary Czerwinski	Microsoft Research, USA
Anind K. Dey	Human-Computer Interaction, Carnegie Mellon University, USA
Paul Fergus	Liverpool John Moores University, UK
Marie Gustafsson-Friberger	Malmö University, Sweden
Eduard Groeller	Vienna University of Technology, Austria
Erik Grönvall	Aarhus University, Denmark
Gourab Sen Gupta	Massey University, New Zealand
Jim Hollan	University of California, San Diego, USA
Maddy Janse	Philips Research, The Netherlands
Ray Jones	University of Plymouth, UK
Henry Kautz	University of Rochester, USA
Shin'ichi Konomi	The University of Tokyo, Japan
Kristof van Laerhoven	Embedded Sensing Systems, Technische Universität Darmstadt, Germany
Christine Lisetti	Florida International University, USA
Lenka Lhotska	Czech Technical University, Czech Republic
Paul Lukowicz	DFKI and University of Kaiserslautern, Germany
Anthony J. Maeder	University of Western Sydney, Australia
Marilyn McGee-Lennon	University of Glasgow, UK
Oscar Mayora	CREATE-NET, Italy

Contents

From Smart Health to Smart Hospitals

Andreas Holzinger[1(✉)], Carsten Röcker[1,2],
and Martina Ziefle[3]

[1] Holzinger Group, Research Unit HCI-KDD, Institute for Medical Informatics,
Statistics and Documentation, Medical University Graz, Graz, Austria
{a.holzinger,c.roecker}@hci-kdd.org
[2] Fraunhofer Application Center Industrial Automation (IOSB-INA),
Lemgo, Germany
carsten.roecker@iosb-ina.fraunhofer.de
[3] Human–Computer Interaction Center, RWTH Aachen University,
Aachen, Germany
ziefle@comm.rwth-aachen.de

Abstract. Prolonged life expectancy along with the increasing complexity of medicine and health services raises health costs worldwide dramatically. Advancements in ubiquitous computing applications in combination with the use of sophisticated intelligent sensor networks may provide a basis for help. Whilst the *smart health* concept has much potential to support the concept of the emerging P4-medicine (preventive, participatory, predictive, and personalized), such high-tech medicine produces large amounts of high-dimensional, weakly-structured data sets and massive amounts of unstructured information. All these technological approaches along with "big data" are turning the medical sciences into a data-intensive science. To keep pace with the growing amounts of complex data, *smart hospital* approaches are a commandment of the future, necessitating context aware computing along with advanced interaction paradigms in new physical-digital ecosystems. In such a system the medical doctors are supported by their smart mobile medical assistants on managing their floods of data semi-automatically by following the human-in-the-loop concept. At the same time patients are supported by their health assistants to facilitate a healthier life, wellness and wellbeing.

Keywords: Smart health · Smart hospital · Ubiquitous computing · Pervasive health · P4 medicine · Context awareness · Computational intelligence

1   Introduction and Motivation

Life expectancy on our planet is still increasing [1, 2]. The World Population Database of the United Nations Population Information Network, POPIN (http://www.un.org/popin) forecasts a further increase in life expectancy through 2050. This prolonged life expectancy along with an increasing survival of acute diseases poses a lot of challenges for health care systems worldwide, making the use of sophisticated technologies not an added value, but a requirement [3].

© Springer International Publishing Switzerland 2015
A. Holzinger et al. (Eds.): Smart Health, LNCS 8700, pp. 1–20, 2015.
DOI: 10.1007/978-3-319-16226-3_1

Along with the worldwide increasing complexity of health care systems and the fact that modern medicine is turning into a data-intensive science, traditional approaches for handling this "big data" can no longer keep pace with demand, also increasing the risk of delivering unsatisfactory results. Consequently, to cope with this rising flood of data, *smart* approaches are vital [4–8].

Particularly, the advent of smart phones, powerful ubiquitous smart sensors and decreasing costs of data storage has led to an ongoing trend to record all sort of personal biomedical data over time [9, 10]. These recordings lead also to a growing amount of so-called longitudinal data, in the engineering domain better known as time series data [11, 12], being of much importance for predictive analytics – one of the cornerstones of P4-medicine (see Sect. 4.1).

The meanwhile "historic" vision by Mark Weiser of ubiquitous computing [13] and smart objects [14] is also true for healthcare: Moore's law [15] is also applicable for biomedical sensors which will be embedded in more devices than we can imagine. The vision is that people will interact seamlessly in both cyberspace and physical space. The power of such cyber-physical systems [16], is in their "intelligence", i.e. smartness, which lies in their adaptive behavior.

A major future trend is moving the human-in-the-loop [17], for a good reason, as both humans and computers have very different strengths, but both together can indeed be more powerful. At large scale this means to combine the best of two worlds: cognitive science with computer science [18, 19].

Recent technological advances in networked sensors, low-power integrated circuits, and wireless communications have enabled the design of low-cost, miniature, light-weight, and intelligent physiological sensor nodes [20]. All these developments leave enormous expectations to our future: Smart environments will be able to automatically track our health and will, to some extend, shift the point of care away from clinician's offices – thus hopefully be of economic relieve of the much overstressed hospital systems and moving the preventive aspect into the foreground. There is a clear paradigm shift from explicit measuring your health vitals to sensors that fade in the background and track important measures. Second, consumers tend to increasingly like becoming their own health managers and actively participate in healthcare. This hypothesis is expressed through a booming movement called "Quantified Self" were consumer constantly track health vitals such as sleep patterns, blood pressure and body fat.

This paper provides a very brief overview about the concept of smart health, discusses the challenge of "big data" driven by the emerging P4-medicine, and debates some aspects of smart hospitals, with a focus on how to deal with the large amounts of data. Finally, we present some open questions and future challenges – only by touching some aspects on the surface just to stimulate the debate.

2 Glossary

Acceptance: A very important concept for the successful integration of any smart health concept, the term goes back to the work of [21].

Ambient Intelligence: This term was coined within the European research community [22], as a reaction to the terms Ubiquitous Computing [13] and Pervasive Computing [23], which were introduced and frequently used by American researchers. In contrast to the more technical terms of Ubiquitous and Pervasive Computing, Ambient Intelligence emphasizes aspects of Human–Computer Interaction and Artificial Intelligence. Hence, the emphasis of Ambient Intelligence is on better usability, more efficient and embedded services, user-empowerment and support for advanced human interactions [24].

Context Awareness: Involves knowledge about how individuals interact within a shared socio-technical environment and includes information about the participants' locations, their present and past actions, and their intentions and possible future actions [25, 26].

Context-aware computing: Integration of multiple diverse sensors for awareness of situational context that can not be inferred from location, and targeted at mobile device platforms that typically do not permit processing of visual context [26, 27].

E-Health: Describes the fusion of medicine and healthcare services through the use of information and communication technologies, with particular focus on everyday life and low cost devices [28].

E-Homecare: Similar to the E-Health, but with a strong focus on preventive care applications in the home domain [29]. E-Homecare services may include patient assessment, supervision of patient care, routine nursing care and health monitoring, medication administration and scheduled injections, management of dietary needs, daily exercise, and lifestyle changes [30].

P4-Medicine: Focusing on the four aspects: predictive, personalized, preventive and participatory, P4-medicine moves from a reactive to a proactive discipline supported by systems approaches to disease, emerging smart technologies and analytical tools [31]; actually "big data" is good for P4-medicine, as machine learning approaches may get better results by more training examples.

Privacy: A must in the health domain is to ensure privacy, data protection, safety and security; a particular necessity in smart health, as main security problems encompass protection Precautions, confidentiality, and integrity, which is a challenge as most of the smart devices are working in a wireless environment [32–34].

Smart: The word synonym for clever, socially elegant, sophisticated, shrewd, showing witty behaviour and ready mental capability, is a term which is intended to replace the overly stressed word "intelligent", mostly due to the fact that research in both human and artificial intelligence is lacking far behind the original expectations when the field of artificial intelligence was formed [35].

Smart Health: A term, inherently integrating ideas from ubiquitous computing and ambient intelligence applied to the future P4-medicine concept, thus tightly connected to concepts of wellness and wellbeing [3, 36], and including big data, collected by large amounts of biomedical sensors (e.g., temperature, heart rate, blood pressure, blood and urine chemical levels, breathing rate and volume, activity levels etc.) and actuators, to monitor, predict and improve patients' physical and mental conditions.

Smart Hospital: An old dream of a highly interactive environment saturated with high-end ubiquitous devices [37], and closely related to the context aware health paradigm [38]; this topic is in the strategic focus of large companies including IBM, Siemens, Google, etc., as it is highly business relevant, as it might help to overcome the worldwide cost problems of health systems.

Smart Multi-agents: consist of n interacting smart agents within an given environment and are used to solve difficult problems, impossible solvable by an individual agent. The goal of an agent based model is to search for explanatory insight into the collective behavior of the agents, which can be software agents, robots, humans or collective human teams. Smart agents are usually active software agents with simple goals (e.g. birds in flocking or wolf-sheep in the prey-predator model), or they can be complex cognitive agents. Such approaches have enormous capacity for solving biomedical problems.

Ubiquitous Computing (UbiComp): A vision by Weiser (1991) [39], who argued, that computers should be integrated into the physical environment, and hence be effectively invisible to the user, rather than distinct objects on the desktop. Making many computers available throughout the physical environment enables people to move around and interact with computers, more naturally than they currently do, leading to the disappearing computer concept [40].

Wellness Technology: A term mainly introduced to correct the negative connotations of 'technology for disability' and associated with technical devices for the prevention of deterioration, the support of changes in lifestyle, and the improvement of social contacts [41], becoming now more important [42].

3   From Ubiquitous Computing to Smart Health Environments

Ubiquitous computing provides enormous possibilities for establishing smart health services as integral parts of future care concepts [43], which are challenged by our ageing society. In this context, in particular smart homecare environments are often propagated as a promising solution for taking care of elderly or disabled people. Sensors and new interaction technologies seamlessly integrated in such environments offer various forms of personalized and context-adapted medial support, including assistance to carry out everyday activities, monitoring personal health conditions, enhancing patient safety, as well as getting access to social, medical and emergency systems. By providing a wide variety of services, smart healthcare applications bear the potential of bringing medical, social and economical benefits to different stakeholders. The goals are from enhancing comfort, supporting autonomy enhancement up to emergency assistance, including detection, prevention, and prediction (Fig. 1).

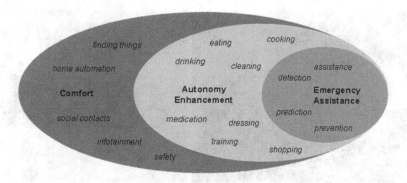

Fig. 1. From emergency assistance (right) to autonomy enhancement and comfort [44].

Technological challenges include mobility, invisibility (smart devices embedded in our daily objects, e.g. clothes as in wearable computing [45], watches [46], glasses [47], etc.), natural communication including voice and gestures instead of keyboard or mouse [48], and most of all adaptivity and context-awareness, as those two important issues "adaptive behavior in context" are key for "intelligence" i.e., capable of reacting to all abnormal and exceptional situations in a flexible way.

3.1 Emergency Support

The majority of existing systems for detecting and preventing medical emergencies focus on falls and congestive heart failures as their main application areas. In particular fall detection becomes more and more important as recent statistics show that over 30 % of the people over 65 years and 50 % of the people over 80 years fall at least once a year [49]. In approximately one fourth of these cases, people suffer serious injuries with sustaining effects on their mobility and independence [50]. As many of these falls happen when people are alone at home, several projects started to develop mobile emergency systems, which should enable users to call for help in an emergency situation [51]. While mobile solutions seem to be a promising approach at first sight, empirical evidence shows that patients often do not carry those devices with them or are simply not able to operate them when medical problems have occurred. Consequently, several research projects developed prototypes of pressure sensitive floor elements allowing the detection of falls without additional technology being worn by the patient. While early systems distributed pressure sensitive floor tiles at specific locations within the environment (e.g. [52, 53]), more recent approaches use distributed sensors to cover an entire room and thereby enable fine-grained location detection [54], see Fig. 2.

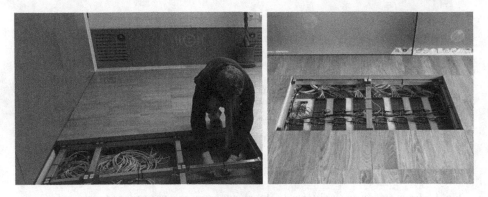

Fig. 2. Smart Floor consisting of an array of pressure sensitive floor tiles for unobtrusively monitoring patients in home environments [54, 55].

3.2   Monitoring of Patients with Chronic Diseases

Long-term treatment of chronic conditions does not only increase the quality of life for patients, it is also expected to bring significant economical benefits compared to traditional care concepts. Hence, it is not surprising that a broad variety of smart health services have been developed for various kinds of chronic diseases. For example, Klack et al. (2011) [56] developed an assistive home monitoring system for patients suffering from end-stage heart failure, which incorporates medical data captured via different biosensors embedded into the patient's physical surrounding. The system focuses particularly on patients with implanted mechanical circulatory support devices, including ventricular assist devices and total artificial hearts and provides an easy and unobtrusive way for monitoring crucial vital parameters over extended periods of time. Figure 3 shows the monitoring system in a home environment. An infrared camera is integrated behind a translucent interactive display, weight sensors are installed under the entire floor and blood pressure and coagulation monitoring devices are implemented in a coffee table next to the sofa.

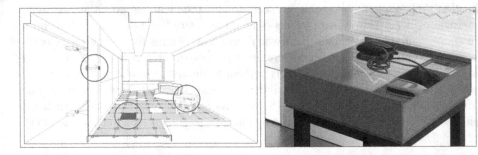

Fig. 3. Medical sensors integrated in a smart home environment (left), blood pressure and coagulation-monitoring device embedded in a coffee table (right), from the RWTH Living Lab

Similar research prototypes have been developed for patients with diabetes [57], (for the importance of diabetes refer to [58]), pulmonary diseases [59], memory loss [60–62], physical impairments [63–65], for the aurally disabled [66, 67] for the elderly [68, 69], or for wellness of the young [42].

An interesting pioneering sample work has been presented by Park et al. (2003) [61]: in their smart home project they devised a set of intelligent home appliances that provided awareness of the end users needs and to improve day-to-day home life with various smart technologies, including smart memories (the smart home learns favourite ambient settings), smart pen (translates and offers additional help on vocabularies during reading of text), gate reminder (reminds you before you leave your house on important issues), smart photo album (see here also [70]), smart wardrobe (looks up the weather forecast and recommends adequate clothing), smart dressing table, smart bed, smart pillow, smart mat, smart table (see here also [71]), smart picture frame, smart furniture (see here particularly [40]), smart refrigerator, smart sofa, smart greenhouse, smart wall, smart window, and smart bathroom.

3.3 Integrated Care Environments

Over the last years, several prototypes of integrated medical care environments have been developed, which incorporate different smart healthcare. For example, the Future Care Lab (Fig. 4) at RWTH Aachen University provides an intelligent care infrastructure, consisting of different mobile and integrated devices, for supporting elderly people in technology-enhanced home environments. The setup of the lab enables in situ evaluations of new care concepts and medical technologies by observing different target user populations in realistic usage situations. As the lab relies on a modular technical concept, it can be expanded with other technical products, systems and functionalities, in order to address different user groups as well as individuals with differences in their cognitive, health-related or cultural needs [43] (Röcker et al. 2010).

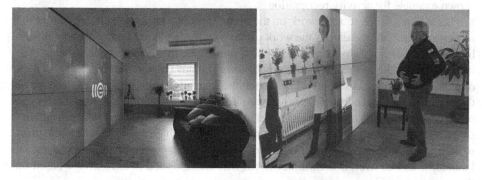

Fig. 4. An example of smart medical technologies integrated into a smart home environment, from the RWTH Living Lab

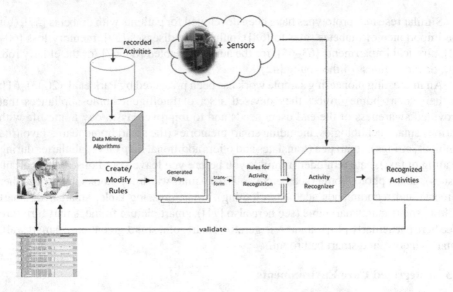

Fig. 5. Concept of Human-in-the-loop (Doctor-in-the-loop), similar to supervised learning. With massive sensor data only machine learning approaches can bring us further.

3.4 Machine Learning: Human-in-the-Loop

Whereas large amounts of data not good for humans, as they are difficult to handle manually, large data sets are good for machine learning algorithms, as the more training data are available the better results are achieved. However, a perfect match of both together is to include the human-in-the-loop. Figure 5 shows an example: a medical-doctor-in-the-loop crates and modifies rules on demand to train the algorithms, in the shown example for activity recognition.

There is not much related work on the human-in-the-loop approach yet, one of the most prominent ones to date is the work of Shyu et al. (1999) [72]: they implemented a human-in-the-loop (a physician-in-the-loop, more specifically) approach in which the medical doctor delineates the pathology bearing regions (regions of interest) and a set of anatomical landmarks in the image when the image is entered into the database. To the regions thus marked, their approach applies low-level computer vision and image processing algorithms to extract attributes related to the variations in gray scale, texture, shape, etc. Additionally their system recorded attributes which captured relational information such as the position of a region of interest with respect to certain anatomical landmarks and an overall multidimensional index is assigned to each image based on these attribute values.

4   From Smart Health to the Smart Hospital

4.1   Future Medicine as a Data Science

Today the design of a drug involves more data science than biological or medical science. The life sciences are increasingly turning into a data intensive science [73–76]. In bioinformatics and computational biology we face not only increased volume and a heterogeneity and diversity of highly complex, multi-dimensional, multivariate and weakly-structured, noisy and dirty data [6, 7, 77–79], but also the growing need for integrative analysis and modeling [80–85]. Due to the increasing trend towards P4-medicine: Predictive, Preventive, Participatory, Personalized [76, 86], even more amounts of large and complex data sets, particularly omics-data [87], including data from genomics, epi-genomics, meta-genomics, proteomics, metabolomics, lipidomics, transcriptomics, epigenetics, microbiomics, fluxomics, phenomics, etc., are becoming available. A recent article on "HCI for Personal Genomics" by [88] gets straight to the point: Recent advances in -omics along with Web technologies have led to a dramatic increase in the amount of available complex data sets to both expert and non-expert users. They emphasize that the HCI community is challenged with designing and developing tools and practices that can help make such data more accessible and understandable. However, the problem is, that despite the fact that humans are excellent at pattern recognition in dimensions of lower than three [89], most of our current data is in dimensions much higher than three, making manual analysis difficult, yet often impossible [90]. Today, biomedical experts both in daily routine and science are no longer capable of dealing with such increasingly large, complex, high-dimensional and weakly-structured data sets. Consequently, efficient, useable computational methods, algorithms and tools to interactively gain insight into such data are a commandment of the time [91].

Consequently, a synergistic combination of methodologies and approaches of two areas offer ideal conditions towards unraveling these problems: Human-Computer Interaction (HCI) and Knowledge Discovery/Data Mining (KDD), with the goal of supporting human intelligence with machine learning – human-in-the-loop – to discover novel, previously unknown insights into the data [18]. Big Data is bad for humans, but good for machines, as machine learning algorithms improve their precision with the amount of training samples, however, what we really need is not more data – but *better* data.

4.2   Mobile Medical Doctors Assistants

The vision of a "mobile medical doctor's assistant" is an example of a cognitive computing project (see Sect. 5) that shall enable a more natural interaction between medical professionals and biomedical data and would be a cornerstone in the development of a smart hospital, and can contribute to enhanced patient safety [92]. One step to reach such a goal is in the application of sophisticated modern technologies such as the Watson Content Analytics. Technologically, "Watson" consists of diverse algorithms, created in the context of cognitive computing research to demonstrate the capability of the DeepQA technology [93]. The challenge to date is, that Watson has "no eyes and no ears", so Watson needs sophisticated user interfaces, to date Watson the current algorithms – sophisticated as they are – are far from being usable for the non-expert end user [5].

A future vision is to make the Watson technology useable from a smart phone – so that a medical professional can ask questions to the data, e.g. "Show me the similarities, differences, anomalies … between patients with symptom X and patients with symptom Y". Why mobility? Medical professionals work in an environment which requires high mobility; within their daily routine their sphere of activity alters frequently between wards, outpatient clinics, diagnostic and therapeutic departments and operating theatres – they rarely sit in an office. Although access to stationary clinical workstations is provided in the hospital, their locations do not always coincide with the user's current workplace. In order to fulfill a high health service standard, the medical staff has an extensive demand for information at a number of locations – which actually only mobile computers can supply [94]. For example: Up-to-the-minute electronic patient record information is not always available at the bedside [95, 96]. New orders or diagnostic results noted during rounds must be transcribed to the electronic patient records via a clinical workstation at a later time – whereas a mobile computer enables direct access [97–100].

4.3 Smart Hospital

Mark Weiser (1991) expressed his vision of invisible computing by his famous sentence: "… the most profound technologies are those that disappear [39]". We interpret this and develop it further: "The best technology is those who is in the direct workflow", and practically not perceived as such. A smart hospital would integrate all aforementioned approaches with the aim to support both professionals and patients.

Approaches to a smart hospital are rare to date, a search in the Web of Science as of December, 30, 2014 returned only 22 hits (title = "smart hospital"). The most prominent example is a project on Activity recognition for the smart hospital, by the group around Jesus Favela [37]: they developed an approach for automatically estimating hospital-staff activities, where they trained a discrete hidden Markov model (HMM) to map contextual information to a user activity. The vision of the authors is called iHospital and includes a highly interactive smart environment saturated with heterogeneous computing devices. At the core of this approach is context aware computing (see Sect. 5).

5   Future Challenges

5.1   Challenge 1: Context Aware Computing

Context is *key* in the development of the smart hospital in the sense that it is any *information* that can be used to characterize the situation of entities (people, places, objects), considered to be relevant to the *interaction* between an end user and an ubiquitous computing application [101]. A classical paper [102] provides a good overview of context in the field of artificial intelligence. If context is redefined continually and ubiquitously, then how can users form an accurate model of a constantly evolving digital world? If system adaptation is negotiated, then how do we avoid disruption in human activities? A clear architecture and a well-founded, explicit relationship between environment and adaptation are the critical factors; indeed, they are the key that will unlock context-aware computing at a global scale [103]. Such approaches require the integration of concepts in User Experience and Context-aware computing in the sense of [26], and [27] and to see our surrounding environment as a Physical-Digital Ecosystem [104–106]. Context aware computing is not only key for the smart hospital, but for the overall smart health principle: Situational awareness can be used to reduce the amount of explicit input a person is required to provide a computer. Contextual information of what and where the user task is, what the user knows, and what the system capabilities are, can simplify the user scenario [107]. Improving the user experience *is not enough;* we need concepts, frameworks, and methods that will enable it to consider humans and computers as part of our complex world full of limitations and opportunities (see also challenge 4).

5.2 Challenge 2: Cognitive Computing

Cognitive computing (cc) is suited to solve medical problems: because it is on how to deal with complex situations and information uncertainty, and dealing with probable information is the key challenge in biomedical informatics [108]. The quest towards a smart hospital requires new breakthroughs in the overlapping area of cognitive science and computer science: Whilst high-dimensionality of our data is often regarded as a curse [109], it is also possible that very high dimensionality actually facilitates processing: for example, numbers (i.e., scalars) can be seen as one-dimensional data, but in a computer they can be represented by strings of bits, i.e. by high-dimensional vectors, so a 32-bit integer can be seen as a binary vector in $\mathbb{R}^{32}$. Such a high-dimensional representation makes simple algorithms and circuits for high-precision arithmetic possible. We can contrast this with one-dimensional representation of numbers. The slide rule represents them one-dimensionally and makes calculating awkward and imprecise. Thus, the dimensionality of an entity (a number) and the dimensionality of its representation for computing purposes (a bit vector) are separate issues – the first with the existence in our world, the other with the manipulation by algorithms in abstract spaces – which is more suitable for computing. Pentti Kanerva (2009) [110] shows a nice example of the advantages of such a hyper-dimensional approach, which we cannot discuss here due to the limited space but we can summarize: A grand challenge of cognitive computing is to explore both hyper-dimensional representation of data and **randomness.** This brings us further beyond Von-Neumann machines and is a core topic of brain informatics [111–113] – which may bring us to both smart health and smart hospitals.

5.3 Challenge 3: Stochastic Computation

Closely related to cognitive computing by emphasizing the aspect of randomness is the concept of stochastic computation [114]. Stochastic computing (sc) was proposed in the 1960s as a low-cost alternative to conventional binary computing. It is unique in that it represents and processes information in the form of digitized probabilities and employs low-complexity arithmetic units which was a primary design concern in the past – due to the limited computing power and inaccurate results [115]. Meanwhile, Bayesian computational techniques such as Markov chain Monte Carlo (MCMC), Sequential Monte Carlo (SMC), and Approximate Bayesian Computation (ABC) methods are well established and have revolutionized the practice of Bayesian statistics, however new grand opportunities have appeared with the emergence of massive, high-dimensional and complex data sets [116, 117]. Stochastic computation is an approach for the design of robust and energy-efficient systems-on-chip (SOC) in nanoscale process technologies [118], which will be vital for smart hospital environments. The reduction of size along with massive parallelization is one step towards implementing stochastic computation approaches, hence to overcome classical von Neumann machines to perform meaningful and accurate computations in neural circuits. Much work is needed here in the future, but there are promising ideas for the realization of smart health and smart hospital particularly in programmable and autonomous stochastic molecular automata, which have been shown to perform direct analysis of disease-related molecular indicators in vitro and may have the potential to provide in situ medical diagnosis and cure [119].

5.4   Challenge 4: Smart Multi-agent Collectives with Experts-in-the-Loop

Multi-agent systems are an extremely interesting research area [120–123] and are becoming continually important for solving medical problems (e.g. [124]). Human–Agent collectives (HAC) are an upcoming class of socio-technical hybrid systems in which both humans and smart agents may develop a flexible relationship to achieve both their individual and collective goals. It is increasingly accepted that it is both necessary and beneficial to involve human experts, working as active information processors, in a concerted effort together with smart agents [125, 126]. Such approaches are completely in line with the goal of combining cognitive science with computer science [19], following the HCI-KDD approach [18]. The challenge in Human-Agent collectives is, that despite relevant work in the AI, HCI and Ubicomp communities a comprehensive scientific foundation is lacking, hence is of urgent need for fundamental research; in particular the challenges are in flexible autonomy (balance control between human experts and smart agents), agile teaming, incentive engineering and most of all on how to provide a necessary infrastructure, and the application of machine learning to network metrics and the human labelling of graphs provide a lot of interesting research challenges [127]. There are several best practice examples from disaster management [128, 129].

5.5   Challenge 5: Beyond Data Mining

As Yvonne Rogers pointed out in the Foreword to this volume: Being smart about health data is not straightforward: Smart health has the potential to enable more people to manage their own health, and in doing so become more aware and better informed. But it also raises many moral questions. Who owns the health data being collected? Who is willing to share their health data? Where do the new streams of health data end up? All these questions must be considered when realizing a smart hospital. These are grand challenges and not easy to tackle and can be summarized as "What comes beyond data mining?", to close with the words of Tim Menzies "Prediction is all well and good – but what about decision making?" [130].

References

1. Oeppen, J., Vaupel, J.W.: Demography - broken limits to life expectancy. Science **296**(5570), 1029 (2002)
2. Mathers, C.D., Stevens, G.A., Boerma, T., White, R.A., Tobias, M.I.: Causes of international increases in older age life expectancy. Lancet **385**(9967), 540–548 (2015)
3. Röcker, C., Ziefle, M., Holzinger, A.: From computer innovation to human integration: current trends and challenges for pervasive HealthTechnologies. In: Holzinger, A., Ziefle, M., Röcker, C. (eds.) Pervasive Health, pp. 1–17. Springer, London (2014)
4. Holzinger, A., Dehmer, M., Jurisica, I.: Knowledge discovery and interactive data mining in bioinformatics - state-of-the-art, future challenges and research directions. BMC Bioinform. **15**(Suppl 6), I1 (2014)
5. Holzinger, A., Stocker, C., Ofner, B., Prohaska, G., Brabenetz, A., Hofmann-Wellenhof, R.: Combining HCI, natural language processing, and knowledge discovery - potential of IBM content analytics as an assistive technology in the biomedical field. In: Holzinger, A., Pasi, G. (eds.) HCI-KDD 2013. LNCS, vol. 7947, pp. 13–24. Springer, Heidelberg (2013)
6. Holzinger, A.: On knowledge discovery and interactive intelligent visualization of biomedical data - challenges in human–computer interaction and biomedical informatics. In: DATA 2012, pp. 9–20 (2012)
7. Holzinger, A.: Weakly structured data in health-informatics: the challenge for human-computer interaction. In: Proceedings of INTERACT 2011 Workshop: Promoting and Supporting Healthy Living by Design, pp. 5–7. IFIP (2011)
8. Duerr-Specht, M., Goebel, R., Holzinger, A.: Medicine and health care as a data problem: will computers become better medical doctors? In: Holzinger, A., Roecker, C., Ziefle, M. (eds.) Smart Health. LNCS, vol. 8700, pp. 21-39. Springer, Heidelberg (2015)
9. Culler, D.E., Mulder, H.: Smart sensors to network the world. Sci. Am. **290**(6), 84–91 (2004)
10. Ghrist, R., de Silva, V.: Homological sensor networks. Notic. Amer. Math. Soc. **54**(1), 10–17 (2007)
11. Esling, P., Agon, C.: Time-series data mining. ACM Comput. Surv. (CSUR) **45**(1), 12 (2012)
12. Holzinger, A., Schwarz, M., Ofner, B., Jeanquartier, F., Calero-Valdez, A., Roecker, C., Ziefle, M.: Towards interactive visualization of longitudinal data to support knowledge discovery on multi-touch tablet computers. In: Teufel, S., Min, T.A., You, I., Weippl, E. (eds.) CD-ARES 2014. LNCS, vol. 8708, pp. 124–137. Springer, Heidelberg (2014)
13. Weiser, M.: Some computer science issues in ubiquitous computing. Commun. ACM **36**(7), 75–84 (1993)
14. Weiser, M., Gold, R., Brown, J.S.: The origins of ubiquitous computing research at PARC in the late 1980s. IBM Syst. J. **38**, 693–696 (1999)
15. Moore, G.E.: Cramming more components onto integrated circuits. Electronics **38**(8), 114–117 (1965)
16. Wu, F.J., Kao, Y.F., Tseng, Y.C.: From wireless sensor networks towards cyber physical systems. Pervasive Mob. Comput. **7**(4), 397–413 (2011)
17. Schirner, G., Erdogmus, D., Chowdhury, K., Padir, T.: The future of human-in-the-loop cyber-physical systems. Computer **46**(1), 36–45 (2013)

18. Holzinger, A.: Human-computer interaction and knowledge discovery (HCI-KDD): what is the benefit of bringing those two fields to work together? In: Cuzzocrea, A., Kittl, C., Simos, D.E., Weippl, E., Xu, L. (eds.) CD-ARES 2013. LNCS, vol. 8127, pp. 319–328. Springer, Heidelberg (2013)
19. Holzinger, A.: Trends in interactive knowledge discovery for personalized medicine: cognitive science meets machine learning. Intell. Inform. Bull. 15(1), 6–14 (2014)
20. Milenkovic, A., Otto, C., Jovanov, E.: Wireless sensor networks for personal health monitoring: issues and an implementation. Comput. Commun. 29(13–14), 2521–2533 (2006)
21. Davis, F.D.: Perceived usefulness, perceived ease of use, and user acceptance of information technology. MIS Q. 13(3), 319–339 (1989)
22. Aarts, E., Harwig, E., Schuurmans, M.: Ambient intelligence. In: Denning, J. (ed.) The Invisible Future, pp. 235–250. McGraw-Hill, New York (2001)
23. Satyanarayanan, M.: Pervasive computing: vision and challenges. IEEE Pers. Commun. 8(4), 10–17 (2001)
24. Ramos, C., Augusto, J.C., Shapiro, D.: Ambient intelligence - the next step for artificial intelligence. IEEE Intell. Syst. 23(2), 15–18 (2008)
25. Abowd, G.D., Dey, A.K.: Towards a better understanding of context and context-awareness. In: Gellersen, H.-W. (ed.) HUC 1999. LNCS, vol. 1707, pp. 304–307. Springer, Heidelberg (1999)
26. Gellersen, H.W., Schmidt, A., Beigl, M.: Multi-sensor context-awareness in mobile devices and smart artifacts. Mob. Netw. Appl. 7(5), 341–351 (2002)
27. Bardram, J.E., Hansen, T.R., Mogensen, M., Soegaard, M.: Experiences from real-world deployment of context-aware technologies in a hospital environment. In: Dourish, P., Friday, A. (eds.) UbiComp 2006. LNCS, vol. 4206, pp. 369–386. Springer, Heidelberg (2006)
28. Yan, H.R., Huo, H.W., Xu, Y.Z., Gidlund, M.: Wireless sensor network based e-health system - implementation and experimental results. IEEE Trans. Consum. Electron. 56(4), 2288–2295 (2010)
29. Demiris, G., Rantz, M.J., Aud, M.A., Marek, K.D., Tyrer, H.W., Skubic, M., Hussam, A.A.: Older adults' attitudes towards and perceptions of 'smart home' technologies: a pilot study. Med. Inform. Internet Med. 29(2), 87–94 (2004)
30. Demiris, G., Tan, J.: Rejuvenating home health care and tele-home care. In: Tan, J. (ed.) E-Health Care Information Systems: An Introduction for Students and Professionals, pp. 267–290. Jossey-Bass, San Francisco (2005)
31. Hood, L., Friend, S.H.: Predictive, personalized, preventive, participatory (P4) cancer medicine. Nat. Rev. Clin. Oncol. 8(3), 184–187 (2011)
32. Weippl, E., Holzinger, A., Tjoa, A.M.: Security aspects of ubiquitous computing in health care. Springer Elektrotechnik und Informationstechnik, e & i 123(4), 156–162 (2006)
33. Holzinger, A., Nischelwitzer, A., Friedl, S., Hu, B.: Towards life long learning: three models for ubiquitous applications. Wirel. Commun. Mob. Comput. 10(10), 1350–1365 (2010)
34. Kieseberg, P., Hobel, H., Schrittwieser, S., Weippl, E., Holzinger, A.: Protecting anonymity in data-driven biomedical science. In: Holzinger, A., Jurisica, I. (eds.) Interactive Knowledge Discovery and Data Mining in Biomedical Informatics. LNCS, vol. 8401, pp. 301–316. Springer, Heidelberg (2014)
35. Minsky, M.: Steps towards artificial intelligence. Proc. Inst. Radio Eng. 49(1), 8–30 (1961)
36. Suryadevara, N.K., Mukhopadhyay, S.C.: Determining wellness through an ambient assisted living environment. IEEE Intell. Syst. 29(3), 30–37 (2014)
37. Sanchez, D., Tentori, M., Favela, J.: Activity recognition for the smart hospital. IEEE Intell. Syst. 23(2), 50–57 (2008)

38. Solanas, A., Patsakis, C., Conti, M., Vlachos, I.S., Ramos, V., Falcone, F., Postolache, O., Perez-Martinez, P.A., Di Pietro, R., Perrea, D.N., Martinez-Balleste, A.: Smart health: a context-aware health paradigm within smart cities. IEEE Commun. Mag. **52**(8), 74–81 (2014)
39. Weiser, M.: The computer for the twenty-first century. Sci. Am. **265**(3), 94–104 (1991)
40. Streitz, N., Magerkurth, C., Prante, T., Röcker, C.: From information design to experience design: smart artefacts and the disappearing computer. Interactions **12**(4), 21–25 (2005)
41. Cowan, D., Turner-Smith, A.: The role of assistive technology in alternative models of care for older people. In: Sutherland, I. (ed.) With Respect To Old Age: The Royal Commission for the Long Term Care of the Elderly, Appendix 4, vol. 2, pp. 325–346. The Stationery Office, London (1999)
42. Holzinger, A., Dorner, S., Födinger, M., Valdez, A.C., Ziefle, M.: Chances of increasing youth health awareness through mobile wellness applications. In: Leitner, G., Hitz, M., Holzinger, A. (eds.) USAB 2010. LNCS, vol. 6389, pp. 71–81. Springer, Heidelberg (2010)
43. Röcker, C., Wilkowska, W., Ziefle, M., Kasugai, K., Klack, L., Möllering, C., Beul, S.: Towards adaptive interfaces for supporting elderly users in technology-enhanced home environments. In: Proceedings of the 18th Biennial Conference of the International Communications Society (2010)
44. Kleinberger, T., Becker, M., Ras, E., Holzinger, A., Müller, P.: Ambient intelligence in assisted living: enable elderly people to handle future interfaces. In: Stephanidis, C. (ed.) UAHCI 2007 (Part II). LNCS, vol. 4555, pp. 103–112. Springer, Heidelberg (2007)
45. Kern, N., Schiele, B., Schmidt, A.: Multi-sensor activity context detection for wearable computing. In: Aarts, E., Collier, R.W., van Loenen, E., de Ruyter, B. (eds.) EUSAI 2003. LNCS, vol. 2875, pp. 220–232. Springer, Heidelberg (2003)
46. Holzinger, A., Searle, G., Prückner, S., Steinbach-Nordmann, S., Kleinberger, T., Hirt, E., Temnitzer, J.: Perceived usefulness among elderly people: experiences and lessons learned during the evaluation of a wrist device. In: International Conference on Pervasive Computing Technologies for Healthcare (Pervasive Health 2010), pp. 1–5. IEEE (2010)
47. Muensterer, O.J., Lacher, M., Zoeller, C., Bronstein, M., Kubler, J.: Google glass in pediatric surgery: an exploratory study. Int. J. Surg. **12**(4), 281–289 (2014)
48. Holzinger, A.: Finger instead of mouse: touch screens as a means of enhancing universal access. In: Carbonell, N., Stephanidis, C. (eds.) UI4ALL 2002. LNCS, vol. 2615, pp. 387–397. Springer, Heidelberg (2003)
49. Overstall, P.W., Nikolaus, T.: Gait, balance, and falls. In: Pathy, M.S.J., Sinclair, A.J., Morley, J.E. (eds.) Principles and Practice of Geriatric Medicine, vol. 2, 4th edn, pp. 1299–1309. Wiley, Chichester (2006)
50. Ruyter, B.D., Pelgrim, E.: Ambient assisted-living research in carelab. Interactions **14**(4), 30–33 (2007)
51. Noury, N., Fleury, A., Rumeau, P., Bourke, A., Laighin, G., Rialle, V., Lundy, J.: Fall detection-principles and methods. In: 29th Annual International Conference of the IEEE Engineering in Medicine and Biology Society, 2007, EMBS 2007, pp. 1663–1666. IEEE (2007)
52. Addlesee, M.D., Jones, A., Livesey, F., Samaria, F.: The ORL active floor. IEEE Pers. Commun. **4**, 35–41 (1997)
53. Orr, R.J., Abowd, G.D.: The smart floor: a mechanism for natural user identification and tracking. In: CHI 2000 Extended Abstracts on Human Factors in Computing Systems, pp. 275–276. ACM (2000)

54. Leusmann, P., Mollering, C., Klack, L., Kasugai, K., Ziefle, M., Rumpe, B.: Your floor knows where you are: sensing and acquisition of movement data. In: 2011 12th IEEE International Conference on Mobile Data Management (MDM), pp. 61–66. IEEE (2011)

55. Ziefle, M., Röcker, C., Wilkowska, W., Kasugai, K., Klack, L., Möllering, C., Beul, S.: A multi-disciplinary approach to ambient assisted living. In: Röcker, C., Ziefle, M. (eds.) E-Health, Assistive Technologies and Applications for Assisted Living: Challenges and Solutions. IGI Global, Hershey (2010)

56. Klack, L., Möllering, C., Ziefle, M., Schmitz-Rode, T.: Future care floor: a sensitive floor for movement monitoring and fall detection in home environments. In: Lin, J. (ed.) MobiHealth 2010. LNICST, vol. 55, pp. 211–218. Springer, Heidelberg (2011)

57. Baker, A.M., Lafata, J.E., Ward, R.E., Whitehouse, F., Divine, G.: A web-based diabetes care management support system. Jt. Comm. J. Qual. Patient Saf. 27(4), 179–190 (2001)

58. Donsa, K., Spat, S., Beck, P., Pieber, T.R., Holzinger, A.: Towards personalization of diabetes therapy using computerized decision support and machine learning: some open problems and challenges. In: Holzinger, A., Roecker, C., Ziefle, M. (eds.) Smart Health. Lecture Notes in Computer Science LNCS, vol. 8700, pp. 235–260. Springer, Heidelberg, Berlin (2015)

59. Morlion, B., Knoop, C., Paiva, M., Estenne, M.: Internet-based home monitoring of pulmonary function after lung transplantation. Am. J. Respir. Crit. Care Med. 165(5), 694–697 (2002)

60. Ávila-Funes, J.A., Amieva, H., Barberger-Gateau, P., Le Goff, M., Raoux, N., Ritchie, K., Carriere, I., Tavernier, B., Tzourio, C., Gutiérrez-Robledo, L.M.: Cognitive impairment improves the predictive validity of the phenotype of frailty for adverse health outcomes: the three-city study. J. Am. Geriatr. Soc. 57(3), 453–461 (2009)

61. Park, S.H., Won, S.H., Lee, J.B., Kim, S.W.: Smart home–digitally engineered domestic life. Pers. Ubiquit. Comput. 7(3–4), 189–196 (2003)

62. Mynatt, E.D., Melenhorst, A.S., Fisk, A.D., Rogers, W.A.: Aware technologies for aging in place: understanding user needs and attitudes. IEEE Pervasive Comput. 3(2), 36–41 (2004)

63. Holzinger, A., Nischelwitzer, A.K.: People with motor and mobility impairment: innovative multimodal interfaces to wheelchairs. In: Miesenberger, K., Klaus, J., Zagler, W.L., Karshmer, A.I. (eds.) ICCHP 2006. LNCS, vol. 4061, pp. 989–991. Springer, Heidelberg (2006)

64. Nischelwitzer, A.K., Sproger, B., Mahr, M., Holzinger, A.: MediaWheelie – a best practice example for research in multimodal user interfaces (MUIs). In: Miesenberger, K., Klaus, J., Zagler, W.L., Karshmer, A.I. (eds.) ICCHP 2006. LNCS, vol. 4061, pp. 999–1005. Springer, Heidelberg (2006)

65. Nischelwitzer, A., Sproger, B., Holzinger, A.: Assistive text input methods: 3D-space writing and other text input methods for powerwheelchair users: best practice examples on the MediaWheelie. In: Kempter, G., Hellberg, P.V. (eds.) Informationen Nutzbar Machen, pp. 75–80. Papst Science Publishers, Lengerich (2006)

66. Debevc, M., Kosec, P., Rotovnik, M., Holzinger, A.: Accessible multimodal web pages with sign language translations for deaf and hard of hearing users. In: 20th International Conference on Database and Expert Systems Application, DEXA 2009, pp. 279–283. IEEE (2009)

67. Debevc, M., Kožuh, I., Kosec, P., Rotovnik, M., Holzinger, A.: Sign language multimedia based interaction for aurally handicapped people. In: Miesenberger, K., Karshmer, A., Penaz, P., Zagler, W. (eds.) ICCHP 2012, Part II. LNCS, vol. 7383, pp. 213–220. Springer, Heidelberg (2012)

68. Holzinger, A., Searle, G., Nischelwitzer, A.K.: On some aspects of improving mobile applications for the elderly. In: Stephanidis, C. (ed.) HCI 2007. LNCS, vol. 4554, pp. 923–932. Springer, Heidelberg (2007)
69. Holzinger, A., Searle, G., Kleinberger, T., Seffah, A., Javahery, H.: Investigating usability metrics for the design and development of applications for the elderly. In: Miesenberger, K., Klaus, J., Zagler, W.L., Karshmer, A.I. (eds.) ICCHP 2008. LNCS, vol. 5105, pp. 98–105. Springer, Heidelberg (2008)
70. Nischelwitzer, A.K., Lenz, F.-J., Searle, G., Holzinger, A.: Some aspects of the development of low-cost augmented reality learning environments as examples for future interfaces in technology enhanced learning. In: Stephanidis, C. (ed.) HCI 2007. LNCS, vol. 4556, pp. 728–737. Springer, Heidelberg (2007)
71. Sproger, B., Nischelwitzer, A., Holzinger, A.: TeamTable: lowcost team-display hardware and tangible user interfaces facilitate interaction & learning. In: Kempter, G., Hellberg, P.V. (eds.) Informationen Nutzbar Machen, pp. 57–60. Papst Science Publishers, Lengerich (2006)
72. Shyu, C.R., Brodley, C.E., Kak, A.C., Kosaka, A., Aisen, A.M., Broderick, L.S.: ASSERT: a physician-in-the-loop content-based retrieval system for HRCT image databases. Comput. Vis. Image Underst. **75**(1–2), 111–132 (1999)
73. Ranganathan, S., Schonbach, C., Kelso, J., Rost, B., Nathan, S., Tan, T.: Towards big data science in the decade ahead from ten years of InCoB and the 1st ISCB-Asia Joint Conference. BMC Bioinform. **12**(Suppl 13), S1 (2011)
74. Dhar, V.: Data science and prediction. Commun. ACM **56**(12), 64–73 (2013)
75. Kolker, E., Özdemir, V., Martens, L., Hancock, W., Anderson, G., Anderson, N., Aynacioglu, S., Baranova, A., Campagna, S.R., Chen, R.: Toward more transparent and reproducible omics studies through a common metadata checklist and data publications. OMICS: A J. Integr. Biol. **18**(1), 10–14 (2014)
76. Holzinger, A., Dehmer, M., Jurisica, I.: Knowledge discovery and interactive data mining in bioinformatics - state-of-the-art, future challenges and research directions. BMC Bioinform. **15**(S6), I1 (2014)
77. Morik, K., Brockhausen, P., Joachims, T.: Combining statistical learning with a knowledge-based approach-a case study in intensive care monitoring. In: ICML 1999, pp. 268–277 (1999)
78. Sultan, M., Wigle, D.A., Cumbaa, C., Maziarz, M., Glasgow, J., Tsao, M., Jurisica, I.: Binary tree-structured vector quantization approach to clustering and visualizing microarray data. Bioinformatics **18**(Suppl 1), S111–S119 (2002)
79. Koch, I.: Analysis of Multivariate and High-Dimensional Data. Cambridge University Press, New York (2014)
80. Olshen, A.B., Hsieh, A.C., Stumpf, C.R., Olshen, R.A., Ruggero, D., Taylor, B.S.: Assessing gene-level translational control from ribosome profiling. Bioinformatics **29**(23), 2995–3002 (2013)
81. Li, W., Godzik, A.: CD-HIT: a fast program for clustering and comparing large sets of protein or nucleotide sequences. Bioinformatics **22**(13), 1658–1659 (2006)
82. Pržulj, N., Wigle, D., Jurisica, I.: Functional topology in a network of protein interactions. Bioinformatics **20**(3), 340–348 (2004)
83. Bullard, J.H., Purdom, E., Hansen, K.D., Dudoit, S.: Evaluation of statistical methods for normalization and differential expression in mRNA-Seq experiments. BMC Bioinform. **11**, 94 (2010)
84. Kiberstis, P.A.: All eyes on epigenetics. Science **335**(6069), 637 (2012)

85. Barrera, J., Cesar-Jr., R.M., Ferreira, J.E., Gubitoso, M.D.: An environment for knowledge discovery in biology. Comput. Biol. Med. **34**(5), 427–447 (2004)
86. Holzinger, A., Ziefle, M., Röcker, C.: Pervasive Health. Springer, London (2014)
87. Huppertz, B., Holzinger, A.: Biobanks – a source of large biological data sets: open problems and future challenges. In: Holzinger, A., Jurisica, I. (eds.) Interactive Knowledge Discovery and Data Mining in Biomedical Informatics. LNCS, vol. 8401, pp. 317–330. Springer, Heidelberg (2014)
88. Shaer, O., Nov, O.: HCI for personal genomics. Interactions **21**(5), 32–37 (2014)
89. Marr, D.: Vision: A Computational Investigation into the Human Representation and Processing of Visual Information. Henry Holt, New York (1982)
90. Donoho, D.L.: High-dimensional data analysis: the curses and blessings of dimensionality. In: AMS Math Challenges Lecture, pp. 1–32 (2000)
91. Holzinger, A.: Extravaganza tutorial on hot ideas for interactive knowledge discovery and data mining in biomedical informatics. In: Ślęzak, D., Tan, A.-H., Peters, J.F., Schwabe, L. (eds.) BIH 2014. LNCS, vol. 8609, pp. 502–515. Springer, Heidelberg (2014)
92. Stocker, C., Marzi, L.-M., Matula, C., Schantl, J., Prohaska, G., Brabenetz, A., Holzinger, A.: Enhancing patient safety through human-computer information retrieval on the example of german-speaking surgical reports. In: TIR 2014 - 11th International Workshop on Text-Based Information Retrieval, pp. 1–5. IEEE (2014)
93. Gondek, D.C., Lally, A., Kalyanpur, A., Murdock, J.W., Duboue, P.A., Zhang, L., Pan, Y., Qiu, Z.M., Welty, C.: A framework for merging and ranking of answers in DeepQA. IBM J. Res. Dev. **56**(3–4), 399–410 (2012)
94. Reuss, E., Menozzi, M., Buchi, M., Koller, J., Krueger, H.: Information access at the point of care: what can we learn for designing a mobile CPR system? Int. J. Med. Inform. **73**(4), 363–369 (2004)
95. Choi, J., Chun, J., Lee, K., Lee, S., Shin, D., Hyun, S., Kim, D., Kim, D.: MobileNurse: hand-held information system for point of nursing care. Comput. Methods Programs Biomed. **74**(3), 245–254 (2004)
96. Young, P.M.C., Leung, R.M.W., Ho, L.M., McGhee, S.M.: An evaluation of the use of hand-held computers for bedside nursing care. Int. J. Med. Inform. **62**(2–3), 189–193 (2001)
97. Moffett, S.E., Menon, A.S., Meites, E.M., Kush, S., Lin, E.Y., Grappone, T., Lowe, H.L.: Preparing doctors for bedside computing. Lancet **362**(9377), 86 (2003)
98. Konstantakos, A.K.: Personal computers versus patient care: at the desktop or at the bedside? Curr. Surg. **60**(4), 353–355 (2003)
99. Holzinger, A., Kosec, P., Schwantzer, G., Debevc, M., Hofmann-Wellenhof, R., Frühauf, J.: Design and development of a mobile computer application to reengineer workflows in the hospital and the methodology to evaluate its effectiveness. J. Biomed. Inform. **44**(6), 968–977 (2011)
100. Holzinger, A., Errath, M.: Mobile computer web-application design in medicine: some research based guidelines. Univ. Access Inf. Soc. Int. J. **6**(1), 31–41 (2007)
101. Dey, A.K., Abowd, G.D., Salber, D.: A conceptual framework and a toolkit for supporting the rapid prototyping of context-aware applications. Hum.-Comput. Inter. **16**(2–4), 97–166 (2001)
102. Brézillon, P.: Context in problem solving: a survey. Knowl. Eng. Rev. **14**(1), 47–80 (1999)
103. Coutaz, J., Crowley, J.L., Dobson, S., Garlan, D.: Context is key. Commun. ACM **48**(3), 49–53 (2005)
104. Harper, R., Rodden, T., Rogers, Y., Sellen, A.: Being Human: Human-Computer Interaction in the Year 2020. Microsoft Research, Cambridge (2008)

105. Sellen, A., Rogers, Y., Harper, R., Rodden, T.: Reflecting human values in the digital age. Commun. ACM **52**(3), 58–66 (2009)

106. Schmidt, A., Pfleging, B., Alt, F., Sahami, A., Fitzpatrick, G.: Interacting with 21st-century computers. IEEE Pervasive Comput. **11**(1), 22–31 (2012)

107. Selker, T., Burleson, W.: Context-aware design and interaction in computer systems. IBM Syst. J. **39**(3–4), 880–891 (2000)

108. Holzinger, A., Stocker, C., Dehmer, M.: Big complex biomedical data: towards a taxonomy of data. In: Obaidat, M.S., Filipe, J. (eds.) Communications in Computer and Information Science CCIS 455, pp. 3–18. Springer, Berlin Heidelberg (2014)

109. Catchpoole, D.R., Kennedy, P., Skillicorn, D.B., Simoff, S.: The curse of dimensionality: a blessing to personalized medicine. J. Clin. Oncol. **28**(34), E723–E724 (2010)

110. Kanerva, P.: Hyperdimensional computing: an introduction to computing in distributed representation with high-dimensional random vectors. Cogn. Comput. **1**(2), 139–159 (2009)

111. Ma, J.H., Wen, J., Huang, R.H., Huang, B.X.: Cyber-individual meets brain informatics. IEEE Intell. Syst. **26**(5), 30–37 (2011)

112. Zhong, N., Liu, J., Yao, Y., Wu, J., Lu, S., Qin, Y., Li, K., Wah, B.W.: Web intelligence meets brain informatics. In: Zhong, N., Liu, J., Yao, Y., Wu, J., Lu, S., Li, K. (eds.) Web Intelligence Meets Brain Informatics. LNCS (LNAI), vol. 4845, pp. 1–31. Springer, Heidelberg (2007)

113. Modha, D.S., Ananthanarayanan, R., Esser, S.K., Ndirango, A., Sherbondy, A.J., Singh, R.: Cognitive computing. Commun. ACM **54**(8), 62–71 (2011)

114. Jones, B., Carvalho, C., Dobra, A., Hans, C., Carter, C., West, M.: Experiments in stochastic computation for high-dimensional graphical models. Stat. Sci. **20**(4), 388–400 (2005)

115. Alaghi, A., Hayes, J.P.: Survey of stochastic computing. ACM Trans. Embed. Comput. Syst. (TECS) **12**(2s), 92 (2013)

116. Yoshida, R., Ueno, G., Doucet, A.: Special issue: bayesian inference and stochastic computation preface. Ann. Inst. Stat. Math. **66**(3), 441–442 (2014)

117. Tehrani, S.S., Mannor, S., Gross, W.J.: Survey of stochastic computation on factor graphs. In: 37th International Symposium on Multiple-valued Logic, 2007, ISMVL 2007, pp. 54–54. IEEE (2007)

118. Shanbhag, N.R., Abdallah, R.A., Kumar, R., Jones, D.L.: Stochastic computation. In: Proceedings of the 47th Design Automation Conference, pp. 859–864. ACM (2010)

119. Adar, R., Benenson, Y., Linshiz, G., Rosner, A., Tishby, N., Shapiro, E.: Stochastic computing with biomolecular automata. Proc. Natl. Acad. Sci. U.S.A. **101**(27), 9960–9965 (2004)

120. Olfati-Saber, R., Fax, J.A., Murray, R.M.: Consensus and cooperation in networked multi-agent systems. Proc. IEEE **95**(1), 215–233 (2007)

121. Wooldridge, M., Jennings, N.R.: Intelligent agents: theory and practice. Knowl. Eng. Rev. **10**(2), 115–152 (1995)

122. Costanza, E., Fischer, J.E., Colley, J.A., Rodden, T., Ramchurn, S.D., Jennings, N.R.: Doing the laundry with agents: a field trial of a future smart energy system in the home. In: Proceedings of the 32nd Annual ACM Conference on Human Factors in Computing Systems, pp. 813–822. ACM (2014)

123. Jennings, N.R., Corera, J.M., Laresgoiti, I.: Developing industrial multi-agent systems. In: ICMAS, pp. 423–430 (1995)

124. Roche, B., Guegan, J.F., Bousquet, F.: Multi-agent systems in epidemiology: a first step for computational biology in the study of vector-borne disease transmission. BMC Bioinform. **9**, 435 (2008)

125. Kamar, E., Gal, Y.K., Grosz, B.J.: Modeling information exchange opportunities for effective human–computer teamwork. Artif. Intell. **195**, 528–550 (2013)
126. Tambe, M., Bowring, E., Jung, H., Kaminka, G., Maheswaran, R., Marecki, J., Modi, P.J., Nair, R., Okamoto, S., Pearce, J.P.: Conflicts in teamwork: hybrids to the rescue. In: Proceedings of the Fourth International Joint Conference on Autonomous Agents and Multiagent Systems, pp. 3–10. ACM (2005)
127. Jennings, N.R., Moreau, L., Nicholson, D., Ramchurn, S.D., Roberts, S., Rodden, T., Rogers, A.: On human-agent collectives. Commun. ACM **57**, 80–88 (2014)
128. Gao, H., Barbier, G., Goolsby, R.: Harnessing the crowdsourcing power of social media for disaster relief. Intell. Syst. IEEE **26**(3), 10–14 (2011)
129. Takeuchi, I.: A massively multi-agent simulation system for disaster mitigation. In: Ishida, T., Gasser, L., Nakashima, H. (eds.) MMAS 2005. LNCS (LNAI), vol. 3446, pp. 269–282. Springer, Heidelberg (2005)
130. Menzies, T.: Beyond data mining. IEEE Softw. **30**(3), 92 (2013)

Medicine and Health Care as a Data Problem: Will Computers Become Better Medical Doctors?

Michael Duerr-Specht[1]([✉]), Randy Goebel[2], and Andreas Holzinger[3]

[1] Duke University Hospital, 40 Duke Medicine Circle, Durham, NC 27710, USA
mikespecht@me.com
[2] Department of Computing Science, University of Alberta, 2-21 Athabasca Hall,
Edmonton, AB, Canada
goebel@cs.ualberta.ca
[3] Institute for Medical Informatics, Statistics and Documentation,
Medical University Graz, Auenbruggerplatz 2/V, 8036 Graz, Austria
a.holzinger@hci-kdd.org

Abstract. Modern medicine and health care in all parts of our world are facing formidable challenges: exploding costs, finite resources, aging population as well as deluge of big complex, high-dimensional data sets produced by modern biomedical science, which exceeds the absorptive capacity of human minds. Consequently, the question arises about whether and to what extent the advances of machine intelligence and computational power may be utilized to mitigate the consequences. After prevailing over humans in chess and popular game shows, it is postulated that the biomedical field will be the next domain in which smart computing systems will outperform their human counterparts. In this overview we examine this hypothesis by comparing data formats, data access and heuristic methods used by both humans and computer systems in the medical decision making process. We conclude that the medical reasoning process can be significantly enhanced using emerging smart computing technologies and so-called computational intelligence. However, as humans have access to a larger spectrum of data of higher complexity and continue to perform essential components of the reasoning process more efficiently, it would be unwise to sacrifice the whole human practice of medicine to the digital world; hence a major goal is to mutually exploit the best of the two worlds: We need computational intelligence to deal with big complex data, but we nevertheless – and more than ever before – need human intelligence to interpret abstracted data and information and creatively make decisions.

Keywords: Medical decision support · Medical reasoning · Big data · Data centric medicine · Medical informatics · Smart health

1 Introduction: The Case of Watson Winning Jeopardy!

> "If our brains were simple enough for us to understand them,
> we'd be so simple that we couldn't."
> Ian Stewart, The Collapse of Chaos: Discovering Simplicity in a Complex World

© Springer International Publishing Switzerland 2015
A. Holzinger et al. (Eds.): Smart Health, LNCS 8700, pp. 21–39, 2015.
DOI: 10.1007/978-3-319-16226-3_2

On January 14th, 2011, the well known game show *Jeopardy!* offered something completely new to their large audience. For the first time since its inception in 1964, one of the participants answering the challenges offered by moderator Alex Trebek was not human – but a computer.

Watson, an IBM computer system, took the central seat between two human champions, Ken Jennings and Brad Rutter. 14 years after the famous victory of "Deep Blue" over Gary Kasparov in chess, a software system – some would describe it rather as artificial intelligence, or smart computing device – beat its human counterparts by a significant margin, though not with a perfect score.

Advances of computer systems have been remarkable since their early beginnings in the 1950's. We have advanced far from arrays of soldered transistors on large circuit boards in air-conditioned rooms shielded with copper plates against interfering electromagnetic radiation. Capacities in computing power and data storage have doubled every 18–24 months over the past decades (Moore's law [1, 2]) and the computing power today has reached a level that allows systems to compete in the human field in complex environments. For proponents of computer technology and artificial intelligence this marks the beginning of a new era in human–computer interaction; and the next battlefield to be conquered by computer technology is human medicine and health – smart health [3].

In fact, the challenges in the medical field are enormous [4] and seem to be increasing daily. Medical knowledge is growing at an exponential rate, far beyond what an individual medical doctor can be expected to absorb. It is estimated that a family physician would have to read new medical literature for more than 600 h per month to stay current [5]. The global availability of information on the press of a button is tempting, but the cognitive capacity reaches its natural limit. More information does not lead automatically to better decisions: the US American Institute of medicine (IOM) estimates that medical errors in the United States alone cost 98,000 lives a year at a financial cost of $29 billion a year [6]. The financial burden of health care on just the US economy is staggering and has been steadily increasing over decades raising some immediate questions:

(1) Are future computer systems going to provide a solution to these issues?
(2) Are we looking at a future where diagnoses and treatment decisions for the majority of health problems will be rapidly, accurately and efficiently made by smart Watson-like systems and their offspring?
(3) Or will computer systems, just like technological medical advances in the past, simply accelerate expenses in the health care arena without significantly impacting life expectancy or well-being for the average person?

Certainly we first need to understand the limitations of the human decision making process to understand how to design and build such systems. We also have to face the challenges of the enormous *complexity* of the medical domain [7].

2   Glossary

Abductive Reasoning: a logical inference that leads from an observation to a hypothesis explaining the observation, seeking to find the simplest and most likely explanation (allows inferring a as an explanation of b; deduction in reverse) [8].

Big Data: a buzz word to describe growing amounts of large data sets, having strong relevance from a socio-technical perspective and economy [9] and a recent important topic in biomedical informatics [10].

Content Analytics: umbrella term for the application of machine intelligence to any form of digital content.

Deductive Reasoning: logical inference that links premises with conclusions (allows deriving b from a, where b is a formal logical consequence of a;) [11].

DeepQA: core of the Watson project at IBM on a grand challenge in Computer Science: to build a computer system, that is able to answer natural language questions over an open and broad range of knowledge [12].

Evidence Based Medicine (EBM): is about the integration of individual clinical expertise with the best external evidence [13], originally coming from medical education for improving decision making strategies [14].

Inductive Reasoning: allows inferring b from a, where b does not necessarily follow from a; this reasoning is inherently uncertain (e.g. Billo is a boxer, Billo is a dog > all dogs are boxer)

Machine Learning: field of study and design of algorithms that can learn from data, operate by building a model based on inputs and using that to make predictions or decisions, rather than following only explicitly programmed instructions. The more data the better, hence big data is good for machine learning [15].

Reasoning: associated with thinking, cognition, and intelligence it is core essence in decision making as it is one of the ways by which thinking comes from one idea to a related idea (cause-effect, truth-false, good-bad, etc.) [16].

Watson: synonym for a cognitive technology system of IBM, using DeepQA that tries to process information more like a human than a computer with the goal of understanding natural language based on hypothesis generation and dynamic learning [17].

Watson Content Analytics: a business solution, based on Watson technology for knowledge discovery from unstructured information aiming to help enterprises to validate what is known and reveal what is unknown, having much potential for medicine and health care [18].

3   What Is This Watson?

In 2007, the IBM Research labs began with the grand challenge of building a computer system that could eventually compete with human champions at the game quiz show *Jeopardy!* In 2011, the open-domain question-answering (QA) system, called Watson (in honor of Thomas J. Watson (1874–1956), CEO of IBM from 1914 to 1956), beat the two highest ranked players in a nationally televised two-game *Jeopardy!* competition.

Technologically, Watson is the result of a systems integration of many diverse algorithmic techniques, performed at champion levels [12, 19], and was created to demonstrate the capability of so-called DeepQA technology [20]: this architecture was designed to be *massively parallel,* with an expectation that low latency response times could be achieved by doing parallel computation on many distributed computing systems. A large set of natural-language processing programs were integrated into a single application, scaled out across hundreds of central processing unit cores, and optimized to run fast enough to compete in a real-world application [21].

Because Watson cannot hear or see, when the categories and clues were displayed on the game board, they were inputted manually (as text) to Watson. The program also monitored signals generated when the buzzer system was activated and when a contestant successfully rang in. If Watson was confident of its answer, it triggered a solenoid to depress its buzzer button and used a text-to-speech system to speak out loud its response – to make the output more appealing. Since it did not hear the host's judgment, it relied on changes to the scores and the game flow to infer whether the answer was correct or not. The Watson interface program had to use what were sometimes conflicting events to determine the state of the game, without any human intervention [22].

Deep Blue, the computer that played chess and beat world champion Garry Kasparov in 1996 first, and in 1997 the six-game match [23], was also impressive, but far not as impressive as Watson [24]. Deep Blue operated in a finite and well specified problem space. Though the chess problem space is large (estimated to be greater than 10^{120} positions) making it impossible for computers to calculate every potential outcome [25] it could certainly calculate the merits of every immediate move and the possible alternatives two or three moves ahead [26]. Combined with some strategic knowledge, it was able to beat any opponent at chess.

The problem space that Watson took on was much less well defined and required the interpretation of natural language to form and select an appropriate answer. Exactly this is the big problem: Whereas chess programs tend towards performing "super-human", i.e. perform better than all humans, natural language processing, i.e. word sense disambiguation is traditionally considered an AI-hard problem [27, 28].

For those of us who study both human and artificial intelligence, the question arises as to what extent to which Watson mimics human intelligence [29, 30]. In the past, human intelligence researchers and many artificial intelligence researchers have dismissed the possibility of any strong similarity between artificial and human intelligence [31]. This was almost certainly correct for any past accomplishment in artificial intelligence, especially which focused on games and search.

Could Watson be different? It is very likely that Watson would do quite well on many test items that compose intelligence tests including general information, vocabulary, similarities, and nearly anything dependent on verbal knowledge. Nevertheless, it is very likely that Watson would do quite poorly on many other kinds of tests that require reasoning or insight. In its current state, it would be difficult for Watson to understand directions for the various and different subtests that usually make up an intelligence test, something that children as young as three or four do easily.

Tests of computer intelligence are as old as computers themselves. The most famous is the Turing test proposed by Alan Turing (1912–1954) more than 60 years ago. Turing suggested that a machine would be intelligent when an observer would have a conversation with a computer and a real person and not be able to distinguish which was which [32].

Numerous other approaches have been proposed, including the construction of a unique battery of tests that would provide an actual IQ score for artificial intelligence systems, similar to the way human IQ scores are determined [33]. This challenge is supported by the editorial board of the journal "Intelligence" and members of the International Society for Intelligence Research.

A recent paper by Rachlin [34] speculates on the abilities Watson would need, in addition to those it has, to emulate true human behaviour: essential human attributes such as consciousness, the ability to love, to feel, to sense, to perceive, and to imagine. Most crucially, such a computer may exhibit self-control and may act altruistically.

At this point, the external perception of Watson's performance in *Jeopardy!* exposes only "question in – single answer out" with no detailed explanation of *how* the answer was found. However, internally, Watson uses a form of hypothetical reasoning called *"probabilistic abduction"*, e.g., see [35], which creates and ranks alternative answers based on the alternatives that can be inferred from a variety of text resources within the time limit for a response.

Currently the IBM team is working on a vision for an evidence-based clinical decision support system, based on the DeepQA technology, that affords exploration of a broad range of hypotheses and their associated evidence, as well as uncovers missing information that can be used in mixed-initiative dialog [17]. Whereas Watson used simple but broad encyclopaedic knowledge for the *Jeopardy!* task, the extended medical Watson uses medical information gleaned from sources also available to the practicing physician: medical journals and textbooks.

Considering the fact that medicine is turning more and more into a data intensive science, it is obvious that integrated machine learning approaches for knowledge discovery and data mining are indispensable [36].

The grand goal of IBM is having the Watson technology ready as a medical doctor's assistant (in German: Arzthelfer) available on a mobile computing device by the year 2020 [37]. This is a grand challenge exactly at the intersection of human-computer interaction (HCI) and knowledge discovery and data mining (KDD) [38].

4 Computers and Medicine

Undeniably, computers offer ever-increasing capabilities in areas where we as humans have trouble competing. Information entered can be reproduced accurately and without degradation innumerable times to as many users as desired. Data elements can be grouped, parsed, abstracted, combined, copied, and displayed in any conceivable way, offering seemingly infinite options to view even very large sets of data. Numeric values can be instantly analyzed and participate in complex calculations, the result of which is immediately available. Network environments allow multiple users to access and share identical information in real time.

Not least, advances in natural language processing allow an increasingly accurate analysis of data contained within unstructured written documents and reports. In fact, IBM's *Jeopardy!* contestant Watson is the first system to show the power of this technology in quasi real time [39, 40].

In medicine, electric and electronic devices as well as computerized systems have an impressive track record. Assistance in diagnosis dates back to 1895 when Conrad Wilhelm Roentgen (1845–1923) demonstrated that the use of electromagnetic radiation, invisible to the naked eye was able to penetrate tissues and visualize the bones [41]. Advances in this basic technology combined with the computing power of modern semiconductors led to the development of sophisticated imaging technology such as computerized tomography offering 2-D and 3-D images of internal tissues and organs as well as real time fluoroscopy, providing essential information for tricky medical interventions. Magnetic resonance imaging provides digital images constructed from atomic nuclear resonance of body tissues allowing for accurate visual diagnoses of many pathological conditions. Computer generated images based on the analysis of ultrasound waves reflected from body tissues have become an indispensable tool in the evaluation of internal organs and prenatal care.

In the realm of therapy, computers led to significant medical advances. Cardiac pacemakers generate a cardiac rhythm in cases of failure of the innate sinus node. Implanted automatic defibrillators continuously analyze the electrical system of the heart and sophisticated algorithms determine the selection of multiple response modes which allow the device to save a failing heart and prolong the patient's life.

The use of electronic medical records has been steadily growing over the past 10 years. Today about 42 % of US hospitals utilize some type of electronic documentation [42]. In 2011 the US government introduced the concept of "Meaningful Use" initially offering financial incentives to increase the adoption of computerized record systems. The advance of electronic documentation has created a fertile basis for diagnostic and therapeutic decision support systems, which have diversified significantly over time. Some projects have taken into account newest findings in neurocognitive research ("cognostics") for their human–computer interface development, and are adapting principles and methods to ideally support the human cognitive process with its interactive analytical and constellatory operations [43]. Most recently, the market penetration with small computing devices such as smart phones and table computers has shifted medical referencing from printed media to electronic devices, though the analysis of accumulated patient data is yet to be abstracted and codified in a manner that would easily amplify the abilities of the clinical decision maker – but that is anticipated to come.

5   The Digital Challenge

In view of these impressive advances in technology and computing it is not surprising that a debate has been sparked as to whether the continuation of this development will lead to a future situation in which computers will eventually outperform human doctors and consequently assume larger roles in medical diagnostics and therapeutic decisions.

The venture capitalist Vinod Khosla states in an interview published by Techcrunch on January 10th, 2012 that

> *"we cannot expect our doctor to be able to remember everything from medical school twenty years ago or memorize the whole Physicians Desk Reference (PDR) and to know everything from the latest research, and so on and so forth. This is why, every time I visit the doctor, I like to get a second opinion. I do my Internet research and feel much better."* [44].

In order to better understand the issues involved in the potential of computing technology and artificial intelligence as it is integrated into medical decision making, it might be worthwhile to differentiate between three different aspects of the process of delivering health care to a patient: data formats and relationships amongst those, the accumulation of large volumes of medical data contained within databases, and the reasoning process used to interpret and apply those data to benefit a specific patient.

6 Data Formats and Relationships

Here we follow the definitions of Boisot & Canals [45], who describe data as originating in discernible differences in physical states of the world. Significant regularities in this data constitute *information*. This implies that the information gained from data, depends on the expectations, called: *hypotheses*. A set of hypotheses is called *knowledge* and is constantly modified by new information. This definition fits well to the human information processing model by Wickens [46]: The physical stimuli (cues) are selected by the attentional resources and the perceived information builds working hypotheses H1, H2, H3 ... etc., which are constantly compared and judged against available hypotheses, already present in the long-term memory. On this basis the best possible alternative will be chosen and actions A1, A2, A3, ... etc., performed according to likelihoods and consequences of the outcomes – which can be perceived again via the feedback loop. Wickens described the input "filter" as the "nebula of uncertainty" and this emphasizes perfectly a general problem in decision making: we deal always with probable information. Each information chunk, item or whatever you call it, has always a certain probability aspect (refer to lecture 7 in [10]).

Based on these definitions, the commonly used term "unstructured data" might just capture random state descriptors – uncertainty – noise [47]. In Informatics, particularly, it can be considered as unwanted non-relevant data without meaning within a given data model – or, even worse, with an interpretation assigned in error, hence modelling of artefacts is a constant danger in medical informatics [48].

The question "what is information?" continues to be an open question in basic research. Any definition depends on the view taken. For example, the definition given by Carl-Friedrich von Weizsäcker (1912–2007): "Information is what is understood," implies that information has both a sender and a receiver who have a common understanding of the representation within a shared modelling system and the means to communicate information using some properties of the physical systems. His addendum: "Information has no absolute meaning; it exists relatively between two semantic levels" implies the necessity of context [49].

There is a distinct and insurmountable difference between human and computer data formats. Computers – at least as current electronic methods of computation on the basis of Von Neumann machines [50] are concerned – operate exclusively with digital data formats. Content is stored as strings of binary data elements. Meaning and relationships between content items are added by method of (human) assignment or (machine) calculation, i.e., they are subsequently provided as additional data layer to the original content data.

All data elements are provided to computer systems by means of human interaction (e.g., keyboard, touch pad, etc.), technical devices (sensors, microphones, cameras, etc.) or secondary data generated through calculation of previously available data. As outlined above, regardless of the original data format, making data available to computer technology has an absolute requirement of translating data into a binary format, regardless of the original complexity. All relationships between data elements are initially stripped from the occurrence observed, though some may be added back and preserved for future use (e.g. machine learning) by adding additional documentation. As such, every pixel of a picture file has no "knowledge" of its neighbor pixel and the composition of the picture is provided by a separate instruction, providing placement of the pixel within a defined grid format. This feature provides the power and flexibility of digital image processing, as individual elements can be altered without affecting the remainder of the composition.

Humans, on the other hand, have the luxury of a primary experience of their environment. We traditionally speak of our five senses, sight, hearing, taste, smell and touch, though other senses also provide data, such as temperature, balance, pain, time and another less well-understood class of senses commonly referred to as "intuition". As we experience life, it appears that the input from the individual senses interact and is stored in a complex fashion with a high degree of connectedness between individual data items. The human subjective experience overrules the (measurable) objective state and data content is difficult to differentiate from data interpretation. This has been demonstrated quite impressively in pictures such as the checker-shadow optical illusion [51, 52]. In spite of the lack of objectivity, however, the skewed data perception by the human observer has advantages, as it puts acquired data content into a *contextual perspective* thereby allowing the all-important differentiation between relevant and irrelevant items.

This ability differentiates human perception from machine analysis. It is used effectively to block automated software responses, e.g. with the so-called CAPTCHA ("Completely Automated Public Turing test to tell Computers and Humans Apart") [53–55]. It is also the basis of the human ability to analyze visual motion in general scenes which – as of now – exceeds the capabilities of even the most sophisticated computer vision algorithms [56].

7   On Data and Context

Regardless of whether examining a computer system or the human brain, calculations and conclusions can only be based on data available to the system. For technical systems this means that the basis of all operations is the availability of binary input data. Though large computer systems such as IBM's Watson have access to databases of many tera-bytes and can process data at the rate of more than 500 gigabytes per second, access is still restricted to data published or digitally available in other formats. This makes these systems vulnerable to the GIGO ("garbage in, garbage out") phenomenon, which plagues large data environments [57].

As in other fields with computerized data entry, medical documentation in health records is biased by documentation guidelines, template requirements and constraints on entry formats, as well as reimbursement requirements, etc., and does not accurately reflect the complete array of signs and symptoms of a patient's presentation.

The human brain, on the other hand, does not rely on single-bit data streams as its input method. We have a complex and analog (not binary digital) experience of our surroundings, which delivers simultaneous perception data from all senses. Acquired information from one sensory organ is therefore never one-dimensional but experi-enced in the multidimensional context of the other senses, thereby adding meaning to the data. In contrast to technical systems however, the human brain reduces the original environmental data quantity, according to principles of interest or "meaningfulness," led by attentional resources [58] though the exact mechanism of information conden-sation and subsequent storage still remains poorly understood.

Some catchy numbers shall highlight the comparison between human and computer (although the following numbers are theoretical and the exact function of human infor-mation processing is not known yet):

The human eye has been estimated to be able to perceive 6 Mbits/s of primary visual information, however less than estimated 1 % of this information reaches the visual cortex of the brain for further cognitive processing [59, 60]. By the time information reaches our consciousness, the rate of information flow has been estimated to shrink to about 100 bits/s for visual sources, 200 bits/s for all sensory sources combined [61]. At this rate it would take about 300,000 years for a human to obtain the data utilized by Watson in the 2011 *Jeopardy!* contest.

8   Reasoning Process

Reasoning is according to the common definition "the process of thinking about some-thing in a logical way in order to form a conclusion or judgment" [62, 63]. In medicine, we apply reasoning to come to a conclusion about which diagnosis would be appropriate for a patient presenting with a certain constellation of signs and symptoms. The reasoning process typically applied by medical doctors has been described to include abductive, deductive and inductive reasoning elements [35]. Upon presentation of the patient, the physician will first generate domain-specific hypotheses based on an initial set of obser-vations (abduction). These initial hypotheses are confirmed and refined by additional observations (induction). Textbook knowledge of the disease entity is then employed to select the appropriate treatment to improve the patient's health (deduction).

Adopting this concept of the medical reasoning process, it can be argued that man and machine have complementary strengths and weaknesses (see Table 1). The abduc-tive component provides the basis for hypothesizing known causes or diseases that imply the observed symptoms. This initiates the diagnostic process and is uniquely supported by the human high dimensional intrinsically correlated mechanism of perception which includes concrete observations that can be measured and documented in the record and is highly supported by soft factors (sense of illness severity and distress, emotional state, social environment, etc.), typically not documented or even consciously recognized. The human brain is capable of rapidly associating this overall picture with known disease patterns and can thereby not only very efficiently postulate the hypotheses within the abductive process but also intuit measures to manage cases in which the observed pattern does not sufficiently match known entities. The medical literature is full of examples of unique presentations in which the treating physician invoked a creative process of expanding hypotheses beyond what had previously been known or documented (as an example and fun reading please refer to a recently published report by Rice et al. [64]).

Table 1. Medical Reasoning: Human vs. Computer

Reasoning Process	Human	Computer
Abductive Hypothesis generation	Uniquely capable of complex pattern recognition and creative thought. "the whole is greater than the sum of its parts"	Matches multiple individual correlations from extensive data banks based on preconceived algorithms. Secondary construction of relationships. "the whole equals the sum of its parts"
Inductive Symptom → Disease	Limited database. Subject to biases - Anchoring bias - Confirmation bias - Premature closure	Extensive database. Probability based on Bayesian statistics, no significant bias. Limitation based on available data.
Deductive Disease → Symptoms, Treatment	Limited database. Personal intuition and experience affect decision making.	Extensive database. Application of rules of evidence based medicine with potential biases.

Computerized systems, on the other hand, only can use data supplied as binary code which is processed in pre-conceived algorithms and have no original perception of "Gestalt." Relationships are based on correlations extracted secondarily from extensive databases, however the whole remains equal to the sum of the parts. What seems elusive is an information model or structure that emulates the emergence of genuinely novel concepts and ideas the human mind is capable of, without succumbing to a reductionist view of acknowledged but unformulated physician insights. At the very least, the information system support would have to consider a wider breadth of feasible hypotheses guided by the deeper experiences of physicians, which would require a much more sophisticated and extensive conceptual underpinning of the language in which hypotheses are expressed.

Human reasoning in the practice of medicine is, however, hampered in the inductive process of confirming and refining abductive hypotheses due to biases and poor understanding of probability calculations. The tendency of physicians to retain their initial hypotheses even in the light of contradicting data is a well-described phenomenon [65, 66].

Multiple concepts of bias are described in this context:

- Anchoring bias: focusing on a single concept before sufficient data is available to support it,
- Confirmation bias: gathering only information to support an hypothesis, and
- Premature closure: terminating the reasoning process and eliminating evaluation of alternative explanations prematurely;

Computer systems are not prone to these biases. The computer has no urge to favor one hypothesis over another but rather uses information from extensive medical databases as entry data for probability calculations, often along the lines of Bayesian statistics. Conceptually this approach is supported by the probabilistic nature of information, and the role of reasoning to calculate and identify the most probable hypotheses. In contrast to computer algorithms, a recent study reports that most physicians misunderstand the underlying probabilistic logic of significance tests and consequently often misinterpret their results. The study concludes that a solid understanding of the fundamental concepts of probability theory is becoming essential to the rational interpretation of medical information per se [48].

One of the earliest software tools in medical reasoning, MYCIN, developed by the Stanford Medical Center in the 1960's was based on the concepts of inductive reasoning [67, 68]. In the same manner, well-designed clinical reasoning software could be of significant value in alerting physicians about possible bias in their decision process, assisting in the probability calculations and helping to minimize or avoid clinical error.

Sophisticated access to the knowledge of large medical databases could also assist in the deductive phase of medical reasoning. In selecting the most likely diagnosis among a selection of differential diagnostic considerations, specific tests and exams are necessary. Physicians generally have a very poor track record in selecting the course of clinical tests that provides for the most efficient information gain. Often studies are ordered according to individual habits with limited understanding or consideration of how the test results affect the likelihood of a disease being present or not. Software with access to extensive data regarding prevalence of disease entities in specific populations as well as the sensitivity and specificity of diagnostic studies would offer guidance to an efficient selection of tests to confirm or refute a diagnosis as it relates to a particular patient presentation.

Once a diagnosis has been established, the decision on therapeutic interventions can also be assisted by medical software. Unlike their human counterparts, computers have access to all published information and recommendations and can suggest the intervention that is most current. In addition, the broader influence of historical data as well as subtle trends can be considered, which is difficult and time challenging for humans. Since 2011, IBM Watson's capabilities in assisting in treatment decisions are being studied by multiple medical facilities, including Columbia University, the Memorial Sloan-Kettering Cancer Center as well as the Cleveland Clinic [69]. In the German speaking world progress has been made particularly at Graz University Hospital [18], and Vienna University Hospital [70] – two of the largest hospitals in Europe.

Computerized assistance in medical treatments are based on the principles of "evidence based medicine," an approach that is led by the idea that the best treatment is one based on the results of published trials and applies findings to the individual patient. While this treatment philosophy represents an understandable ideal, it is subject to significant limitations, among others: selection of study population, publication bias, bias based on financial incentives and errors in study results due to incomplete understanding of the biological system (e.g., Simpsons paradox [71]). In addition, computer generated treatment recommendations exclude the personal experience and intuition of the treating physician. Recent research further elaborates on the dual processing theory of human cognition [72] and a recent study reports that reasoning and decision-making can be described as a function of both an intuitive, experiential and affective system (system 1) and/or an analytical, deliberative processing system (system 2) [73].

9   Future Challenges

Faced with unsustainable costs and enormous volumes of under-utilized data, health care needs more efficient practices, research, and tools. It is our opinion that there is tremendous potential in harnessing the power of modern information technology and applying it to the medical sciences.

We believe that the challenges and future work needed to support medicine, health and well-being with software products can be categorized in three distinct areas: organizational (including administrative and political), technological and educational:

Area 1: Organizational/administrative/political

- data access and data ownership issues;
- balancing legitimate privacy concerns with the benefits of access to large amounts of anonymized open clinical data for public and personal health assessment;

Area 2: Technological

- building new software products based on existing technology and using available digitally stored data elements, with a special focus on visual representation of complex clinical data, trending of individual health parameters and weak signal detection;
- developing intuitive medical record systems to allow for improved documentation of the process of care and medical reasoning and promoting continuity of care during the hand-off process between health care providers
- enhancing digital data capture through newly designed intelligent user interfaces and/ or secondary processing by means of natural language processing and content tagging
- developing new hardware products to automatically capture relevant physiological data, e.g. along the lines of the quantified self movement
- promoting preventative care by analyzing large amount of high quality clinical data to detect weak signals that serve to risk stratify for future health events
- continuing research in artificial intelligence and machine learning and testing concepts of software systems acting as legitimate sparring partners in sophisticated medical decision making, which is still the core area of biomedical informatics [56].

Area 3: Educational

- promoting and supporting interdisciplinary events in which software engineers and medical professionals exchange ideas and concepts and develop a common language in describing domain specific needs.

We envision a future where medical doctors can ask questions to the available data and have an integrative overview of both the clinical patient data and -omics data (e.g. genomics, proteomics, metabolomics, etc.) [74]. Software support in personal and global health data would allow the expert to find and diagnose diseases in advance, before symptomatically apparent. In this form of *data-centric medicine,* prevention could really become efficient, and the dream of a personalized medicine approach can become true [75]. Although both science and engineering are making significant progress, a lot of work remains to be done within the coming years for this vision to become a reality.

The integration of technology into clinical medicine includes at least three broad classes of challenges. In our discussion regarding the role of Artificial Intelligence, it is clear that there are a large variety of technologies that can begin by augmenting and amplifying the value of clinical practioners:

(1) improvements in diagnostic sensing and imaging; capture and rapid deployment of new medical knowledge,
(2) logistics and management improvements in both small clinics and hospitals, and
(3) improvement in the capture, security, and use of medical data.

Not all of these challenges are technical. In fact 2 and 3 are largely organizational challenges, partly due to educational lag and the pace with which modern medical management adopts technologies that are already available. These include not just actionable medical knowledge and technology, but operational management and technology procurement. Challenge 3 is largely about the development and exploitation of patient data, where two major impediments exist. One is simply the evolutionary adoption of standards of data capture and use, partly at capture time, where capture, storage and open access must be addressed. Subsequent to that, medical ontology systems, which provide the foundation for aggregating data, and using analytics (machine learning) to find trends and help improve clinical practice.

A more serious challenge is the development and deployment of medical data governance models, into which public, government, and medical organizations can collaborate to develop the trust to actually use medical data. Many jurisdictions are recognizing that data security methods have never been better, so that the governance of medical data, and building public trust for its value is the key.

Thus, in the effort to achieve superior and cost-effective medical care by virtue of integration of physician expertise and computerized clinical decision support systems (CDSS), the following issues need to be addressed:

Issue 1. Negotiating the contradiction between structured digital data capture and the expressive narrative in clinical documentation: Whereas downstream use and reuse of clinical data in decision support systems requires data that is highly structured and standardized, practicing clinicians demand documentation systems that afford flexibility and efficiency and easily integrates into busy and hectic workflows [76]. In order to successfully implement computerized clinical support systems, EHR solutions will have to be developed in a way that satisfy the needs for clinical workflow support, documentation of unsuspected circumstances, machine readability and structured data capture.

Issue 2. Development and adoption of a standardized biomedical "language". Automated data capture processes and electronic health records are producing data sets too large to be manually analyzed or processed. Therefore it is important that clinical data can be tagged according to a common biomedical ontology to allow for widespread international data sharing and analysis [77].

Currently several competing ontologies are being used, serving various interests in the biomedical domain (e.g. UMLS, MeSH, GALEN, SNOMED, ICD), however, all these are difficult to use and rather impossible to map to each other due to inconsistent representation.

Issue 3. Regulatory and legal framework. Legal exposure to practicing physicians can result from errors due to flawed design or functionality of computerized clinical support systems, or their improper use. Currently there exist few standards for the design and development of automated decision support systems and there have been calls to enhance current functionalities and create tools to avoid automation associated errors [78]. Changes to the regulatory framework have been recommended [79]. Furthermore, as recommendations based on computerized algorithms and decision support systems become part of the practice reality in the medical field, legal structures need to be adapted to allow physicians to base diagnostic and treatment decisions on their individual acumen and expertise, even if in disagreement with machine recommendations, without immediate legal exposure.

Issue 4. Inhibitory medical data protection regulations. While patients have a valid interest in protecting confidential medical data, overly protective limitation to access community health care data thwarts medical research and knowledge development and can harm general public health interests. In the interest of advancing medical knowledge and quality of care it will be necessary to increase access to biomedical information whilst at the same time protecting legitimate individual privacy interests.

Issue 5. Creating a dynamic educational system. It is shocking that the average transfer time for medical knowledge from initial research to widespread implementation in medical practice has been estimated to be between 12 and 17 years [80]. As we increase our ability to fuel computerized clinical decision support systems with real time date, processes need to be developed to extract knowledge regarding diagnoses and optimal treatment and make this available to the medical practitioners. Adjusting to this dynamic decision environment will require a new mind set in programmers, policy makers and practitioners.

10   Summary

Since their early beginnings, more than half a century ago, computer systems have evolved into highly complex data environments that are able to rapidly deliver vast amounts of information. It has been postulated that the computing power of advanced systems will be able to provide medical care to patients in the near future that will be more efficient and of higher quality and lower cost than currently offered by physicians. While this is probably overly enthusiastic, current developments in medical software promise an exciting future for physicians. Needed information will be delivered to our fingertips without delay. Intelligent selection algorithms will allow us to rapidly review case-relevant studies and protocols.

Unusual constellations of signs and symptoms will be screened for rare diseases and suggested for consideration. Our electronic medical records will be smart in prompting us to answer only the questions that are relevant for case-specific decision-making. Graphical user interfaces will make it easy to detect and review even subtle trends and compare symptom constellations of the differential diagnoses under consideration.

Software capabilities have graduated to the professional league of medical care. As the pilots in the diagnostic and therapeutic process, we as physicians are now called to step up to the plate and engage in active conversations with software developers and IT departments. Mustering this initiative will allow us to leverage the unique strengths and capabilities of both information technologies and medical sciences into powerful and effective health care services of the future in which doctors will be able to navigate the complex landscape of a patient's health information similar to how an airline pilot manages a complex flying machine with the assistance of a the sophisticated flight data display of a computerized glass cockpit.

Computers cannot become better medical doctors. Medical doctors can become better medical doctors with the support of smart hospital systems [3]. Information technology and medical sciences are not battling for territory in a zero sum game. If we approach it correctly, everyone wins, most importantly: our patients!

11 Epilogue

As for the triumph of IBM Watson in the *Jeopardy!* game show: the amazing observation, one may argue, is not that Watson won, employing its database of four terabytes, cluster of 90 IBM Power 750 serves each using a 3.5 GHz Power7 eight core processor and able to push the response button within 5 ms, 20 times the human response time. The amazing thing is that the human contestants scored. Just imagine what the two forces combined could achieve [38].

References

1. Moore, G.E.: Cramming more components onto integrated circuits. Electronics **38**(8), 114–117 (1965)
2. Cavin, R., Lugli, P., Zhirnov, V.: Science and engineering beyond Moore's Law. IEEE Proc. **100**(13), 1720–1749 (2012)
3. Holzinger, A., Röcker, C., Ziefle, M.: From smart health to smart hospitals. In: Holzinger, A., Röcker, C., Ziefle, M. (eds.) Smart Health. LNCS, vol. 8700, pp. 1–19. Springer, Heidelberg (2015)

 4. Holzinger, A., Dehmer, M., Jurisica, I.: Knowledge discovery and interactive data mining in bioinformatics - state-of-the-art, future challenges and research directions. BMC Bioinform. **15**(S6), I1 (2014)
 5. Alper, B.S., Hand, J.A., Elliott, S.G., Kinkade, S., Hauan, M.J., Onion, D.K., Sklar, B.M.: How much effort is needed to keep up with the literature relevant for primary care? J. Med. Lib. Assoc. **92**(4), 429–437 (2004)
 6. Kohn, L.T., Corrigan, J., Donaldson, M.S.: To err is human: building a safer health system. National Academy Press, Washington (DC) (2000)
 7. Patel, V.L., Kahol, K., Buchman, T.: Biomedical complexity and error. J. Biomed. Inform. **44**(3), 387–389 (2011)
 8. Poole, D.: Explanation and prediction: an architecture for default and abductive reasoning. Comput. Intell. **5**(2), 97–110 (1989)
 9. Dong-Hee, S., Min Jae, C.: Ecological views of big data: Perspectives and issues. Telematics Inform. **32**(2), 311–320 (2015)
10. Holzinger, A.: Biomedical Informatics: Discovering Knowledge in Big Data. Springer, New York (2014)
11. Johnson-Laird, P.N.: Deductive reasoning. Ann. Rev. Psychol. **50**, 109–135 (1999)
12. Ferrucci, D., Brown, E., Chu-Carroll, J., Fan, J., Gondek, D., Kalyanpur, A.A., Lally, A., Murdock, J.W., Nyberg, E., Prager, J.: Building Watson: An overview of the DeepQA project. AI Mag. **31**(3), 59–79 (2010)
13. Sackett, D.L., Rosenberg, W.M., Gray, J., Haynes, R.B., Richardson, W.S.: Evidence based medicine: what it is and what it isn't. BMJ. Br. Med. J. **312**(7023), 71 (1996)
14. Guyatt, G.: Evidence based medicine - a new approach to teaching the practice of medicine. JAMA-J. Am. Med. Assoc. **268**(17), 2420–2425 (1992)
15. Holzinger, A.: Trends in interactive knowledge discovery for personalized medicine: cognitive science meets machine learning. Intell. Inf. Bull. **15**(1), 6–14 (2014)
16. Holzinger, A.: Lecture 8 biomedical decision making: reasoning and decision support. In: Biomedical Informatics, pp. 345–377. Springer (2014)
17. Ferrucci, D., Levas, A., Bagchi, S., Gondek, D., Mueller, E.T.: Watson: Beyond jeopardy! Artif. Intell. **199–200**, 93–105 (2013)
18. Holzinger, A., Stocker, C., Ofner, B., Prohaska, G., Brabenetz, A., Hofmann-Wellenhof, R.: Combining HCI, natural language processing, and knowledge discovery - potential of IBM content analytics as an assistive technology in the biomedical field. In: Holzinger, A., Pasi, G. (eds.) HCI-KDD 2013. LNCS, vol. 7947, pp. 13–24. Springer, Heidelberg (2013)
19. Ferrucci, D.A.: Introduction to "This is Watson". IBM J. Res. Develop. **56**, 3–4 (2012)
20. Gondek, D.C., Lally, A., Kalyanpur, A., Murdock, J.W., Duboue, P.A., Zhang, L., Pan, Y., Qiu, Z.M., Welty, C.: A framework for merging and ranking of answers in DeepQA. IBM J. Res. Develop. **56**, 3–4 (2012)
21. Epstein, E.A., Schor, M.I., Iyer, B.S., Lally, A., Brown, E.W., Cwiklik, J.: Making Watson fast. IBM J. Res. Develop. **56**, 3–4 (2012)
22. Lewis, B.L.: In the game: The interface between Watson and Jeopardy! IBM Journal of Research and Development 56(3–4), (2012)
23. Newborn, M.: Deep Blue's contribution to AI. Ann. Math. Artif. Intell. **28**(1–4), 27–30 (2000)
24. Campbell, M., Hoane, A.J., Hsu, F-h: Deep blue. Artif. Intell. **134**(1), 57–83 (2002)
25. Newell, A., Shaw, J.C., Simon, H.A.: Chess-playing programs and the problem of complexity. IBM J. Res. Dev. **2**(4), 320–335 (1958)
26. Ensmenger, N.: Is chess the drosophila of artificial intelligence? A social history of an algorithm. Soc. Stud. Sci. **42**(1), 5–30 (2012)

27. Navigli, R., Velardi, P.: Structural semantic interconnections: A knowledge-based approach to word sense disambiguation. IEEE Trans. Pattern Anal. Mach. Intell. **27**(7), 1075–1086 (2005)

28. Bhala, R.V.V., Abirami, S.: Trends in word sense disambiguation. Artif. Intell. Rev. **42**(2), 159–171 (2014)

29. Tesauro, G., Gondek, D.C., Lenchner, J., Fan, J., Prager, J.M.: Simulation, learning, and optimization techniques in Watson's game strategies. IBM J. Res. Develop. **56**, 3–4 (2012)

30. Tesauro, G., Gondek, D.C., Lenchner, J., Fan, J., Prager, J.M.: Analysis of WATSON's strategies for playing jeopardy! J. Artif. Intell. Res. **47**, 205–251 (2013)

31. Simon, H.A.: Studying human intelligence by creating artificial intelligence. Am. Sci. **69**(3), 300–309 (1981)

32. Turing, A.M.: Computing machinery and intelligence. Mind **59**(236), 433–460 (1950)

33. Detterman, D.K.: A challenge to Watson. Intelligence **39**(2–3), 77–78 (2011)

34. Rachlin, H.: Making IBM's computer, watson, human. Behav. Anal. **35**(1), 1–16 (2012)

35. Sun, Z.H., Finnie, G., Weber, K.: Abductive case-based reasoning. Int. J. Intell. Syst. **20**(9), 957–983 (2005)

36. Holzinger, A., Jurisica, I.: Knowledge discovery and data mining in biomedical informatics: the future is in integrative, interactive machine learning solutions. In: Holzinger, A., Jurisica, I. (eds.) Interactive Knowledge Discovery and Data Mining in Biomedical Informatics. LNCS, vol. 8401, pp. 1–18. Springer, Heidelberg (2014)

37. Chip. http://business.chip.de/news/IBM-Watson-Sein-erster-Job-ist-Arzthelfer_51623616. html

38. Holzinger, A.: Human-computer interaction and knowledge discovery (HCI-KDD): What is the benefit of bringing those two fields to work together? In: Cuzzocrea, A., Kittl, C., Simos, D.E., Weippl, E., Xu, L. (eds.) CD-ARES 2013. LNCS, vol. 8127, pp. 319–328. Springer, Heidelberg (2013)

39. Nadkarni, P.M., Ohno-Machado, L., Chapman, W.W.: Natural language processing: an introduction. J. Am. Med. Inform. Assoc. **18**(5), 544–551 (2011)

40. Murdock, J.W., Fan, J., Lally, A., Shima, H., Boguraev, B.K.: Textual evidence gathering and analysis. IBM J. Res. Dev. **56**(3–4), 1–14 (2012)

41. Röntgen, W.C.: On a new kind of rays. Science **3**(59), 227–231 (1896)

42. Robert Wood Johnson Foundation (RWJF). http://www.rwjf.org/en/about-rwjf/newsroom/ newsroom-content/2013/07/hospitals–physicians-make-major-strides-in-electronic-health- re.html

43. Miller, R.A.: Medical diagnostic decision support systems - past, present and future. J. Am. Med. Inform. Assoc. **1**(1), 8–27 (1994)

44. Techcruch. http://techcrunch.com/2012/01/10/doctors-or-algorithms/

45. Boisot, M., Canals, A.: Data, information and knowledge: have we got it right? J. Evol. Econ. **14**(1), 43–67 (2004)

46. Wickens, C.D.: Engineering Psychology and Human Performance. Charles Merrill, Columbus (1984)

47. Holzinger, A., Stocker, C., Dehmer, M.: Big complex biomedical data: towards a taxonomy of data. In: Obaidat, M.S., Filipe, J. (eds.) Communications in Computer and Information Science CCIS 455, pp. 3–18. Springer, Berlin Heidelberg (2014)

48. Holzinger, A.: On knowledge discovery and interactive intelligent visualization of biomedical data: Challenges in human–computer interaction & biomedical informatics. In: Helferd, M., Fancalanci, C., Filipe, J. (eds.) DATA - International Conference on Data Technologies and Applications, pp. 5–16. INSTICC, Rome (2012)

49. Marinescu, D.C.: Classical and Quantum Information. Academic Press, Burlington (2011)
50. von Neumann, J.: Electronic methods of computation. Bull. Am. Acad. Arts Sci. **1**(3), 2–4 (1948)
51. Adelson, E.H.: Checkershadow illusion. http://web.mit.edu/persci/people/adelson/checker shadow_illusion.html (last Accessed 24 November 2014) (1995)
52. Geisler, W.S., Kersten, D.: Illusions, perception and Bayes. Nat. Neurosci. **5**(6), 508–510 (2002)
53. von Ahn, L., Blum, M., Hopper, N.J., Langford, J.: CAPTCHA: Using hard AI problems for security. In: Biham, E. (ed.) EUROCRYPT 2003. LNCS, vol. 2656. Springer, Heidelberg (2003)
54. Rusu, A., Govindaraju, V., Soc, I.C.: Handwritten CAPTCHA: Using the difference in the abilities of humans and machines in reading handwritten words. IEEE Computer Society, Los Alamitos (2004)
55. Belk, M., Germanakos, P., Fidas, C., Holzinger, A., Samaras, G.: Towards the personalization of CAPTCHA mechanisms based on individual differences in cognitive processing. In: Holzinger, A., Ziefle, M., Hitz, M., Debevc, M. (eds.) SouthCHI 2013. LNCS, vol. 7946, pp. 409–426. Springer, Heidelberg (2013)
56. Weiss, Y., Simoncelli, E.P., Adelson, E.H.: Motion illusions as optimal percepts. Nat. Neurosci. **5**(6), 598–604 (2002)
57. Leunens, G., Verstraete, J., Vandenbogaert, W., Vandam, J., Dutreix, A., Vanderschueren, E.: Human errors in data transfer during the preparation and delivery of radiation treatment affecting the final reasult - garbage in, garbage out. Radiother. Oncol. **23**(4), 217–222 (1992)
58. Kahneman, D.: Remarks on attention control. Acta Psychologica **33**, 118–131 (1970)
59. Shiffrin, R.M., Gardner, G.T.: Visual processing capacity and attention control. J. Exp. Psychol. **93**(1), 72 (1972)
60. Duncan, J.: Selective attention and the organization of visual information. J. Exp. Psychol. Gen. **113**(4), 501–517 (1984)
61. Anderson, C.H., Van Essen, D.C., Olshausen, B.A.: Directed visual attention and the dynamic control of information flow. In: Itti, L., Rees, G., Tsotsos, J.K. (eds.) Neurobiology of Attention, pp. 11–17. Academic Press/Elservier, Burlington (2005)
62. Patel, V.L., Arocha, J.F., Zhang, J.: Thinking and reasoning in medicine. Cambridge Handb. Think. Reason. **14**, 727–750 (2005)
63. Alfaro-LeFevre, R.: Critical Thinking, Clinical Reasoning, and Clinical Judgment: A Practical Approach. Elsevier Saunders, Philadelphia (2013)
64. Rice, S.P., Boregowda, K., Williams, M.T., Morris, G.C., Okosieme, O.E.: A Welsh-sparing dysphasia. Lancet **382**(9904), 1608 (2013)
65. Croskerry, P.: The importance of cognitive errors in diagnosis and strategies to minimize them. Acad. Med. **78**(8), 775–780 (2003)
66. Berner, E.S., Graber, M.L.: Overconfidence as a cause of diagnostic error in medicine. Am. J. Med. **121**(5), S2–S23 (2008)
67. Shortliffe, E.H., Buchanan, B.G.: A model of inexact reasoning in medicine. Math. Biosci. **23**(3), 351–379 (1975)
68. Shortliffe, E.H., Buchanan, B.G.: Rule-Based Expert Systems: The MYCIN Experiments of the Stanford Heuristic Programming Project. Addison-Wesley, Reading (1984)
69. Washington Technology. http://washingtontechnology.com/articles/2011/02/17/ibm-watson-next-steps.aspx

70. Stocker, C., Marzi, L.-M., Matula, C., Schantl, J., Prohaska, G., Brabenetz, A., Holzinger, A.: Enhancing patient safety through human-computer information retrieval on the example of german-speaking surgical reports. In: TIR 2014 - 11th International Workshop on Text-based Information Retrieval, pp. 1–5. IEEE (2014)

71. Simpson, E.H.: The interpretation of interaction in contingency tables. J. R. Stat. Soc. Ser. B-Stat. Methodol. **13**(2), 238–241 (1951)

72. Croskerry, P., Nimmo, G.: Better clinical decision making and reducing diagnostic error. J. R. Coll. Physicians Edinb. **41**(2), 155–162 (2011)

73. Djulbegovic, B., Hozo, I., Beckstead, J., Tsalatsanis, A., Pauker, S.: Dual processing model of medical decision-making. BMC Med. Inform. Decis. Mak. **12**(1), 94 (2012)

74. Huppertz, B., Holzinger, A.: Biobanks – A source of large biological data sets: open problems and future challenges. In: Holzinger, A., Jurisica, I. (eds.) Interactive Knowledge Discovery and Data Mining in Biomedical Informatics. LNCS, vol. 8401, pp. 317–330. Springer, Heidelberg (2014)

75. Downing, G., Boyle, S., Brinner, K., Osheroff, J.: Information management to enable personalized medicine: stakeholder roles in building clinical decision support. BMC Med. Inform. Decis. Mak. **9**(1), 1–11 (2009)

76. Rosenbloom, S.T., Denny, J.C., Xu, H., Lorenzi, N., Stead, W.W., Johnson, K.B.: Data from clinical notes: a perspective on the tension between structure and flexible documentation. J. Am. Med. Inf. Assoc. **18**(2), 181–186 (2011)

77. Lenfant, C.: Clinical research to clinical practice — lost in translation? N. Engl. J. Med. **349**(9), 868–874 (2003)

78. Love, J.S., Wright, A., Simon, S.R., Jenter, C.A., Soran, C.S., Volk, L.A., Bates, D.W., Poon, E.G.: Are physicians' perceptions of healthcare quality and practice satisfaction affected by errors associated with electronic health record use? J. Am. Med. Inf. Assoc. **19**(4), 610–614 (2011)

79. Bowman, S.: Impact of electronic health record systems on information integrity: quality and safety implications. Perspect. Health Inf. Manage. **10**, 1–19 (2013)

80. Morris, Z.S., Wooding, S., Grant, J.: The answer is 17 years, what is the question: understanding time lags in translational research. J. R. Soc. Med. **104**(12), 510–520 (2011)

Spatial Health Systems
When Humans Move Around

Björn Gottfried[1]([⊠]), Hamid Aghajan[2,3], Kevin Bing-Yung Wong[2,3],
Juan Carlos Augusto[4], Hans Werner Guesgen[5], Thomas Kirste[6],
and Michael Lawo[1]

[1] Centre for Computing and Communication Technologies,
University of Bremen, Bremen, Germany
{bg,mlawo}@tzi.de
[2] AIR (Ambient Intelligence Research) Lab, Stanford University, Stanford, USA
{aghajan,kbw5}@stanford.edu
[3] iMinds, Ghent University, Ghent, Belgium
[4] Research Group on the Development of Intelligent Environments,
Middlesex University, London, UK
J.Augusto@mdx.ac.uk
[5] School of Engineering and Advanced Technology, Massey University,
Palmerston North, New Zealand
h.w.guesgen@massey.ac.nz
[6] Department of Computer Science, University of Rostock, Rostock, Germany
thomas.kirste@uni-rostock.de

Abstract. This chapter outlines spatial health systems and discusses issues regarding their technical implementation and employment. This concerns in particular diseases which manifest themselves in the spatiotemporal behaviours of patients, showing patterns that enable conclusions about their underlying well-being. While a general overview is given, as an example the case of patients suffering from Alzheimer's disease is examined more carefully in order to treat different aspects detailed enough. Especially, wearable and ambient technologies, activity recognition techniques as well as ethical aspects are discussed. The given literature review ranges from basic methods of Artificial Intelligence research to commercial products which are already available from the industry.

1 Introduction

In the last two decades significant progress has been made in pervasive computing technologies and Artificial Intelligence research. Many application areas benefit from these developments and encounter their challenges with new technologies. One such area is the field of health that itself divides into many subareas, one of which being concerned with the application of pervasive technologies.

The employment of pervasive computing technologies in the health sector motivated the introduction of the dichotomy between *health information systems* and *spatial health systems* [38–40]: While the former enables health organisations to interchange information and provide patients information about health

© Springer International Publishing Switzerland 2015
A. Holzinger et al. (Eds.): Smart Health, LNCS 8700, pp. 41–69, 2015.
DOI: 10.1007/978-3-319-16226-3_3

care, spatial health systems are about the gathering and evaluation of information about the spatial behaviours of patients. In particular the spatiotemporal dimension of the behaviours of patients gain support by these technologies which monitor, interpret, or even directly aid patients acting in space and time. Indeed, the way how humans move around shows to be the fundamental objective for spatial health systems and is therefore of great importance for the design of spatial health systems.

2   Glossary

- Activities of daily living (ADL): common activities, usually self care activities, that an individual performs during a day. Typical activities include eating, bathing, dressing, grooming, working, and homemaking.
- Ambient intelligence (AmI): refers to environments that are sensitive and responsive to the activities of people; AmI is realised by a diversity of methods it brings together from different areas like pervasive computing, ubiquitous computing, context awareness, profiling, and human-centric computing.
- Ambient technologies: a collection of technologies that are placed in the environment for monitoring occupants; it is conceived of as one of the subareas of AmI. In the present paper this notion is employed in order to make the distinction between ambient and wearable technologies.
- Context information: spatial, temporal, or other information, such as vital signs, relevant for interpreting a specific situation, for example to recognise ADLs. Context information is either obtained through sensors or other sources. Artificial intelligence research investigates methods for reasoning about context information.
- Intelligent biomedical clothing (IBC): clothes with sensors that are close to or in contact with the skin, measuring vital signs, such as the heartbeat. Intelligent biomedical clothing fall within the scope of wearable technologies.
- Mini-mental state examination (MMSE) or Folstein test: a 30-point questionnaire test which is employed to detect cognitive impairments, in particular dementia. It is employed for both to determine the severity of impairment and to monitor its course of changes.
- Neurodegenerative disorders: disorders of the central nervous system, for example Alzheimer's disease (AD), Parkinson's disease (PD), or multiple sclerosis (MS) all of which affecting motor behaviours.
- Sensory impairments: visual and hearing impairments. Both kinds of impairments do influence the spatiotemporal behaviours of individuals to a particularly high degree. They are therefore of interest for spatial health systems.
- Spatial health systems: those systems that monitor and evaluate the spatiotemporal behaviours of patients. This notion is to be distinguished from health information systems which are basically about the management of health information.
- Wearable technologies: mobile technologies attached to the mobile patient. An example is intelligent biomedical clothing. One of the most common application areas of wearable technologies is the monitoring of movements.

3   State-of-the-Art

In the following, an overview is provided about typical diseases affecting the motion behaviours of patients. To get a more comprehensive view on how the analysis of motion behaviours can be analysed, the succeeding section presents a study about the detection of changes in the motion of patients suffering from Alzheimer's disease. Besides the analysis of motion behaviours there are also technologies that can be worn by patients in order to monitor their vital signs while moving around. Such technologies are shown in the next section. Typical interpretation methods of motion behaviours are presented afterwards. Eventually, ethical aspects are discussed which are of particular importance when it comes to the monitoring of how and where patients move around.

3.1   Diseases Affecting Motion Behaviours

Worldwide, the population is aging and the number of persons above the age of 60 years was estimated at 605 million in 2000 to increase to 2 billion in 2050 [75]. With age the cognitive and sensory functions change as observed in longitudinal studies [26]. The number of persons with dementia was estimated at about 25 million in 2000 [110]. About 6.1 % of the population 65 years of age and older suffered from dementia. The predictions indicated a considerable increase in the number of demented elderly from 25 million in the year 2000 to 63 million in 2030 (41 million in less developed regions) and to 114 million in 2050 [110].

The WHO's International Classification of Functioning, Disability and Health recognises a broad definition of mobility, including both indoor and outdoor movement as well as the use of assistive devices and transportation [58,72]. The following key determinants of mobility have been detected by [29]: cognitive, psychosocial, physical, environmental, and financial influences. The relative impact of these factors depends on the specific mobility context for each individual. Moreover an important role in the mobility context is played by the chronic medical conditions and the cognitive or sensory impairment caused by the chronic condition. That is, in cognitively, visually, or hearing impaired people, the level of mobility particularly decreases, affecting the ability to travel independently and to conduct activities in daily life outside the house [23].

The three main groups of these disorders, namely neurodegenerative disorders, sensory impairments, as well as chronic diseases are discussed in turn.

Neurodegenerative Disorders. In particular motor behaviours encompass a range of phenomena which are observable in spacetime at different levels of detail, ranging from the spatiotemporal trajectories of body parts during a motion act – such as the motion of the knee joint while walking – to the causal structure of a composite activity such as commuting from home to work using multiple modes of transport.

Several neurodegenerative disorders of the central nervous system, for instance Alzheimer's disease (AD), Parkinson's disease (PD), or multiple sclerosis (MS) affect motor behaviours. Depending on the specific disorder, the changes express themselves at different levels of detail. The characteristic tremor caused by PD affects motion trajectories of body parts (where the tremor can be considered a superimposed high frequency signal). Spastic palsies caused by diseases such as MS reduce the range of motion of affected limbs and joints, and show a specific correlation between joint motion and EMG data (cp. [102,103]). Wandering episodes caused by AD affect the spatial structure of indoor motion paths [38,56]. Finally, disorientation during outdoor activities causes discrepancies between predicted and observed geographic positions in transport routines – such discrepancies can be used by assistive systems supporting outdoor navigation for detecting disorientation and for providing appropriate orientation hints [48,79].

Sensory Impairments. Another aspect of functional decline is the visual impairment with a significant increased prevalence with the age. Worldwide, about 314 million adults are visually impaired: 82 % of them are aged 50 years and older and it is expected that this number will double in the next 25 years [15]. Moreover, individuals with visual impairments caused by aging have frequent hearing impairments as well. Loss of hearing acuity is part of the natural aging process: hearing impairment was experienced by approximately 24 % of those aged 65 to 74 and almost 40 % of the persons over age 75 [105]. In addition, declines in cognition, vision or hearing are associated with decline in functional status [105] and mobility [69].

Chronic Diseases. Chronic diseases are long-term, which is usually defined as lasting more than 6 months, and might have a significant effect on a person's life. Management to reduce the severity of both the symptoms and the impact is possible in many conditions. This includes medication or lifestyle changes, such as diets, exercises, and stress management. At the same time, it should be noted that chronic diseases may get worse, lead to death, be cured, remain dormant, or require continual monitoring.

Chronic disease management tools are mainly home care systems, which focus on vital sign monitoring and the reports of patients on specific situations. Fewer of them are accompanied with patient interfaces for communication and education purposes. The generic system architecture of *Chronious* [4,114] supports chronic disease management: Apart from vital sign monitoring and patient reporting, the system exploits significant environmental measurements, such as those concerning the context of the patient in order to classify events as alerts or not. *Chronious* developed a smart wearable platform, based on multi-parametric sensor data processing and fusion for monitoring people suffering from chronic diseases in long-stay setting. In addition, the proposed platform offers interfaces for monitoring, drug intake, dietary habits, and bio-chemical parameters concerning the health situation. Although not investigated yet, the correlation of those parameters with motion behaviours of patients can be seen as another application of spatial health systems.

3.2 Motion Behaviours of Patients Suffering from Alzheimer's Disease

After having summarised a number of disease patterns which influence observable behaviours, this section outlines a recent study [57] that provides evidence that the spatiotemporal structure of activities is indeed affected by AD. Interestingly, those activities are measured at a stage where such behavioral changes are not evident to a human observer. This is a fundamental argument for the employment of monitoring technologies in spatial health systems.

Background. AD leads to significant changes in the temporal structure of activities. Abnormal motion behaviour and degeneration of the sleep-waking cycle are among the most severe behavioral symptoms [32]. An early detection and even a prediction of these behaviours would allow a timely onset of interventions that aim to delay the manifestation or exacerbation of symptoms and reduce the need of institutionalized care [99]. To date, medical history and behavioral rating scales are the main diagnostic instruments to detect abnormal motion behaviours [60].

It is therefore of interest to establish behavioral measures that are less dependent on human observers. Although there is a substantial number of actigraphical studies aiming at establishing behavioral markers at the population level, cp. [25, 61, 73], these studies did not yet analyse the capabilities of the identified markers to reliably classify *individuals* as "AD" or "not AD". Using behavioral cues as determined by automated sensor-based monitoring as diagnostic instruments is interesting for three reasons:

- data can be acquired in the everyday environment of a person without observer interaction,
- behavioral cues may be predictive for the manifestation of behavioral disturbances,
- once behaviour analysis is in place, assistive functionality can be added for compensating errors in daily routine activities and for other forms of ambient assisted living [13, 46–48].

Subjects and Data. A conducted study was based on 23 dyads ($n = 46$ subjects) with one partner diagnosed with AD and one partner with no cognitive abnormality detected (healthy controls, HC). By using a dyad setup, we intended to ensure that for every lifestyle present in the study one subject diagnosed with AD and one healthy control were available, thus alleviating the variance induced by differences in lifestyle. Severity of cognitive impairment was assessed by a comprehensive set of instruments including the MMSE score [33], which serves as widely established measure for the severity of overall cognitive impairment.

The partners in a dyad were asked to simultaneously record about 50 continuous hours of everyday activity using an ankle-mounted 3 axes accelerometric sensor with 50 Hz sampling rate. This schedule guaranteed that we were able to record a complete day-night cycle (from 22:00 at day 1 to 22:00 at day 2) for each subject. The average recording duration for the accelerometric motion protocols was 53.4 h ($SD = 8.9$ h), resulting in an average number of 9.61×10^6 samples ($SD = 1.61 \times 10^6$ samples) in a data set. In total, 2455.8 h of data were recorded, with a total data volume of 18.4 GByte.

Signal Processing. For building a discrimination model we chose to use spectral features of the activity level obtained from the recorded motion protocols. This activity level is given by the envelope curve of the acceleration magnitude. Analysis of the envelope curve is a well established method for activity analysis based on accelerometric data, cp. [104]. We converted the three-axes acceleration sample vectors (x, y, z) to a scalar signal by computing the acceleration magnitude $m = \sqrt{x^2 + y^2 + z^2}$. In order to remove gravitational artifacts and high frequency noise from the magnitude signal, we applied a sinc band-pass filter with band edges of 0.5 Hz and 5 Hz (cp. [104]). (We chose an upper band edge of 5 Hz rather than 11 Hz as [104] because the main carrier signal component is created by the individual's walking motion, which will have a frequency well below 2.5 half-steps per second, being the Nyquist limit induced by the 5 Hz upper band-pass edge.) The resulting signal can be considered as a carrier for the activity level, which we recovered by rectifying and low-pass filtering using a sinc low-pass. Two examples for the resulting envelope curve signals are given in Fig. 1.

We assumed that behavioral episodes specific to AD could occur at any point in time. We therefore needed a time-invariant feature set, which is for instance provided by the magnitude values of the complex coefficients given by the envelope signal's discrete Fourier transform. Assuming an upper band limit of 50 mHz for the envelope (20 s per cycle), the discrete Fourier transform of the envelope signal in the 22:00-22:00 window will contain coefficients X_0 to X_{4320}. Coefficient X_0 can be dropped (it contains the constant offset, known as "DC offset"). The remaining coefficient vector $X_{1:4320}$ was scaled to unit energy. Thus, any effects of "more" or "less" activity (including variances in sensor sensitivity and sensor bias) are removed from the data, leaving just the relevant spectral structure for further consideration by the classification methodology. The magnitudes of the scaled coefficients span a feature space of 4320 dimensions. We observed that neither individual Fourier coefficients nor simple derived scalar

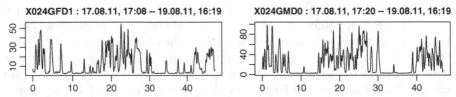

Left: female person, diagnosis AD (GFD1). Right: male person, diagnosis HC (GMD0). X axis: recording hours, Y axis: activity level. Grey regions signify night (22:00–7:00).

Fig. 1. Preprocessed data sample from a dyad

features (entropy, spectral centroid, bandwidth) did show a significant group separation, requiring the use of discrimination models with higher dimensionality for achieving reasonable classification performance.

The number of samples (46 subjects, 23 per class) is much lower than the number of Fourier coefficients (4320). Therefore, we used principal component analysis (PCA) to reduce the number of dimensions. PCA computes eigenvectors of the correlation matrix, which intuitively can be understood as independent "activity structures" from which daily routines are composed. Each eigenvector is a dimension of the transformed feature space. We refer to the coefficients of a transformed feature vector as "PC features".

Classification Models. Our core objective was to determine the association of motion behaviours with a diagnosis of AD. We reframed this into the problem to classify a given subject into the AD or HC group, based on his/her PC features. We built classification models for several popular classifiers that were allowed to use up to five PC features to discriminate between AD and HC subjects. We limited the number of features to five to avoid an overfitting of the limited number of samples [35]. Quadratic discriminant analysis (QDA) achieved a classification accuracy of 91 % in leave-one-out cross-validation (specificity $= 0.96$, sensitivity $= 0.87$; see also Fig. 2). In absolute numbers: 22 true positives (AD subjects classified as AD), 20 true negatives, 3 false positives, and 1 false negative. QDA achieves the highest performance considering ROC plots, accuracy, F_1 score, and AUC (cp. Fig. 2).

Regression Models. We were additionally interested in the association between the MMSE score and the activity envelopes.

Based on the Fourier coefficients as predictor variables, we built linear models using MMSE as regression target. Predictor variables for the model were selected by applying the step function of the statistics system R to an initially empty model. Again we restricted the number of predictor variables to at most five to avoid overfitting.

With respect to predicting the MMSE, we found Fourier coefficients to perform better than PC features. This mode explains 70.3 % of the variance in MMSE ($R^2 = 0.703$, $F_{(5,40)} = 18.9$, $p < 0.001$). For the AD subset values of R^2 up to 0.95 (22:00–22:00 window, $\sqrt{\text{MMSE}}$ target) were achieved. A comparison of predicted and true MMSE using is given in Fig. 3.

Discussion. Our data indicate a high classification accuracy over a range of classification approaches and parameters based on spectral motion features, suggesting that the spectral structure of activity is associated with a clinical diagnosis of AD. Although the resulting surrogate markers of motion behaviours do not easily offer themselves to a clinical interpretation, the overall concept of an impairment of the temporal structure of everyday motion behaviours agrees with a range of neurobiological and clinical studies in AD. AD patients exhibit altered synchronisation among multiple circadian oscillators associated with altered clock gene

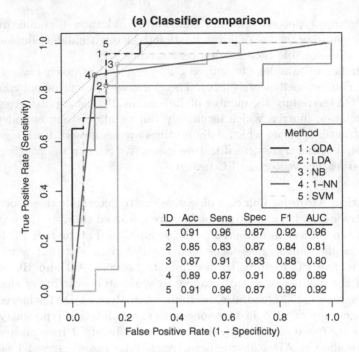

Fig. 2. ROC plots for selected classifiers. QDA = quadratic discriminant analysis, LDA = linear discriminant analysis, NB = naive Bayes, 1-NN = nearest neighbor (we evaluated k-NN for $k = 1, 3, 5, 7$, with $k = 1$ giving best performance.), SVM = support vector machine.

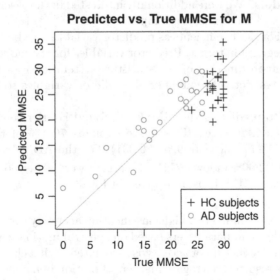

Fig. 3. Regression model for MMSE

expression [100,116]. In particular, degeneration of the suprachiasmatic nucleus (SCN) of the hypothalamus, the master clock of the brain, and its disconnection with other circadian pace makers, such as the pineal gland, has been documented in AD dementia [113].

The available signal resolution is high enough to discriminate individual steps in a motion protocol, thus providing the option to recreate the spatial trajectory followed by the subject during the recording period. For instance, Foxlin [34] has developed an algorithmic approach for reconstructing such trajectories from foot-mounted accelerometers and gyroscopes. Using a different sensor modality, Kearns et al. [56] show that spatial trajectories can be employed for analysing wandering behaviours of dementia patients.

In summary, behavioral consequences of AD manifest themselves as impairments in everyday behaviours. They are important determinants of further disease course and institutionalisation. However, semiquantitative rating scales, such as the CMAI [108] or the NPI [24], only detect the late stages of these behaviours when they lead to social and clinical disabilities. Our findings are encouraging as they suggest that the easily accessible assessment of early signs of forthcoming decline of motion behaviours using automated sensors may be possible and could have a major impact on the development and application of interventions to prevent or attenuate behavioral impairments in AD.

Note that providing on-line assistance – the last point mentioned in the Background section – requires fine-grained analysis with high temporal resolution, as such systems have to react within minutes or seconds after the onset of specific motor behaviours. The envelope curve analysis used in the study presented here does not provide the required detail. Although we have shown that the *spatial* level of motion detail does not necessarily enforce a specific methodological approach, there remains a gap at the *temporal* level – the gap between gross motor behaviour analysis required for the purposes of behaviour detection and prediction as well as detailed motion behaviour analysis for assistive purposes such as presented in [47].

3.3 Moving Around with Wearable Technologies

Wearable sensors, such as activity sensors used in fitness monitoring devices, have been in use for quite some time. For example, the pedometer, perhaps the most simple physical activity sensor, was invented in 1780 by Abraham-Louis Perrelet [1]. However, commercial activity monitoring technology that employs modern integrated electronics is a relatively recent invention and has been largely targeted toward the fitness market [5,7,8]. These technologies rely on a combination of accelerometers and gyroscopes to determine the type of movement the user is performing and act as data loggers to monitor the activity level of a person throughout the day. Most newer devices also offer wireless synchronisation with other devices, such as smartphones, typically using Bluetooth for the purposes of visualising and tracking fitness levels and setting fitness goals [5,7,8]. Some of these wearable fitness monitors [5] also act as sleep monitors, which measure the duration and quality of sleep by detecting movements or sleep interruptions at night.

Current research into using wearable sensors for movement detection have mainly concentrated on extracting useful characteristics from wearable accelerometers and gyroscopes [36,51,54,68,101,118–120]. These sensors are typically part of a wireless sensing module attached to multiple points on the body of a person to track the movement characteristics of that person as she goes about her daily activities. One of the most important characteristics that researchers have focused on is the gait of a person, with a specific interest in the gait of the elderly and those suffering from Parkinson's disease [36,51,68,81,82,91,94,118]. The importance of gait measurements lies in the fact that gait is an important indicator of frailty and fall risk for the elderly [90]. There have been a number of studies [45,70] which suggest gait variability as a key predictor of falls and that reduced gait velocity can be seen as an indicator of cognitive impairments [19,94]. Additionally, activity patterns of the sensorimotor cortex which are involved in movements have been analysed [49]; such studies become important in the context of rehabilitation in order to investigate the reorganisation of the cortex after a stroke.

More complex wearable GPS tracking systems can generate data from which the mobility patterns of individuals can be derived, which would provide more context for the physical activities of an individual [77]. These small devices typically contain a GPS receiver with a data logger, for example obtaining location information every 10 s, inertial motion trackers, and a haptic indicator able to generate acceleration. These sensors are present in most smart phones, which enables a person not only to be tracked but also allows for the integration with other devices [80]. Such systems not only give information on specific locations and provide assessment of individual trips into the community, but enable the assessment of mobility patterns, such as the day and time of walking to specific places, the number of steps, or the walking frequency [88]. Further technical solutions even enhance the mobility of specific target groups, for example, tracking combined with electronic tagging assist patients suffering from dementia [72] and others have developed devices that assist visually impaired elderly [55].

In addition to wearable devices that measure the positions or movements of an individual, there is a great deal of commercial wearable sensor platforms targeted at measuring physiological signals to monitor various medical conditions. These are relevant for spatial health systems since vital signs are normally correlated with body motions and locomotion. Measuring these vital signs is possible through intelligent biomedical clothing (IBC) which refers usually to clothes with sensors that are close to or in contact with the skin. The sensors are enclosed in the layers of fabric or it is the fabric itself that is used as the sensors. To such sensors pertain piezo-resistive yarns, optic fibers, and coloured multiple layers. IBCs have several advantages, starting with removing the task of placing the sensors by nurses or other experts, providing a natural interface with the body. Commonly, IBC is understood as the integration of sensors, actuators, computing, and power sources into textiles, with the whole being part of an interactive communication network. Major prototypes are VTAM and WEALTHY [78,107] as well as the Lifeshirt and SmartShirt [65,98]:

- *VTAM* is a T-shirt made from textile with woven wires, dry ECG electrodes, a breath rate sensor, a shock/fall detector, and two temperature sensors [107].
- *Wealthy* is a wireless-enabled garment with embedded textile sensors for simultaneous acquisition and continuous monitoring of biomedical signs like ECG, respiration, EMG, and physical activity. It embeds a strain fabric sensor based on piezo-resistive yarns and fabric electrodes realised with metal-based yarns [78].
- *LifeShirt* is a miniaturised, ambulatory version of respiratory inductance plethysmography. The garment is a lightweight, machine washable, formfitting shirt with embedded sensors to measure respiration. A modified limb two-lead ECG quantifies cardiac performance and a three-axis accelerometer measures posture and activity [65].
- *SmartShirt* is a garment equipped with wearable computing devises that measure human heart rhythm and respiration using a three lead ECG shirt. The conductive fiber grid and sensors are fully knitted in the garment [98].

Wearable sensors are able to capture personal physiological data from patients, however the key limitation of such sensors is power and context. Since they are typically battery powered, wearable sensors require regular maintenance to ensure functionality. Additionally, any wearable device requires the compliance of the person wearing it, to ensure that the sensors are used as intended. Accelerometer and gyroscope base sensors also cannot directly observe the world around them, so that the context of the actions of a person in the environment is difficult to infer. To compensate for this weakness, some researchers have tied accelerometers to other more capable sensors to get context, such as outward facing video cameras [66] and smart phones [67] to capture the locations and actions of a person. There have also been hybrid approaches that use both wearable and ambient sensors to detect falls [28] with the ability to verify falls using cameras. Such ambient technologies are discussed in the following section.

3.4   Moving Around with Ambient Technologies

Ambient sensors are a collection of technologies that are designed to be placed in the environment for the purposes of monitoring any occupants by measuring how the occupants interact with or change that environment. For the purpose of understanding human health and well-being, we will limit our discussion to technologies that focus on detecting the characteristics of how the occupants move around in the environment. Even with this narrow scope, a wide variety of sensors can be used, depending on the granularity of data that is desired. For example, one could equip the environment with motion sensors in order to sense what areas a person occupies during the day and to determine the level of motion in those areas for the purposes of activity recognition. This type of ambient sensor deployment has been extensively researched in academia for the purposes of detecting Activities of Daily Living (ADL), defined as common activities that a person performs to care for themselves [22,53,83,84,87].

On the other side of the spectrum, rich sensors such as cameras can be employed to capture the motion of occupants in some environment. Human motion capture is perhaps the most comprehensive way of capturing movement characteristics, as such systems are designed to track points on a human body with high fidelity instead of just determining the regions being occupied. Using commercially available technology, it is possible to recover the position and orientation of all parts of the body of a person and her location in the environment. These commercial technologies are commonly used for performance capture for computer graphics animations [2, 9, 10] and leverage a variety of different technologies.

A commercial optical motion capture system to track key points on the body of a user is deployed in [10]. This particular system uses a motion capture suit that has optical registration devices embedded, which can be seen as the glowing dots on the face and suit of the person. Systems that rely on this type of motion capture require complex configurations of multiple cameras since each glowing dot must be seen by several cameras in order for its position to be calculated. Marker based motion capture systems can be highly accurate, since the points they are tracking have a known appearance and simplistic motion capture suits provide a uncomplicated background for tracking. In contrast, commercial technologies exist that do not require optical registration devices. Instead, such systems typically work by fitting a model of a human body to visual data acquired by a computer vision system [95, 106]. The last type of common commercial motion tracking hardware uses wearable inertial sensors that sense acceleration and rotation and does not use optical tracking at all. This type mounts the sensors in a close fitting suit, both for repeatability and to prevent the sensors from shifting away from where they are attached [2].

On the research side, much effort has been devoted to novel applications of consumer grade technologies [16, 89, 94]. For instance, there are platforms which were originally created for the video game market to provide a way for users to interact with their games without a controller [6]. The result was an inexpensive depth camera, which is a camera that can measure the distances of the viewable environment in front of the camera. Using a depth camera allows applications to easily segment and extract a person from the background of an image for applications such as gait analysis [6, 94]. Other researchers employed such platforms for activity recognition as well as for tele-medicine [121] in the context of remote evaluation of mobility [16] and supervised rehabilitation exercises [3, 89]. Additionally, other researchers leveraged more conventional multiple camera configurations in order to capture the positions and postures of users for gait analysis and tele-therapy applications [18, 94, 111, 115].

Ambient sensing technologies enable researchers to gather movement characteristics and behaviours of a person and her interactions with the environment. Thus, ambient sensors can be used to detect the context of the actions of a user by measuring where she is moving in space and what she is interacting with. Additionally, for optical based sensing systems, recordings can be kept for later analysis by researchers to characterise more nuanced movements and behaviours. Unfortunately, since the sensors are not attached to a person, physiological information is typically not detectable, which limits detailed medical observations and the capturing of fine movements. But researchers at MIT's Media Lab have developed a system that detects the heartbeat of a person through variations of the colour of the skin that correlates with the pulse; this provides a method to add limited medical sensing to existing movement tracking systems [112].

3.5 Interpreting Motion Behaviours

The approaches to behaviour recognition that have been developed over the last ten years range from logic-based to probabilistic machine learning approaches [11,21,31,37,86,96]. Although the reported successes are promising, determining the correct behaviour from sensor data alone is often impossible, since sensors can only provide very limited information and human behaviours are inherently complex. This holds especially for the behaviours of patients suffering from neurodegenerative disorders which significantly affect the motor behaviours. Instead of discussing the broad area of interpretation methods investigated in Artifitical Intelligence research, we shall here focus on a number of approaches which are of particular interest in spatial health systems.

Several researchers have realised that context information, in particular spatial and temporal information, can be useful to improve the behaviour recognition process [14,43,44,52,97]. It is then not a precise motor behaviour which needs to be accurately determined but rather the location where it takes place, in order to come to meaningful conclusions. A simple example is the intake of breakfast that usually occurs in the kitchen, which means that if something is happening in the kitchen, it is more likely to be breakfast than taking a shower.

Context information can be represented in a number of ways. Since it is often imprecise or uncertain, the representations need to be of a probabilistic or fuzzy nature. In the following, we discuss the advantages and disadvantages of several approaches. We argue that using a probabilistic approach has shortfalls, due to incomplete context information, and that using an approach based on the concept of beliefs fails due to its complexity. We then make a case for fuzzy logic, which not only provides a simple and robust mechanism for reasoning about context information but also provides a means to represent imprecise information.

Behaviours often take place in particular contexts, but there is usually no one-to-one relationship between a behaviour and the context it occurs in. Rather, given a certain behaviour, context information is determined according to some probability distribution. If B is a behaviour (e.g. making breakfast) and C some context information (e.g. in the kitchen), then $P(C|B)$ is the probability that C is true if B occurs (e.g. the behaviour takes place in the kitchen if we know that the behaviour is making breakfast).

Given the conditional probabilities $P(C|B)$, we can calculate conditional probabilities $P(B|C)$ using Bayes' rule. This assumes that we know the conditional probability for each context and behaviour. Moreover, we not only need $P(B|C)$ but also $P(B|C_1,\ldots,C_n)$, since context information is usually correlated. For example, an activity in the kitchen usually takes place while the person is standing (e.g. to prepare a meal), but an activity in the living room is usually performed in a sitting position (e.g. to watch TV). Assuming that we have knowledge of all the necessary conditional probabilities is unrealistic. In addition, the result of using conditional probabilities might be counterintuitive, as it does not align with how humans combine evidence.

Another shortcoming of probability theory is that probabilities have to add up to 100 %. In cases where we have perfect information, this is not a problem. However, when we do not have complete knowledge, this may lead to counterintuitive results. For example, if we do not have any information that a behaviour normally occurs in the kitchen, we cannot assign a probability of 0 % to $P(B|C)$, since this would imply that $P(\neg B|C)$ equals 100 %, which would mean that the behaviour happens outside the kitchen (if it happens at all). From the viewpoint of probability theory, $P(B|C) = 0$ does in fact not suggest lack of knowledge about B occuring in C but the perfect knowledge that B never occurs in C. It is therefore more adequate to assign a probability of 50 % to both $P(B|C)$ and $P(\neg B|C)$. However, this trick might produce inconsistencies in cases where there are more than two hypotheses.

The Dempster-Shafer theory [27,92] offers a way out of this dilemma. It uses the concept of belief (Bel) and plausibility (Pl) instead of probability to formulate uncertainty, where classical probability lies between belief and plausibility:

$$Bel(B|C) \leq P(B|C) \leq Pl(B|C)$$

Belief and plausibility is defined in the Dempster-Shafer theory on the basis of a mass function, which assigns basic probabilities to the power set of the frame of discernment.

Although the Dempster-Shafer theory has been applied successfully in the context of activity recognition in smart homes [71], it is not a solution to reasoning about context information in general, since the Dempster-Shafer theory is an even more complex framework than probability theory. In the following, we discuss a simpler framework, which is not as rigorous from the mathematical point of view but which provides a simple and robust way to deal with context information. This framework is based on Zadeh's fuzzy set theory [117].

Unlike traditional sets, fuzzy sets allow their elements to belong to the set with a certain degree. Rather than deciding whether an element d does or does not belong to a set A of a domain D, we determine for each element of D the degree with which it belongs to the fuzzy set $\tilde{A}$. In other words, a fuzzy subset $\tilde{A}$ of a domain D is a set of ordered pairs, $(d, \mu_{\tilde{A}}(d))$, where $d \in D$ and $\mu_{\tilde{A}} : D \rightarrow [0,1]$ is the membership function of $\tilde{A}$. The membership function replaces the characteristic function of a classical subset $A \subseteq D$.

Rather than asking the question of what is the probability of a certain behaviour occurring in a particular context, we now pose the question as follows. Given some context information C, to which degree is a particular behaviour a C-behaviour? For example, if C is the day of the week, then we can ask for the degree of the behaviour to be a Monday behaviour, Tuesday behaviour, and so on. In terms of fuzzy sets, we define D as the set of the seven days of the

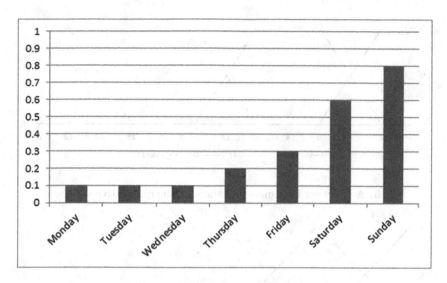

Fig. 4. Graphical representation of a membership functions that determines the degree
to which the visit of a relative falls on a particular day of the week.

week and $\mu_{\tilde{A}}$ as the membership function that determines to which degree the
behaviour or event occurs on a particular day.

For example, we might want to define a fuzzy set that reflects the degree to
which an AD patient is visited by a relative falls on a particular day, influencing his behaviour that is different when he stays home alone. The membership
function of such a fuzzy set is shown graphically in Fig. 4. Unlike probabilities,
the membership grades do not need to add up to 100 %.

In the example above, the context information is still crisp information,
despite the fact that it is used in a fuzzy set: for any visit, we can determine
precisely on which day of the week it occurs. Other context information might
not be precise, but rather conveys some vague information. For example, if we
know that a behaviour occurs near the kitchen, we usually do not know exactly
how many metres away from the kitchen the behaviour occurs. In this case, we
can represent the context information itself as a fuzzy set, as illustrated in Fig. 5.

Similarly, we can define a fuzzy set that expresses distances by rounding them
to the closest half metre – something we as humans often do when we perceive
distances, although not necessarily always on the same scale (see Fig. 6).

As the examples have shown, fuzzy sets can be used for associating behaviours
with context information and for representing imprecise context information.
Fuzzy set theory also provides us with a means to convert fuzzy sets back to
crisp sets, which is achieved with the notion of an α-level set. Let $\tilde{A}$ be a fuzzy
subset in D, then the (crisp) set of elements that belong to the fuzzy set $\tilde{A}$ with
a membership grade of at least α is called the α-level set of $\tilde{A}$:

$$A_\alpha = \{d \in D \mid \mu_{\tilde{A}}(d) \geq \alpha\}$$

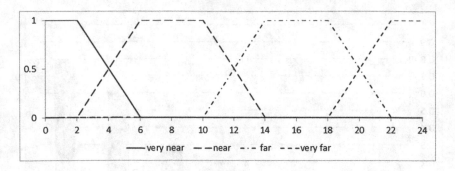

Fig. 5. A fuzzy set that maps distances to the qualitative values.

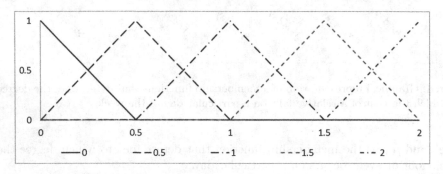

Fig. 6. A fuzzy set that approximates distances with a granularity of half a metre.

If the membership grade is strictly greater than α, then the set is referred to as strong α-level set.

When reasoning with context fuzzy sets, we need to address the potential problem of accumulating values, which we encounter in probability theory and the Dempster-Shafer theory. To avoid this problem, we choose one of the schemes for combining fuzzy sets that was originally proposed by Zadeh [117]. Given two fuzzy sets $\tilde{A}_1$ and $\tilde{A}_2$ with membership functions $\mu_{\tilde{A}_1}(d)$ and $\mu_{\tilde{A}_2}(d)$, respectively, then the membership function of the intersection $\tilde{A}_3 = \tilde{A}_1 \cap \tilde{A}_2$ is pointwise defined by:

$$\mu_{\tilde{A}_3}(d) = \min\{\mu_{\tilde{A}_1}(d), \mu_{\tilde{A}_2}(d)\}$$

Analogously, the membership function of the union $\tilde{A}_3 = \tilde{A}_1 \cup \tilde{A}_2$ is pointwise defined by:

$$\mu_{\tilde{A}_3}(d) = \max\{\mu_{\tilde{A}_1}(d), \mu_{\tilde{A}_2}(d)\}$$

The membership grade for the complement of a fuzzy set $\tilde{A}$, denoted as $\neg\tilde{A}$, is defined in the same way as the complement in probability theory:

$$\mu_{\neg\tilde{A}}(d) = 1 - \mu_{\tilde{A}}(d)$$

In [117], Zadeh stresses that the min/max combination scheme is not the only scheme for defining intersection and union of fuzzy sets, and that it depends on the context which scheme is the most appropriate. While some of the schemes are based on empirical investigations, others are the result of theoretical considerations [30,59]. However, [74] proved that the min/max operations are the most robust operations for combining fuzzy sets, where robustness is defined in terms of how much impact uncertainty in the input has on the error in the output.

To summarise, context information is often incomplete and imprecise. Probabilistic approaches are widespread but frequently impractical and therefore sometimes not useful in real-world applications. Fuzzy logic can offer a way out of this problem, as it provides robust mechanisms for dealing with uncertainty. While it is the purpose of this section to outline a number of methods employed in order to interpret behaviours of moving people under imprecise conditions, the specific conditions might significantly vary from application context to application context [17,20,42], requiring adapted methods coping with specific application constraints. Here, context information of locations are considered as a vehicle to deal with the interpretation of behaviours. Another option is to precisely analyse the trajectory of moving people [41,85]. However, this requires much more precise sensor data which are often difficult to acquire.

3.6 Ethical Aspects When Monitoring Humans Moving Around

The fact that tracking systems such as GPS or Radio-frequency identification (RFID) [50] are used in elderly population arise an ethical dilemma and an impact on family or professional caregiver. Regarding this subject studies are focused on:

- the attitude of the caregivers and the decision about the use of a tracking system for people with cognitive impairments [62,64],
- the attitudes of older people towards the use of tracking devices [93],
- reflexions on different devices used in daily care of persons with dementia [76], and
- providing recommendations for the question about who should decide about the usage of tracking technology [63].

Findings were reported based on questionnaires in [62–64,93], and a qualitative approach based on individual interviews [76]. One example of such a questionnaire included 23 items, each ranked on a 4-point Likert scale (1 = "do not agree at all", 4 = "very much agree"). The items covered several factors such as: respect for the elderly person's autonomy ("An individual has the right not to be tracked."), use of the device for patient safety ("Use the device as it protects patients from risk."), support for restricted use ("Tracking devices should be used only if there are no alternatives".). The qualitative approach based on individual interviews included initial interview questions, a presentation of information and communication technology devices, and a second round of interview questions.

First, caregivers' views ranged from feeling obligated to use the tracking device for the sake of patients' safety through support of the use of the device for the sake of the caregivers' peace of mind and restricted support, to objection to the use of the device and respect for a person's autonomy. Family caregivers provide higher support for the use of GPS and RFID, in the contrary professionals attached higher value to respect to the person's autonomy [64]. The study was done on two groups: family caregivers (N = 69, age 61.26 SD 12.91 years) and professionals (N = 96, age 43 SD 12.89 years) such as family physicians, psychiatrists, neurologists, geriatrists, social workers, or legal guardians.

Regarding who should decide about the use of electronic tracking, persons inside the family were perceived significantly more important in the decision-making process than other persons outside the family [62]. The study groups in this case included cognitively intact elderly (N = 44, age 70.94 SD 7.69 years), family caregivers (N = 94, age 59.62 SD 14.11 years), social workers (N = 51, age 33.76 SD 10.92 years), other professionals (N = 48, age 44.52 SD 10.89 years), and social work students (N = 59, age 24.88 SD 2.29 years). Overall, in order to reach a balance between the wishes and interest of both people with dementia and their family caregivers, the professionals need to be more involved in order to facilitate the family decision-making process.

Furthermore, cognitively intact older people favour the idea of tracking people with dementia. To facilitate family decision-making on the use of tracking devices, structured meetings guided by professionals and including persons with dementia and their family caregivers were suggested [93]. Data were collected from cognitively intact older people, from two sources: 42 participants completed a structured questionnaire and 23 participants provided qualitative data. Qualitative data was gathered from two focus groups of cognitively intact older people in Israel: the first focus group was based in an upscale retirement home (N = 11, age 84.9 SD 4.25 years) and the second one in a more modest home (N = 12, age 83.3 SD 6.8 years). The relatives of the persons with dementia were most likely to be informed about various kinds of information communication technology devices. The central issue from the perspective of the relative and the perceived of the person with dementia is the need for safety and security [76]. Participants of the individual interviews consisted of 14 spouses of persons with dementia (age 73 SD 10 years).

Finally, the main recommendations derived from the mentioned study regarding the patients and caregivers are:

- it is important to maintain balance between the needs for protection and safety and the need for autonomy and privacy [109];
- the decision on using tracking technology should be made jointly by the patient and caregivers and prior attitudes and values of both people with dementia and family caregivers must be considered;
- from the beginning of the treatment program for dementia formal structured meetings should be conducted in which all involved persons make together important decisions (i.e. the use of a GPS tracking system should be made in the early stage of the disease [63]).

Overall, this discussion focuses on ethical issues from a qualitative point of view, as derived from the feedback of users. A complete analysis would have to consider also legal aspects, such as guidelines provided by governments and their practicability. But this is outside the scope of this paper.

4   Open Problems

The development of areas like pervasive and ubiquitous computing brought computing science and in particular Artificial Intelligence research more closely in touch with real life problems which affect directly the everyday life of patients [12]. A substantial part of the creation of automated services in this area rely on the need to precisely locate humans and to determine what their relation with the surroundings is, has been and is likely to be. The previous sections provided insights into the basic concepts of this challenge and on how the understanding of this challenging process enables us to build services in the real world. However, as a relatively recent area there are still more questions than answers, but some progress has been achieved in terms of understanding the use of different technologies available.

Although technology has been made significant advances in the last decade, there are limitations in the infrastructure we can use today, some of which take the level of a barrier. An example of this is tracking the location of a person. Outdoors the best tools available are GPS services offered through satellite support. One problem is that it does not work in certain areas like wilderness and tunnels and even in some places near towns and cities. To this we need to add that in occasions when it works it is not necessarily accurate. Inside homes and buildings there are many devices which are capable to offer information on the whereabouts of individuals with different degrees of precision, from worn devices to triangulation techniques for mobile devices and video cameras.

A further complication is that many services will strongly benefit with the possibility to track an individual trajectory inside and outside the home seamlessly. This will allow to make sure that people with cognitive frailty do not get lost or can find their way through the city, including a way back home, more safely. It also allows a more comprehensive understanding of the activity levels of a person, which provide important information on the health and well-being of an individual. However, technology which tracks people outdoors and indoors are quite different and it will be unrealistic to ask people experiencing cognitive decline to become technical experts and to remember to switch technologies as leaving or entering home. "Change" is a notion which brings interesting challenges, in this cases managing transitions between regions reliably.

The infrastructure available and its intrinsic limitations affects how much we can aspire to do with our theories and algorithms. It is not easy to influence technology with our theories and algorithms and expect industry will implement the devices which make lazy methods workable as there are powerful market forces governing what devices are materialised. If we have to fill in the technological gaps with clever algorithms, what should they be like? Should there be a cloud service which has built in increased capability for inter-operability? A user can have more than one device registered to track her whereabouts. Those devices can recognise where a registered person is, as long as one of those devices provides information, which can have a smaller or bigger circle of uncertainty. The level of certainty might degrade under a certain threshold, for example, when going out of the home without a phone means the person cannot be identified being at home by home devices nor outside as the phone is left behind.

Despite the interesting range of technology available this is a problem which will remain for the foreseeable future. No current technology ensures continuous tracking, even a wearable device which is equipped with technology for both indoor and outdoors cannot guarantee the person in question will wear it, like no current pill dispensers can guarantee the person has swollen the medicine pill. May be a solution to this problem will be implants but this is still a far fetched scientific option, not because it is not possible but because people in general are not accepting this level of body intrusion at this time in history. Given the current limitations discussed above, software is the only apparent way to temporarily ameliorate the problem.

5 Future Outlook

Future challenges have been outlined implicitly in the previous sections. Two particularly challenging factors, at the technological level as well as at the level of the users, can be identified from the previous discussions and summarised as follows:

- **The technological factor:** The realtime gathering of enough context information as well as appropriate fast interpretation methods pose great challenges. Thereby, the main questions concern the kind of context information to collect and how to interpret it in a sufficiently precise and robust way despite of imprecise or even incomplete location and context information. Though advances in Artificial Intelligence research, in particular in spatiotemporal reasoning have been made, these have not yet sufficiently translated into popular tools used by other communities like in Ambient Intelligence in order to exploit them for assistive technologies.
- **The human factor:** Apart from ethical issues another problem with the use of wearable technologies for managing the life of people who, for example, suffer from dementia arises. Such patients often have difficulties in accepting anything new in their environment, and even much more, any foreign objects which are attached to their body. This concerns the notion of unobtrusiveness regarding a particular sensitive issue, inasmuch at some state, patients are not anymore able to let other people know about their anxieties. It is a major challenge beyond the development of new technologies to appropriately deal with such issues.

References

1. Abraham Louis Perrelet. http://en.wikipedia.org/wiki/Abraham-Louis_Perrelet. Accessed 14 Jan 2014
2. Animazoo motion capture. http://www.animazoo.com/products/igs-180-range. Accessed 15 Dec 2013

3. Basque country reaches out to the elderly. http://www.cnbc.com/id/101198944. Accessed 15 Dec 2013
4. Chronious. http://www.chronious.eu. Accessed 29 Dec 2013
5. Fitbit. http://www.fitbit.com/. Accessed 15 Dec 2013
6. Kinect. http://www.microsoft.com/en-us/kinectforwindows/develop/. Accessed 15 Dec 2013
7. Misfit wearables. http://www.misfitwearables.com/. Accessed 15 Dec 2013
8. Nike fuelband. http://www.nike.com/us/en_us/c/nikeplus-fuelband. Accessed 15 Dec 2013
9. Openstage. http://www.organicmotion.com/products/openstage. Accessed 15 Dec 2013
10. Vicon — markers and suits. http://www.vicon.com/System/Markers. Accessed 15 Dec 2013
11. Augusto, J., Nugent, C.: The use of temporal reasoning and management of complex events in smart homes. In: Proceedings of the ECAI 2004, Valencia, Spain, pp. 778–782 (2004)
12. Augusto, J.C., Huch, M., Kameas, A., Maitland, J., McCullagh, P., Roberts, J., Sixsmith, A., Wichert, R.: Handbook on Ambient Assisted Living - Technology for Healthcare Rehabilitation and Well-Being. The AISE Book Series, vol. 11. IOS Press, Amsterdam (2012)
13. Augusto, J.C., Nakashima, H., Aghajan, H.: Ambient intelligence and smart environments: a state of the art. In: Nakashima, H., Aghajan, H., Augusto, J.C. (eds.) Handbook of Ambient Intelligence and Smart Environments, pp. 3–31. Springer, New York (2010)
14. Aztiria, A., Augusto, J., Izaguirre, A., Cook, D.: Learning accurate temporal relations from user actions in intelligent environments. In: Proceedings of the 3rd Symposium of Ubiquitous Computing and Ambient Intelligence, Salamanca, Spain, pp. 274–283 (2008)
15. Ballemans, J., Kempen, G.I., Zijlstra, G.R.: Orientation and mobility training for partially-sighted older adults using an identification cane: a systematic review. Clin. Rehabil. **25**, 880–891 (2011)
16. Bengalur, M.D.: Human activity recognition using body pose features and support vector machine. In: 2013 International Conference on Advances in Computing, Communications and Informatics (ICACCI), pp. 1970–1975 (2013)
17. Bohlken, W., Neumann, B., Hotz, L., Koopmann, P.: Ontology-based realtime activity monitoring using beam search. In: Crowley, J.L., Draper, B.A., Thonnat, M. (eds.) ICVS 2011. LNCS, vol. 6962, pp. 112–121. Springer, Heidelberg (2011)
18. Callejas Cuervo, M., Olaya, A., Salamanca, R.: Biomechanical motion capture methods focused on tele-physiotherapy. In: Health Care Exchanges (PAHCE), 2013 Pan American, pp. 1–6 (2013)
19. Camicioli, R., Howieson, D., Oken, B., Sexton, G., Kaye, J.: Motor slowing precedes cognitive impairment in the oldest old. Neurology **50**(5), 1496–1498 (1998)
20. Chakraborty, B., Bagdanov, A.D., Gonzàlez, J., Roca, F.X.: Human action recognition using an ensemble of body-part detectors. Expert Syst. **30**(2), 101–114 (2013)
21. Chua, S.-L., Marsland, S., Guesgen, H.: Unsupervised learning of patterns in data streams using compression and edit distance. In: Proceedings of IJCAI, Barcelona, Spain, pp. 1231–1236 (2011)
22. Cook, D.: Learning setting-generalized activity models for smart spaces. IEEE Intell. Syst. **27**(1), 32–38 (2012)

23. Crews, J.E., Campbell, V.A.: Vision impairment and hearing loss among community-dwelling older Americans: implications for health and functioning. Am. J. Public Health **94**(5), 823–829 (2004)
24. Cummings, J.L.: The neuropsychiatric inventory: assessing psychopathology in dementia patients. Neurology **48**(Suppl 6), S10–S16 (1997)
25. David, R., Rivet, A., Robert, P.H., Mailland, V., Friedman, L., Zeitzer, J.M., Yesavage, J.: Ambulatory actigraphy correlates with apathy in mild Alzheimer's disease. Dementia **9**(4), 509–516 (2010)
26. DeCarli, C.: Mild cognitive impairment: prevalence, prognosis, aetiology, and treatment. Lancet Neurol. **2**, 15–21 (2003)
27. Dempster, A.: Upper and lower probabilities induced by a multivalued mapping. Ann. Math. Stat. **38**(2), 325–339 (1967)
28. Doukas, C., Maglogiannis, I.: Emergency fall incidents detection in assisted living environments utilizing motion, sound, and visual perceptual components. IEEE Trans. Inf. Technol. Biomed. **15**(2), 277–289 (2011)
29. Downs, S.H., Black, N.: The feasibility of creating a checklist for the assessment of the methodological quality both of randomised and non-randomised studies of health care interventions. J. Epidemiol. Commun. Health **52**, 377–384 (1998)
30. Dubois, D., Prade, H.: Fuzzy Sets and Systems: Theory and Applications. Academic Press, London (1980)
31. Duong, T., Bui, H., Phung, D., Venkatesh, S.: Activity recognition and abnormality detection with the switching hidden semi-Markov model. In: Proceedings of CVPR 2005, San Diego, California, pp. 838–845 (2005)
32. Fernandez-Martinez, M., Molano, A., Castro, J., Zarranz, J.J.: Prevalence of neuropsychiatric symptoms in mild cognitive impairment and Alzheimer's disease, and its relationship with cognitive impairment. Curr. Alzheimer Res. **7**(6), 517–526 (2010)
33. Folstein, M.F., Folstein, S.E., McHugh, P.R.: Mini-mental-state: a practical method for grading the cognitive state of patients for the clinician. J. Psychiatr. Res. **12**, 189–198 (1975)
34. Foxlin, E.: Pedestrian tracking with shoe-mounted inertial sensors. IEEE Comput. Graph **25**(6), 38–46 (2005)
35. Friedman, J.H.: Regularized discriminant analysis. J. Am. Statist. Assoc. **84**(405), 165–175 (1989)
36. Giuberti, M., Ferrari, G., Contin, L., Cimolin, V., Cau, N., Galli, M., Azzaro, C., Albani, G., Mauro, A.: On the characterization of Leg Agility in patients with Parkinson's Disease. In: 2013 IEEE International Conference on Body Sensor Networks, pp. 1–6, May 2013
37. Gopalratnam, K., Cook, D.: Active LeZi: an incremental parsing algorithm for sequential prediction. Int. J. Artif. Intell. Tools **14**(1–2), 917–930 (2004)
38. Gottfried, B.: Spatial health systems. In: Bardram, J.E., Chachques, J.C., Varshney, U. (eds.) 1st International Conference on Pervasive Computing Technologies for Healthcare (PCTH 2006), November 29–December 1, Innsbruck, Austria, pp. 7. IEEE Press (2006)
39. Gottfried, B.: Modelling spatiotemporal developments in spatial health systems. In: Olla, P., Tan, J. (eds.) Mobile Health Solutions for Biomedical Applications. IGI Global (Idea Group Publishing), April 2009
40. Gottfried, B.: Locomotion activities in smart environments. In: Nakashima, H., Aghajan, H.K., Augusto, J.C. (eds.) Handbook of Ambient Intelligence and Smart Environments, pp. 89–115. Springer, Heidelberg (2010)

41. Gottfried, B.: Interpreting motion events of pairs of moving objects. GeoInformatica **15**(2), 247–271 (2011)
42. Gottfried, B., Aghajan, H.: Behaviour Monitoring and Interpretation - Smart Environments. IOS Press, Amsterdam (2009)
43. Gottfried, B., W. Guesgen, H., Hübner, S.: Spatiotemporal reasoning for smart homes. In: Augusto, J.C., Nugent, C.D. (eds.) Designing Smart Homes. LNCS (LNAI), vol. 4008, pp. 16–34. Springer, Heidelberg (2006)
44. Guesgen, H., Marsland, S.: Spatio-temporal reasoning and context awareness. In: Nakashima, H., Aghajan, H., Augusto, J. (eds.) Handbook of Ambient Intelligence and Smart Environments, pp. 609–634. Springer, New York (2010)
45. Hausdorff, J.M., Rios, D.A., Edelberg, H.K.: Gait variability and fall risk in community-living older adults: a 1-year prospective study. Arch. Phys. Med. Rehabil. **82**(8), 1050–1056 (2001)
46. Hoey, J., Plötz, T., Jackson, D., Monk, A., Pham, C., Olivier, P.: Rapid specification and automated generation of prompting systems to assist people with dementia. Pervasive Mob. Comput. **7**(3), 299–318 (2011)
47. Hoey, J., Poupart, P., Bertoldi, A.V., Craig, T., Boutilier, C., Mihailidis, A.: Automated handwashing assistance for persons with dementia using video and a partially observable Markov decision process. Comput. Vision Image Underst. **114**(5), 503–519 (2010)
48. Hoey, J., Yang, X., Quintana, E., Favela, J.: LaCasa: location and context-aware safety assistant. In: 6th International Conference Pervasive Computing Technologies for Healthcare (PervasiveHealth), pp. 171–174 (2012)
49. Holzinger, A., Scherer, R., Seeber, M., Wagner, J., Müller-Putz, G.: Computational sensemaking on examples of knowledge discovery from neuroscience data: towards enhancing stroke rehabilitation. In: Böhm, C., Khuri, S., Lhotská, L., Renda, M.E. (eds.) ITBAM 2012. LNCS, vol. 7451, pp. 166–168. Springer, Heidelberg (2012)
50. Holzinger, A., Schwaberger, K., Weitlaner, M.: Ubiquitous computing for hospital applications: Rfid-applications to enable research in real-life environments. In: 29th Annual International Computer Software and Applications Conference (COMPSAC 2005), 25–28 July 2005, Edinburgh, Scotland, UK, pp. 19–20. IEEE Computer Society (2005)
51. Ito, T.: Walking motion analysis using 3D acceleration sensors. In: 2008 Second UKSIM European Symposium on Computer Modeling and Simulation, EMS 2008, pp. 123–128 (2008)
52. Jakkula, V., Cook, D.: Anomaly detection using temporal data mining in a smart home environment. Methods Inf. Med. **47**(1), 70–75 (2008)
53. Jakkula, V.R., Cook, D.J.: Detecting anomalous sensor events in smart home data for enhancing the living experience. In: Artificial Intelligence and Smarter Living, volume WS-11-07 of AAAI Workshops. AAAI (2011)
54. Jung, P.-G., Lim, G., Kong, K.: A mobile motion capture system based on inertial sensors and smart shoes. In: 2013 IEEE International Conference on Robotics and Automation (ICRA), pp. 692–697 (2013)
55. Kammoun, S., Macé, M.J.-M., Oriola, B., Jouffrais, C.: Towards a geographic information system facilitating navigation of visually impaired users. In: Miesenberger, K., Karshmer, A., Penaz, P., Zagler, W. (eds.) ICCHP 2012, Part II. LNCS, vol. 7383, pp. 521–528. Springer, Heidelberg (2012)
56. Kearns, W., Algase, D., Moore, D., Ahmed, S.: Ultra wideband radio: a novel method for measuring wandering in persons with dementia. Gerontechnology **7**(1), 48–57 (2008)

57. Kirste, T., Hoffmeyer, A., Koldrack, P., Bauer, A., Schubert, S., Schröder, S., Teipel, S.: Detecting the effect of Alzheimer's disease on everyday motion behavior. J. Alzheimer's Dis. **38**(1), 121–132 (2014)
58. Kleinberger, T., Becker, M., Ras, E., Holzinger, A., Müller, P.: Ambient intelligence in assisted living: enable elderly people to handle future interfaces. In: Stephanidis, C. (ed.) UAHCI 2007 (Part II). LNCS, vol. 4555, pp. 103–112. Springer, Heidelberg (2007)
59. Klir, G., Folger, T.: Fuzzy Sets, Uncertainty, and Information. Prentice Hall, Englewood Cliffs (1988)
60. Koss, E., Weiner, M., Ernesto, C., Cohen-Mansfield, J., Ferris, S.H., Grundman, M., Schafer, K., Sano, M., Thal, L.J., Thomas, R., Whitehouse, P.J.: Assessing patterns of agitation in Alzheimer's disease patients with the Cohen-Mansfield Agitation Inventory. The Alzheimer's disease cooperative study. Alzheimer Dis. Assoc. Disord. **11**(Suppl 2), S45–50 (1997)
61. Kuhlmei, A., Walther, B., Becker, T., Müller, U., Nikolaus, T.: Actigraphic daytime activity is reduced in patients with cognitive impairment and apathy. Eur. Psychiatry **28**(2), 806–814 (2011)
62. Landau, R., Auslander, G.K., Werner, S., Shoval, N., Heinik, J.: Who should make the decision on the use of GPS for people with dementia? Aging Ment. Health **15**, 78–84 (2011)
63. Landau, R., Werner, S.: Ethical aspects of using GPS for tracking people with dementia: recommendations for practice. Int. Psychogeriatr. **24**, 358–366 (2012)
64. Landau, R., Werner, S., Auslander, G., Shoval, N., Heinik, J.: Attitudes of family and professional care-givers towards the use of GPS for tracking patients with dementia: an exploratory study. Br. J. Soc. Work **39**(4), 670–692 (2009)
65. Levy, E., Kalis, M., Vo, M., Lindisch, D., Cleary, K.: Feasibility of simultaneous respiratory function monitoring and determination of respiratory-related intrahepatic vessel excursion using the lifeshirt system. In: Lemke, H.U., Inamura, K., Doi, K., Vannier, M.W., Farman, A.G., Reiber, J.H.C. (eds.) Proceedings of the 18th International Congress and Exhibition Computer Assisted Radiology and Surgery, Chicago, USA, June 23–26, vol. 1268, International Congress Series, pp. 764–769. Elsevier (2004)
66. Li, L., Zhang, H., Jia, W., Nie, J., Zhang, W., Sun, M.: Automatic video analysis and motion estimation for physical activity classification. In: Bioengineering Conference, Proceedings of the 2010 IEEE 36th Annual Northeast, pp. 1–2 (2010)
67. Li, Q., Chen, S., Stankovic, J.A.: Multi-modal in-person interaction monitoring using smartphone and on-body sensors. In: 2013 IEEE International Conference on Body Sensor Networks, pp. 1–6, May 2013
68. Lo, G., Suresh, A., Stocco, L., Gonzalez-Valenzuela, S., Leung, V.C.M.: A wireless sensor system for motion analysis of parkinson's disease patients. In: 2011 IEEE International Conference on Pervasive Computing and Communications Workshops (PERCOM Workshops), pp. 372–375 (2011)
69. Long, R.G., Boyette, L.W., Griffin-Shirley, N.: Older persons and community travel: the effect of visual impairment. J. Visual Impairment Blindness **90**(4), 302–313 (1996)
70. Maki, B.E.: Gait changes in older adults: predictors of falls or indicators of fear. J. Am. Geriatr. Soc. **45**(3), 313–320 (1997)
71. McKeever, S., Ye, J., Coyle, L., Bleakley, C., Dobson, S.: Activity recognition using temporal evidence theory. J. Ambient Intell. Smart Environ. **2**(3), 253–269 (2010)

72. Miskelly, F.: A novel system of electronic tagging in patients with dementia and wandering. Age Ageing **33**, 304–306 (2004)
73. Nagels, G., Engelborghsand, S., Vloeberghs, E., Van Dam, D., Pickut, B.A., De Deyn, P.P.: Actigraphic measurement of agitated behaviour in dementia. Int. J. Geriatr. Psychiatry. **21**(4), 388–393 (2006)
74. Nguyen, H., Kreinovich, V., Tolbert, D.: On robustness of fuzzy logics. In: Proceedings of the 2nd IEEE International Conference on Fuzzy Systems, San Francisco, California, pp. 543–547 (1993)
75. Nissenbaum, H.: Privacy as contextual integrity. Wash. Law Rev. **79**(1), 119–158 (2004)
76. Olsson, A., Engstrm, M., Skovdahl, K., Lampic, C.: My, your and our needs for safety and security: relatives' reflections on using information and communication tech-nology in dementia care. Scand. J. Caring Sci. **26**, 104–112 (2012)
77. Oswald, F., Wahl, H.-W., Voss, E., Schilling, O., Freytag, T., Auslander, G., Shoval, N., Heinik, J., Landau, R.: The use of tracking technologies for the analysis of outdoor mobility in the face of dementia: first steps into a project and some illustrative findings from Germany. J. Hous. Elderly **24**, 55–73 (2010)
78. Paradiso, R., Loriga, G., Taccini, N.A.: A wearable health care system based on knitted integrated sensors. IEEE Trans. Inf. Technol. Biomed. **9**, 337–344 (2005)
79. Patterson, D.J., Liao, L., Gajos, K., Collier, M., Livic, N., Olson, K., Wang, S., Fox, D., Kautz, H.: Opportunity knocks: a system to provide cognitive assistance with transportation services. In: Mynatt, E.D., Siio, I. (eds.) UbiComp 2004. LNCS, vol. 3205, pp. 433–450. Springer, Heidelberg (2004)
80. Plaza, I., Martín, L., Martin, S., Medrano, C.: Mobile applications in an aging so-ciety: status and trends. J. Syst. Softw. **84**, 1977–1988 (2011)
81. Pogorelc, B., Gams, M.: Diagnosing health problems from gait patterns of elderly. In: 2010 Annual International Conference of the IEEE Engineering in Medicine and Biology Society (EMBC), pp. 2238–2241 (2010)
82. Pogorelc, B., Gams, M.: Medically driven data mining application: recognition of health problems from gait patterns of elderly. In: 2010 IEEE International Conference on Data Mining Workshops (ICDMW), pp. 976–980 (2010)
83. Rashidi, P., Cook, D.J.: Mining and monitoring patterns of daily routines for assisted living in real world settings. In: Proceedings of the 1st ACM International Health Informatics Symposium, IHI 2010, pp. 336–345. ACM, New York (2010)
84. Rashidi, P., Cook, D.J., Holder, L.B., Schmitter-Edgecombe, M.: Discovering activities to recognize and track in a smart environment. IEEE Trans. Knowl. Data Eng. **23**(4), 527–539 (2011)
85. Renso, C., Baglioni, M., de Macêdo, J.A.F., Trasarti, R., Wachowicz, M.: How you move reveals who you are: understanding human behavior by analyzing trajectory data. Knowl. Inf. Syst. **37**(2), 331–362 (2013)
86. Rivera-Illingworth, F., Callaghan, V., Hagras, H.: Detection of normal and novel behaviours in ubiquitous domestic environments. Comput. J. **53**(2), 142–151 (2010)
87. Roley, S.S., DeLany, J.V., Barrows, C.J., Brownrigg, S., Honaker, D., Sava, D.I., Talley, V., Voelkerding, K., Amini, D.A., Smith, E., Toto, P., King, S., Lieberman, D., Baum, M.C., Cohen, E.S., Cleveland, P.A., Youngstrom, M.J.: Occupational therapy practice framework: domain & practice. Am. J. Occup. Ther. **62**(6), 625–683 (2008). (2nd edn)
88. Rosso, A.L., Auchincloss, A.H., Michael, Y.L.: The urban built environment and mobility in older adults: a comprehensive review. J. Aging Res. **2011**, 10 (2011)

89. Roy, A., Soni, Y., Dubey, S.: Enhancing effectiveness of motor rehabilitation using kinect motion sensing technology. In: 2013 IEEE Global Humanitarian Technology Conference: South Asia Satellite (GHTC-SAS), pp. 298–304 (2013)

90. Runge, M., Hunter, G.: Determinants of musculoskeletal frailty and the risk of falls in old age. J. Musculoskelet. Neuronal Interact. 6(2), 167–173 (2006)

91. Salarian, A., Russmann, H., Vingerhoets, F.J.G., Dehollaini, C., Blanc, Y., Burkhard, P., Aminian, K.: Gait assessment in parkinson's disease: toward an ambulatory system for long-term monitoring. IEEE Trans. Biomed. Eng. 51(8), 1434–1443 (2004)

92. Shafer, G.: A Mathematical Theory of Evidence. Princeton University Press, Princeton (1976)

93. Shoval, N., Auslander, G., Cohen-Shalom, K., Isaacson, M., Landau, R., Heinik, J.: What can we learn about the mobility of the elderly in the GPS era? J. Transport Geogr. 18, 603–612 (2010)

94. Stone, E., Skubic, M.: Evaluation of an inexpensive depth camera for in-home gait assessment. J. Ambient Intell. Smart Environ. 3(4), 349–361 (2011)

95. Sundaresan, A., Chellappa, R.: Markerless motion capture using multiple cameras. Comput. Vision Interact. Intell. Environ. 2005, 15–26 (2005)

96. Tapia, E.M., Intille, S.S., Larson, K.: Activity recognition in the home using simple and ubiquitous sensors. In: Ferscha, A., Mattern, F. (eds.) PERVASIVE 2004. LNCS, vol. 3001, pp. 158–175. Springer, Heidelberg (2004)

97. Tavenard, R., Salah, A., Pauwels, E.: Searching for temporal patterns in ami sensor data. In: Mühlhäuser, M., Ferscha, A., Aitenbichler, E. (eds.) Constructing Ambient Intelligence. Communications in Computer and Information Science, vol. 11, pp. 53–62. Springer, Heidelberg (2007)

98. Tay, F.E.H., Nyan, M.N., Koh, T.H., Seah, K.H.W., Sitoh, Y.Y.: Smart shirt that can call for help after a fall. Int. J. Softw. Eng. Knowl. Eng. 15(2), 183–188 (2005)

99. Teri, L., Larson, E.B., Reifler, B.V.: Behavioral disturbance in dementia of the Alzheimer's type. J. Am. Geriatr. Soc. 36(1), 1–6 (1988)

100. Thome, J., Coogan, A.N., Woods, A.G., Darie, C.C., Hassler, F.: CLOCK genes and circadian rhythmicity in Alzheimer disease. J. Aging Res. Article ID 383091, 4 (2011)

101. Vahdatpour, A., Amini, N., Sarrafzadeh, M.: On-body device localization for health and medical monitoring applications. In: 2011 IEEE International Conference on Pervasive Computing and Communications (PerCom), pp. 37–44 (2011)

102. van den Noort, J.C., Scholtes, V.A., Becher, J.G., Harlaar, J.: Evaluation of the catch in spasticity assessment in children with cerebral palsy. Arch. Phys. Med. Rehabil. 91(4), 615–623 (2010)

103. van den Noort, J.C., Scholtes, V.A., Harlaar, J.: Evaluation of clinical spasticity assessment in cerebral palsy using inertial sensors. Gait Posture 30(2), 138–143 (2009)

104. van Someren, E.J.W., Lazeron, R.H.C., Vonk, B.F.M., Mirmiran, M., Swaab, D.F.: Gravitational artifact in frequency spectra of movement acceleration: implications for actigraphy in young and elderly subjects. J. Neurosci. Methods 65, 55–62 (1996)

105. Wallhagen, M.I., Strawbridge, W.J., Shema, S.J., Kurata, J., Kaplan, G.A.: Comparative impact of hearing and vision impairment on subsequent functioning. J. Am. Geriatr. Soc. 49, 1086–1092 (2001)

106. Wan, C., Yuan, B., Wang, L. Miao, Z.: Model-based markerless human body motion capture using active contour. In: 2008 9th International Conference on Signal Processing, ICSP 2008, pp. 1342–1345 (2008)

107. Weber, J.L., Blanc, D., Dittmar, A., Comet, B., Corroy, C., Noury, N., Baghai, R., Vaysse, S., Blinowska, A.: VTAM - a new "biocloth" for ambulatory telemonitoring. In: 4th International IEEE EMBS Special Topic Conference on Information Technology Applications in Biomedicine, pp. 299–301 (2003)

108. Weiner, M.F., Koss, E., Patterson, M., Jin, S., Teri, L., Thomas, R., Thal, L.J., Whitehouse, P.: A comparison of the Cohen-Mansfield agitation inventory with the CERAD behavioral rating scale for dementia in community-dwelling persons with Alzheimer's disease. J. Psychiatr. Res. **32**, 347–351 (1998)

109. Weippl, E., Holzinger, A., Tjoa, A.M.: Security aspects of ubiquitous computing in health care. e & i. Elektrotechnik und Informationstechnik **123**(4), 156–161 (2006)

110. Wimo, A., Winblad, B., Aguero-Torres, H., von Strauss, E.: The magnitude of dementia occurrence in the world. Alzheimer Dis. Assoc. Disord. **17**, 63–67 (2010)

111. Wong, C., Zhang, Z., McKeague, S., Yang, G.-Z.: Multi-person vision-based head detector for markerless human motion capture. In: 2013 IEEE International Conference on Body Sensor Networks (BSN), pp. 1–6 (2013)

112. Wu, H.-Y., Rubinstein, M., Shih, E., Guttag, J., Durand, F., Freeman, W.: Eulerian video magnification for revealing subtle changes in the world. ACM Trans. Graph. **31**(4), 65:1–65:8 (2012)

113. Wu, Y.-H., Fischer, D.F., Kalsbeek, A., Garidou-Boof, M.-L., van der Vliet, J., van Heijningen, C., Liu, R.-Y., Zhou, J.-N., Swaab, D.F.: Pineal clock gene oscillation is disturbed in Alzheimer's disease, due to functional disconnection from the "master clock". FASEB J. **20**(11), 1874–1876 (2006)

114. Xing, X., Langer, H.: Medical knowledge representation and reasoning in the CHRONIOUS project. In: Behavior Monitoring and Interpretation - Well Being, Workshop on KI-2009, Paderborn (2009)

115. Ye, Y., Ci, S., Katsaggelos, A., Liu, Y.: A multi-camera motion capture system for remote healthcare monitoring. In: 2013 IEEE International Conference on Multimedia and Expo (ICME), pp. 1–6 (2013)

116. Yesavage, J.A., Noda, A., Hernandez, B., Friedman, L., Cheng, J.J., Tinklenberg, J.R., Hallmayer, J., O'Hara, R., David, R., Robert, P., Landsverk, E., Zeitzer, J.M.: Circadian clock gene polymorphisms and sleep-wake disturbance in Alzheimer disease. Am. J. Geriatr. Psychiatry **19**, 635–643 (2011)

117. Zadeh, L.: Fuzzy sets. Inf. Control **8**(3), 338–353 (1965)

118. Zhang, B., Jiang, S., Wei, D., Marschollek, M., Zhang, W.: State of the art in gait analysis using wearable sensors for healthcare applications. In: 2012 IEEE/ACIS 11th International Conference on Computer and Information Science (ICIS), pp. 213–218 (2012)

119. Zhang, Z., Wong, L., Wu, J.-K.: 3D upper limb motion modeling and estimation using wearable micro-sensors. In: 2010 International Conference on Body Sensor Networks (BSN), pp. 117–123 (2010)

120. Zhang, Z.-Q., Wong, W.-C., Wu, J.-K.: Ubiquitous human upper-limb motion estimation using wearable sensors. IEEE Trans. Inf. Technol. Biomed. **15**(4), 513–521 (2011)

121. Ziefle, M., Klack, L., Wilkowska, W., Holzinger, A.: Acceptance of telemedical treatments – a medical professional point of view. In: Yamamoto, S. (ed.) HCI 2013, Part II. LNCS, vol. 8017, pp. 325–334. Springer, Heidelberg (2013)

Reading

- **Behaviour Monitoring and Interpretation – Well-Being**, Editors: B. Gottfried and H. Aghajan, IOS Press, 2011.

This volume offers state-of-the-art contributions in the application area of well-being. The notion of well-being has been treated in diverse disciplines such as engineering, sociology, psychology, and philosophy. With this book a perspective is offered to the latest trends in this field from a few different viewpoints. Well-being is an omnipresent concept that reaches out to a myriad of aspects of our daily lives. In addition to supporting a healthy lifestyle, the concept of well-being extends to the selections involving the type of the environment we live in, the interactions we have with other humans, and the practices we engage in to achieve our plans for future. Well-being concerns us in our daily life, and hence, plays a fundamental role at all times and places. This fact in turn needs to be taken into account when designing ubiquitous computing technologies that pervade our life. With the presented articles the book provides a survey of different research projects that aim to address the many influential aspects of well-being that are considered in todays designs or play an essential role in the designs of the future.

- **Handbook of Ambient Assisted Living – Technology for Healthcare, Rehabilitation and Well-being**, Editors: J. C. Augusto et al., IOS Press, 2012.

The world's population is aging dramatically, and in most countries the cost of care is rising rapidly. We need a system which helps to minimize the onset of chronic conditions which are costly to treat and diminish quality of life, rather than one primarily directed towards the care of the sick. Innovative use of new technologies may be the only way to provide care affordably in future, and to scale that care to far greater numbers as our societies adapt to change. Ambient Assisted Living (AAL) can provide a solution. More integration between the health system and life at home and work will benefit everybody, providing better, more holistic lifelong care at lower cost.

This book presents and summarizes the achievements of an accomplished group of researchers around the globe and from diverse technical backgrounds. They use a wide range of approaches to optimize the use of healthcare technology and integrate such technology into human lives in a way that will benefit all. The book is divided into seven main sections:

- AAL in the health space
- Devices and infrastructure to facilitate AAL
- AAL in gerontology
- Smart homes as a vehicle for AAL
- Applications of AAL in rehabilitation
- AAL initiatives
- Novel developments and visions for the area.

Developing technologies which cater for the broad range of individuals in our complex societies is a major challenge which poses many problems.

The research described here pushes the boundaries, and will inspire other researchers to continue their exploration of technologies to improve lives.

- **Situational Awareness for Assistive Technologies**, Editors: M. Bhatt and H. W. Guesgen, IOS Press, 2012.

The development of smart assistive technology for personal living and public environments is an opportunity that has been recently recognised by research labs across the world. A particular theme that has garnered attention in many countries is the problem of an aging population. The combination of a much larger elderly population and the ever increasing cost of providing full-time human care for them means that finding practical assisted living solutions for this group is becoming increasingly important. Computing is the obvious choice to provide an answer to this growing problem, but to have a real impact, computer-based assistive technologies will need to possess the ability to interact with, and interpret, the actions and situations of those they are designed to assist.

The papers in this book explore the diversity of the field of ambient intelligence, as well as the wide range of approaches and variety of applications that may prove to be possible. Consideration is given to how space, action, time, and other contexts can be represented and reasoned about for use in sensory mapping, multi-agent interactions, assisted living, and even emergency responses. Many techniques are examined; variety represents one of the most important strengths of this area, meaning that the weakness of one approach can be offset by the capability of others.

The book consists of research contributions dealing with the crucial notion of situational awareness within assistive smart systems emerging as an overarching concept. An applied computer science character has been retained, whilst bringing to the fore research projects where formal knowledge representation and reasoning techniques have been demonstrated to be applicable to areas within the broader field of ambient intelligence and smart environments.

Towards Pervasive Mobility Assessments in Clinical and Domestic Environments

Melvin Isken[1]($\boxtimes$), Thomas Frenken[1], Melina Frenken[2], and Andreas Hein[3]

[1] OFFIS Insitute for Information Technology, Escherweg 2,
26127 Oldenburg, Germany
{melvin.isken,thomas.frenken}@offis.de
http://www.offis.de

[2] Institute of Technical Assistance Systems, Jade-University of Applied Sciences,
Westerstr. 10-12, 26121 Oldenburg, Germany

[3] Devision Automation and Measurement Technology, University of Oldenburg,
Ammerlaender Heerstr. 140, 26121 Oldenburg, Germany

Abstract. This paper provides an overview of current research and open problems in sensor-based mobility analysis. It is focused on geriatric assessment tests and the idea to provide easier and more objective results by using sensor technologies. A lot of research has been done in the field of measuring personal movement/mobility by technical approaches but there are few developments to measure a complete geriatric assessment test. Such automated tests can very likely offer more accurate, reliable and objective results than currently used methods. Additionally, those tests may reduce costs in public health systems as well as set standards for comparability of the tests. New sensor technologies and initiatives for data standardization in health processes offer increased possibilities in system development. This paper will highlight some open problems that still exist to bring automated mobility assessment tests into pervasive clinical and domestic use.

Keywords: Assessment · Geriatrics · Clinical · Domestic · Body-worn · Ambient · Sensor · Technology

1 Introduction

1.1 Medical Background

Personal mobility, i.e., the ability to move around and get into and keep up certain body positions, is known to be an important prerequisite for pursuing an independent lifestyle [40]. Mobility normally changes during age. There is no pathological reason for that change at all. Starting at the age of 60 years, elderly peoples' mobility characteristics change [14], i.e., the self-selected gait velocity decreases each decade by 12 %–16 % during self-imposed activities. The decrease is often caused by a reduced step length whereas the step frequency remains stable. This age-related change in gait patterns contributes to a more

© Springer International Publishing Switzerland 2015
A. Holzinger et al. (Eds.): Smart Health, LNCS 8700, pp. 71–98, 2015.
DOI: 10.1007/978-3-319-16226-3_4

stable gait and it is not pathological [52]. If there are pathological reasons for an impairments of mobility the changes of gait parameters are more significant than in age-related changes [52]. Neurological diseases, especially dementia where mobility impairments are an early indicator [111], are one of the most frequent pathological reasons for mobility impairments. In general, severity of gait and balance disorders increases with severity of neurological disorders [100]. Gait and balance disorders have shown being related to a higher risk of falling. Especially slow self-selected gait velocity has found being related to an increased risk for falls and need of care [75]. Due to their often severe gait and balance disorders dementia patients suffer from an increased risk of falling [110].

Costs due to the high need of care of demented people [3] and fall-related costs are two of the major factors influencing the proportionally higher costs to the health care system caused by elderly people. From a clinical perspective long-term monitoring of changes in mobility has a high potential for early diagnosis of various diseases and for assessment to determine the risk to fall [8]. This may help delaying need of care or preventing acute incidents like falls and may thus help saving costs. On a more personal level early detection may help supporting an independent lifestyle by enabling early and purposeful prevention and may therefore increase quality of life for affected people, relatives, and carers.

Therefore, assessment of mobility is an important part of treatments in various medical branches. In the medical domain, mobility is diagnosed in terms of gait and balance respectively in spatio-temporal parameters quantifying these domains. Today, those parameters are either assessed by a medical professional performing a visual analysis or by using highly specialized technical equipment performing either kinetic or kinematic gait or balance analysis. Both alternatives are often not available in less specialized wards and a visual gait analysis is known to be dependent on the subjective capabilities of the analyzing professional. Therefore, some branches of medicine have developed so-called assessment tests in order to enable less specialized physicians to assess a patient's mobility to a certain degree. Geriatrics, the branch of medicine that deals with the illnesses of elderly and multimorbid patients, is such a branch that uses standardized assessment tests in the field of mobility. However, execution of such assessment tests also yields several problems like the required time effort due to manual documentation and the need to deliberately ignore details of a patient's mobility in order to keep the tests easy to use. Additionally, if physicians want to provide prevention and rehabilitation in patients homes most of such assessment tests are not suitable for being executed in domestic environments and cannot be easily executed unsupervised or at least lose their reliability if executed without supervision. Therefore, research was pursued in biomedical engineering of devices for supporting mobility assessment (tests) in clinical and domestic environments.

1.2   Scope of This Paper

The general analysis of personal movement is a wide area (for example sports movement analysis). This paper explicitly focuses on measuring mobility (or single parameters of mobility) in elderly persons using sensor technologies. Since this can be done in various ways, three gold-standard assessment tests are taken as measure for checking the state-of-the-art in technical assessment execution. These three belong to the most common assessment tests used in judging personal mobility: the Timed-up-and-Go test [88], Tinetti test [108] and Berg-Balance-Scale test [10]. A common ground of these tests is to observe people doing several mobility-related tasks like walking, standing or balancing. The tests gain scores which lead to an estimation of the mobility state of a person. More details can be found in the original test descriptions, an extensive selection of those tasks (which are, or can be broken down into, so-called components) is listed in Table 2. This state-of-the-art overview first lists the technologies available and then is matched against the requirements the assessment tests are setting up.

2 Glossary

- Ambient Sensors - Sensors that are attached in the environment of the user, usually installed in homes etc. For example presence detectors, motion detectors or cameras.
- Berg-Balance-Scale (BBS) - Assessment test invented by Katherine Berg et al., detailed description see [10].
- Body-worn Sensors - Sensors that are attached directly to the body or integrated in clothing etc. For example accelerometers, gyroscopes or strain gauges.
- Clinical Document Architecture (CDA) - standardized XML-based markup format for specifying the encoding, structure and semantics of clinical documents for exchange.
- International Classification of Functioning, Disability and Health (ICF) - classification of the health components of functioning and disability coordinated by World Health Organization WHO.
- Kinematic (approaches) - classical mechanics describing the motion of points, and objects without consideration of the causes of motion.
- Kinetic (approaches) - classical mechanics concerned with the relationship between forces and torques.
- Light Detection And Ranging (LIDAR) - sensor measuring distance by calculating times between emitting and receiving light (laser) impulses.
- Mobility - in this context the term mobility relates to personal mobility, i.e., the ability of a person to change its body position. Infrastructural mobility in terms of being able to change places e.g., by using transport systems is not considered here.
- Personal Health Record (PHR), Electronic Health Record (EHR); record where health data and information related to the care of a patient is stored and made accessible to involved third parties.
- Three Dimensional Layer Context Model (3DLC), model which defines the appropriate level of abstraction of data generated by medical applications to be stored inside the PHR, for details see [46].
- Timed Up & Go (TUG) - Assessment test requiring both static and dynamic balance, detailed description see [88].

– Tinetti-Test (TTI) - Assessment test invented by Mary Tinetti et al., detailed description see [108]. Also known as Tinetti Gait and Balance Examination, Tinettis Mobility Test, Tinetti Balance Test or Performance Oriented Mobility Assessment (POMA).
– Ultrasonic sensor (US) - Sensor measuring distance by calculating times between emitting and receiving high-frequency sound waves.

3   State-of-the-Art

3.1   Overview

This state-of-the-art will try to give an overview of current sensor technologies and approaches to measure personal movement parameters. In [33], sensor technologies for measuring single or multiple mobility parameters have been evaluated. Those technologies have been divided into kinetic and kinematic sensors as well as body-worn/ambient usage. An overview is given in Table 1. This section is followed by a comparison of requirements of assessment tests and which requirements are matched by these sensor technologies up to now.

Table 1. Classification of approaches for mobility analysis [33]

	Body worn	Ambient
Kinetic	1. **Pressure and force sensors** in shoes [59, 21, 7, 50, 107, 83, 95, 44, 127]	1. **Pressure and force sensors** on the ground [107, 29] / in treadmills [57, 29] / in furniture [16, 76, 123, 58] / in walkers [20, 86, 2, 109]
Kinecmatic	1. **Time of flight** ultrasound [114, 60, 1, 53, 51, 118] 2. **Visual** marker based [6, 79, 106, 29] 3. **Electrical impulse** electromyography [105, 29] 4. **Inertial forces** (accelerometers, gyroskopes) body worn [69, 28, 12, 92, 47, 71, 128, 74, 129, 5, 77, 13, 121, 4, 24, 54, 72, 122, 26] in clothing [65, 92] 5. **Bending forces** electro-goniometer [105, 29, 19]	1. **Time of flight** RADAR [64, 124, 32, 112, 49, 90, 130, 81, 39] LIDAR [82, 93, 37] 2. **Visual** marker less [61, 98, 102, 63, 116, 41] fluoroscopic [6] 3. **Presence sensors** home automation [84, 85, 92, 87, 15, 17, 113, 94, 18] RFID [22]

Commonly used technical approaches to the assessment of mobility like marker-based vision systems, force plates, and electromyographs, are very expensive, time-intensive in use and not mobile. This means that they are only available in specialized wards, can only be used by trained personal, and cannot be executed at point of care which makes their use time-intensive. Therefore, new technical approaches were developed which either use body-worn or ambient, i.e., integrated into the environment, sensor systems. Body-worn sensor, i.e., accelerometers and gyroscopes, are used more widely due to their advantage of being clearly linked to a single person in any environment. Several approaches (e.g., [65,129]) have demonstrated the ability to support the execution of mobility assessment tests and to compute spatio-temporal parameters of gait and balance using body-worn sensors. Some research projects meanwhile made their way into products. However, results of all approaches are very sensitive to sensor placement and even small misplacements can invalidate all assessment results. Over longer time periods assessment results perish due to sensor drift. Additionally, regarding unsupervised use in domestic environments it is questionable whether layman and especially elderly or demented people may be able to handle those sensors on their own or will be willing to wear those sensors in their daily life. Only a single approach to executing mobility assessments in domestic environments unsupervised by use of body-worn sensors, called Directed Routine (DR), has been proposed so far but was not evaluated yet [126]. Ambient sensors are placed in the environment and do thus not require any explicit handling by patients and results are not dependent on correct sensor placement. Sensors used for mobility analysis include home automation sensors [22,84], cameras [61,104], and laser range scanners [34,84] and have been evaluated in domestic environments several times. However, ambient sensor data are not assigned to a certain person and often sophisticated algorithms are required to filter those sensor recordings which represent a person to be monitored. Currently, there is neither a body-worn nor an ambient sensor system available that supports the execution of mobility assessment (tests) in supervised clinical and unsupervised domestic environments. However, some approaches are currently evaluated and will be available in the near future.

3.2 Kinetic Approaches

The following sections give a short overview of sensor technologies that are used in mobility analysis, for references to current research, see Table 1.

Pressure and Force Sensors. Three types of sensors can be distinguished: binary switches, pressure sensors and force reaction systems. Binary switches are the simplest form using binary information e.g., if a step was made or not. Pressure sensors can provide more detailed information, e.g., the weight distribution and sequence of movements. Force reaction systems are usually mounted on ground plates and not only measure weight forces but shear forces as well which is especially interesting in balance analysis. The most common use of body-worn pressure and force sensors is integration of those sensors in shoes. In ambient setups the sensors can be placed in furniture or moving aids so that pressure information is generated. Pressure and force sensors are relatively cheap and easy to use so they are adequate for being used in pervasive systems.

3.3 Kinematic Spproaches

Time-of-Flight Sensors. Time-of-flight sensors use a system of sending and receiving signals and calculating distance information. Classical types are ultra-sound (US), light detection and ranging (LIDAR) and radio detection and rang-ing (RADAR) sensors. US sensors emit an ultrasound impulse and record the reflection of that impulse. Typically the sound beam has a quite broad disper-sion so detection of small objects is difficult. Additionally detected objects can not exactly be localized (using one sensor), because the exact direction of the reflected signal is not known. The same holds for RADAR sensors which use an electromagnetic wave impulse. The advantage of RADAR sensors is that they are able to measure through walls for example. LIDAR sensors usually emit a laser beam which is quite narrow and so a relatively detailed environment recognition can be performed.

Since LIDAR and RADAR sensors are usually not suitable to be worn at the body up to now, only ultrasound sensors are available in the body worn category. This normally means that US markers are attached at the body and a fixed base-station is used to provide exact localization [53,60,114]. Ambient approaches attach US sensors e.g., to the ceiling and try to recognize persons and their movements [99]. Multiple sensors have to be used to be able to calculate an exact position of an object. RADAR sensors are rarely used compared to US and LIDAR but some researchers were able to extract gait information from RADAR data [97,117]. LIDAR sensors are quite common in robotics and industry mostly for navigation and safety purposes. Due to the exact data object recognition and tracking is relatively easy. In contrast, most systems are producing only 2D information, 3D-LIDAR sensors are quite expensive at the moment.

Visual Sensors. Visual observation of movement is based on video-frame data where movement is calculated by comparing each frame and checking for moved objects. In general this can be divided into tracking based on markers (body-worn, e.g., [29,106]) or marker-less (ambient, e.g., [38,89,102,103]) approaches. Marker-based systems extract movement by tracking active or passive mark-ers that are attached to the observed body parts. The advantage is the exact and defined recognition of the selected moving objects. The attachment of the markers can be a drawback as well because the position is crucial and should not change during a test. Since human skin is not fixed to the bone structure it may be necessary to attach the markers to the bones directly which is inva-sive. Marker-less techniques use image recognition algorithms to extract moving objects without the need of invasive marker positioning. On one hand this is easier to set up but on the other hand the recognition precision is usually not as high as marker systems provide. Visual sensors are a common tool for movement observation, the cost heavily depends on the accuracy.

Electrical Impulse. Electromyography detects activity by measuring electrical power/impulses that are used to contract muscles. The measurement can be performed by attaching either non-invasive electrodes or needle electrodes which are able to measure in deeper muscle areas but also cause pain during muscle movement. The attachment of the electrodes though requires good expertise of the investigator. Since there is no general correlation of electrical energy and muscle movement, electromyography is only used in combination with a second modality to observe the actual movement (e.g., camera systems). In general this setup is only suited for laboratory (clinical) environments.

Inertial Forces. Inertial forces are detected by accelerometers and gyroscopes. Since such sensors are small and use few energy, a lot of research has been done on using inertial forces for movement analysis (see Table 1; e.g., [5,92,121]). Those developments and products nearly completely belong to the category of body-worn sensors because inertial forces can't be measured from distance (using accelerometers or gyros). Sensors can be directly attached to the body or integrated in clothing. Multiple sensors can be integrated into sensor networks (e.g., body area network). Developed systems mainly differ in number of sensors and area of attachment. The accuracy of measurements depends on correct attachment of the sensors and in general only relative movement can be measured because no absolute position is available. These sensors are also relatively low priced and wide spread.

Bending Forces. Bending forces as used in electro-goniometers are mostly used to measure angles of extremities (arm, leg). Since the sensors are attached to the joints directly, they are filed to body-worn sensors. Electro-goniometers are precise in general but not all joint movements of the body can be measured. Most common use is on elbow and knee joints (e.g., [55]). Since there is only relative information, a second modality is necessary to get absolute position information.

Presence Sensors. Presence sensors are ambient sensors that can be placed in a variety of environments. Common presence sensors are cheap but normally inaccurate as there is the information about a detected movement but no directional information is provided. By adding more sensors positions can be determined more accurately. Single body parts can't be observed so information is reduced to movement of a person through an environment (e.g., gait speed) [18,43]. Such sensors are often included in smart home setups.

3.4   From Assessment Test to Assessment Components

To be able to track and quantify assessment tests with technical approaches it makes sense to break a single assessment test down into different components. These components are sequences of movements that can be distinguished from other movements within the same test. In case of the TUG test this means that a set of small components are combined to a complete test: Stand up - walk there - turn around - walk back - sit down. Each of those components can be analyzed separately to gain more information than the complete test itself. A usual TUG test only provides the duration of the complete test in seconds. The division into single components enables the measurement system to provide much more detailed information: time duration of single components, movements, movement speeds, balance parameters etc. are a few examples of such information. Each of such movements can be measured by one or more of the sensor technologies mentioned above. Up to now, no approach is able to track all required components with a single sensor setup. Table 2 therefore provides a classification of identified components, technologies that are currently used to measure them and references to research work.

3.5   Assessment Components and Measurement Approaches

Systems to perform a complete mobility assessment test either in a clinical or domestic environment are rare. As shown before, a lot of research has been done in using different kinds of sensors to measure individual movement parameters. Few systems use one single or a combination of sensors to measure a complete assessment test. Table 2 shows the components that are assessed during the tests and recent approaches to observe them. It also includes a list of sensor technologies that are used to measure the according physical movement. The list of commercial systems is used as an example, more systems exist that mostly have at least a slight different focus (like rehabilitation or sports movement analysis). Four main categories of movement have been identified: transfer sit/stand, gait, balance and turning/moving (body motion). It is obvious that the three selected mobility assessment tests focus on different types of movement but are overlapping in most areas. A combination of all three tests covers the whole spectrum of movements. It can be observed as well that there is no system that is capable of measuring all components and consequently there is no system that could perform all three assessments even if they have quite an overlap in necessary components. Additionally, there are some movement components that are currently not explicitly considered by any research the authors know of. Though technically most of them are measurable.

A result of this overview is the obvious fact that some movement parameters are more intensive investigated than others. It seems that instead of concentrating on single movement analysis, an overall effort should be made to coordinate a complete assessment setup. For example gait analysis is quite common in mobility analysis whereas 'reaching with arm forward' is not tracked by any approach. In some cases it may even be necessary to adapt the test descriptions to match the requirements of technical analysis. But since the less examined components are not completely out of reach from a technical point of view it seems possible to develop a system that is capable of analyzing the used group of assessment tests. Regarding sensor types there is a distribution as well (e.g., preferred usage of accelerometers and pressure sensors) this might be an indication of availability (price, usage) of such sensor technologies.

Table 2. Overview of the most relevant components of the selected mobility assessment tests and current approaches to automated measurement (see Sect. 3.5 for more details). TUG = Timed Up and Go Test, TTI = Tinetti-Test, BBS = Berg Balance Scale, aTUG = automated Timed Up and Go [33], BM = Smart/Basic Balance Master (NeuroCom) [62], iTUG = instrumented Timed Up and Go [91], ETGUG = Expanded Timed Get-up-and-Go [115], ISway = instrumented test of postural sway [67], iWalker = instrumented rollator [109], Simi = Simi Motion (Simi Reality Motion Systems GmbH), Gaitrite = GAITRite (CIR Systems Inc.), OT = OrthoTrak (Motion Analysis), Sensfloor (Future Shape GmbH) ACC = accelerometer, PRES = pressure sensor, RAD = radar, LS = laser scanner, US = ultrasound, CAM = visual/camera, SmH = smart home

Type	No.	Component	Test	Tec. Approach	Sensors	Sources
Transfer sit-stand	1	Stand up	TUG, BBS, TTI	aTUG, iTUG	ACC, PRES	[12,16,33,66,77,78,91,119,120,125]
	2	Sit down	TUG, BBS, TTI	aTUG, iTUG	ACC, PRES	[16,33,66,77,78,91,119,120,125]
Gait	3	Gait speed	(TUG) ETGUG	aTUG, iTUG, iWalker, Simi, Sensfloor, Gaitrite. OT	ACC, PRES, RAD, LS, US, SmH, RFID, CAM	[4,5,7,20,26,33,42,49,51,59,70,74,78,82–84,86,91,93,98,101,102,109,119,120,122,124,125,128,129]
	4	Step initiation	TTI	aTUG, Simi, Gaitrite, OT	ACC	[4,5,7,21,33,42,63,70,78,91,119,120,125]
	5	Step height	TTI	Simi, OT		
	6	Step length	TTI	aTUG, iTUG	PRES, RAD, LS, US, RFID, CAM	[5,7,20,22,26,33,38,39,42,51,53,63,70,74,82,91,93,98,102,119,125]

(Continued)

Table 2. (*Continued*)

Type	No.	Component	Test	Tec. Approach	Sensors	Sources
	7	Step continuity	TTI	aTUG, iTUG, Simi, OT	ACC, CAM	[5,33,42,59,74,91,98,125]
	8	Path deviation	TTI	aTUG	LS	[33]
	9	Trunk stability	TTI	iTUG, iWalker, OT	ACC, PRES, CAM	[20,70,91,98,109,116,125]
	10	Step width	TTI	aTUG, Gaitrite, OT	LS,US	[5,33,60]
Balance	11	Balance (5 sec)	TTI	aTUG, BM, ISway, OT	ACC, PRES, LS	[23,33,54,67,68,109]
	12	Stand stability	BBS, TTI	ISway	ACC	[23,25,66-68,72,116]
	13	Balance w/closed eyes	BBS, TTI	BM, ISway	ACC, PRES	[23,54,66-68]
	14	Balance sitting	BBS	aTUG	PRES	[33,66]
	15	Balance feet side by side	BBS	ISway	ACC	[23,67]
	16	Tandem standing	BBS			
	17	Standing on one foot	BBS		PRES	[25]
	18	Force against trunk	TTI	BM	ACC	[66]
Turning, Moving	19	Turn 360°	BBS, TTI		ACC	[66]
	20	Turn 180°	TUG	aTUG, iTUG	ACC, LS	[33,42,78,91,120,125]
	21	Turn around, look backwards	BBS			
	22	Reach arm forward	BBS			
	23	Retrieve object from floor	BBS			
	24	Stool stepping	BBS		ACC	[78,120]

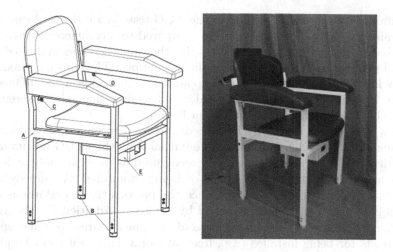

Fig. 1. aTUG apparatus as approach to offer standardized TUG assessments in clinical environments

3.6 Own Approach and Work Conducted

Our own novel approach, called Automated Timed Up & Go (aTUG, see Fig. 1), to supporting the execution of mobility assessment tests in clinical and domestic environments utilizes exclusively ambient sensor technologies and may be performed in domestic environments without creating a test situation. Compared to approaches using body-worn sensors, aTUG saves more time since no calibration or donning of sensors is required. Patients are not directly aware of being technically measured. Additionally, the technical support provides more details about the patients than a manually executed test by performing a gait and balance analysis, if requested.

Part of the aTUG approach is the aTUG apparatus which was developed from sketch starting in 2008 by demand of physicians from the field of geriatrics in order to make the aTUG approach applicable in daily clinical practice. The general idea of the apparatus is to integrate required sensor technologies with a battery and a display in order to enable physicians to transport all required equipment for performing an assessment and gait analysis at point of care. The basis of the apparatus is a blood withdrawal chair. A laser range scanner is used for performing kinematic gait analysis and is installed under the seat of the apparatus. Four force sensors are integrated into the legs of the chair and enable performing kinetic balance analysis while standing up and sitting down. The apparatus may be accompanied with a set of home automation sensors i.e., light barriers in order to provide even more details and to validate computations. For long-term use at home those sensors can be placed in the environment. After an initial proof of concept, the prototype was used as a basis for a complete redesign with the objective of putting the aTUG chair into circulation as a medical product. After a risk analysis, the construction, and safety tests, a new prototype was technically validated for support of the TUG tests in a residential care facility [36] and its gait analysis results were compared to a commercially available marker-based tracking system. Additionally, the approach was evaluated in a field trial in order to demonstrate the ability to perform TUG unsupervised during daily life [35]. Currently, the aTUG apparatus is in a clinical trial of medical products [56] in which it is clinically validated against manual measurements and the GaitRite system at the Charité in Berlin.

The aTUG device can easily be placed and used in clinical environments. Regarding the integration into domestic environments the aTUG has its drawbacks. First of all, the device is certainly recognized as medical analytic device. Persons using the apparatus are aware of being monitored. As already mentioned, this can lead to biased results since the persons try to perform as good as possible in the case they are observed by someone. Additionally, the aTUG device has a (somewhat) fixed position and recognition area so it has special requirements for being installed (e.g., free path of 3–4 m) so it can't be placed in narrow spaces. As a consequence of these drawbacks the idea of the aTUG apparatus was extended to use the same algorithms on a mobile robot platform (see Fig. 2). The main task of doing gait analysis with aTUG is accomplished by using a LRF sensor. This type of sensor is used in most of current state-of-the-art mobile robot systems for navigation purposes. So this sensor is already available on most robot systems and can easily be used to do the same gait analysis. The major difference to aTUG is the mobility of the platform. The robot is able to follow a person through the home, monitoring gait at various places, under dif-

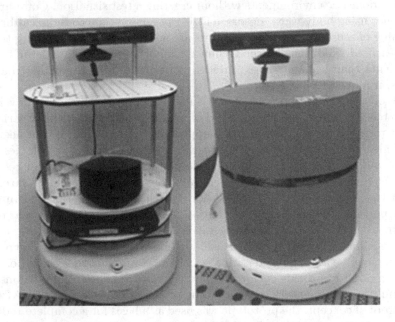

Fig. 2. Mobile robot platform equipped with LRF and Kinect sensor. Approach to bring the aTUG idea to domestic environments.

ferent circumstances and over longer distances even if there is no straight line to perform a classic TUG test. To extend the system even more, 3D sensor information was added to analyze balance parameters and movement characteristics. In this case, the well known Microsoft Kinect sensor was used. The idea is to enable every typical mobile service robot to do such analysis, not to create a new type of robot. So people buy the robot to fulfill any type of service (e.g., cleaning, personal assistance, telepresence) and the mobility monitoring is done in the background (with approval by the user) and after some time the user is not aware of the test situation anymore. So the results of the measured mobility parameters are much more realistic than any test can provide. Using this system, the following major advantages are gained: (1) mobile data acquisition (no need to place many sensors at different locations in the home), (2) gait and full body movement analysis, (3) monitoring over long periods of time, (4) getting mobility data in everyday life, no test situation.

The robot is designed to record the observed movements in a data base so that further analysis can be done by e.g., medical personnel. Open questions are still the communication with medical personnel in terms of data standards and comparability of test results. See Sect. 4 for a more detailed analysis of problems.

4   Open Problems

aTUG and some other body-worn approaches are close to being available as medical products. In daily clinical practice their main advantage will be to provide more detailed and more objective results than manual assessment tests and to save time by digital documentation of results. However, in order to save costs in the future, only more effective procedures in clinical environments are not sufficient. One possibility to save more costs is by early prevention and more sustainable rehabilitation on an individual basis for which domestic assessments may provide the required data. Currently, there are three main open problems in this field: (1) How to implement clinical assessment tests in domestic environments unobtrusively, (2) how to document domestic assessment results in a standardized manner and (3) how to compare these to clinical assessment results.

4.1   Acceptance of Technical Innovations

First of all - if a system shall be used either in clinical or in domestic environments, without acceptance by the users the system will fail. This is even more crucial in the case of domestic environments. It is very hard to predict reactions of users to new technologies brought into their own homes. If there is no real use-case and obvious benefit the system will be rejected usually. In professional environments this is not as serious as in home environments but especially medical personnel is used to work with common tools and new tools are accepted mostly if there is also a benefit for the operator (e.g., faster execution, less stress). So the selection of sensors has to be made in the first place based on acceptance, prices are less important and get even less important due to price decreases through industrial developments.

General Technology Acceptance. Of course all conclusions of acceptance research have to consider the fact that technical developments in recent years also changed the way people react to them [48]. People that will reach the age of the target group of geriatric treatment in 10 or 20 years will have a totally different perspective to new technology than people that are in need of care at present. For example even today's elderly people are used to computer systems etc. since they already worked with them. Ten years ago, this was not the case. The more experience people have, the better they can estimate how this could effect their lives. Perspectively, the group of technically experienced elderly will grow and the other group will scale down [27]. Anyhow, technology is accepted to a greater extend if the benefit of usage is clearly visible [27,73].

In a meta study called *Body-Worn Sensor Design: What Do Patients and Clinicians Want?* Bergmann and McGregor examined the results of multiple studies regarding sensor and technology acceptance of body-worn sensors in medical application areas [11]. They identified 11 studies that provide information about this specific user acceptance. Since the focus of such studies was broad they ware able to draw some overall conclusions like *one of the main recurring factors was the preference for small and embedded sensors, indicating that user are keen to minimize the physical impact of any wearable system*, as well as *the less notable the device is the higher the patient's acceptance will be, which in turn will improve the quality of gathered data, as patient's behavior will then be closer to his/her normal routines.* As already mentioned, this has to be taken into account when designing person monitoring systems. On the other hand, *clinicians were concerned with issues such as restricted recording time due to a limited storage capacity, techniques for attaching the device to the patient and the fact that data should be available in real-time to make instant diagnosis possible.* Which again sets some crucial requirements for hardware and software design.

Robotic Acceptance. An intense study regarding acceptance of robots was conducted in 2011 [9]. It was not focused on elderly but on a broader selection of people. The result of this study was a list of open questions for robot development which also included age dependent acceptance as open problem.

In 2009 there was a survey of the acceptance of service robots comparing different age groups (ages 18–25 and 65–86) [31]. There was no significant difference between these groups as long as the benefit is sufficiently visible. However, elderly persons were more open-minded regarding critical functionality (emergency services) of robots. Another study of the same research group revealed similar results [30].

Smarr et al. gave an overview of robotic assistance systems for elderly people in 2011 [96]. Especially robots assisting at activities of daily living were selected. The study was based on internet and database research which lead to, depending on usage of the system, from 61 to 147 different robot systems. This shows high interest in technological assistance however one conclusion was that there is no comprehensive study that concentrates directly on needs and requests of elderly people.

Concluding this short selection of acceptance research it can be stated that acceptance is crucial for (medical) technical systems but there is still a lack of comprehensive studies which can provide a general guideline for designing such systems. This does not mean that there is no research of acceptance in general, there is a lot, but the diversity of technical solutions is huge and it is hard to create general statements by studying single applications. So every system has to be elaborated carefully for meeting the expectations users have in each case.

4.2 Clinical Assessment Tests in Domestic Environments

Today, several technical approaches to conduct domestic (mobility) assessments have been implemented and are currently evaluated in the field - many will still follow. The most important remaining technical problem is how to implement tests in a way that patients accept these in their daily life. Tests will have to be unobtrusive and should ideally be performed continuously without requiring patients to perform an explicit test. Some researcher i.e., our own work [35] and the work of Stone and Skubic [104] have already shown that assessment tests may be implemented without creating a test situation and thus can be implemented unobtrusively. Some of the lessons learned from the first real world experiences are considered here.

If sensors are used to precisely analyze personal movements those should be broken down into single movement aspects (e.g., the before mentioned components) this will allow better comparability between established test scenarios. The measurement results itself should not remain on a detailed technical level, they should be classified into categories. The ICF already provides a framework for such classification (see next section). Another aspect is data integration. In clinical environments there are established data communication and sharing standards but in home environments there is no such infrastructure. This needs to be considered when systems shall be deployed at home environments but still be useful in the complete medical service environment.

It should not be the goal to try to recreate established tests completely. In fact the original test descriptions have been designed in such a way (being simple) to compensate the lack of technical capabilities. So it is more important to understand the ideas behind the tests and to transfer these to the new circumstances (e.g., home environment). Technical approaches can deliver much more detailed analysis which may provide new insights whereas classical approaches are not able to.

Working within the health sector is often driven by the need of reducing costs. This can be accomplished by introducing automated assessment tests both in preventive as well as actual care scenarios. Though this heavily depends on the costs of the final automated measurement system. Additionally, as mentioned above, in professional medical environments a two-step approach seems to be more realistic. Firstly common techniques should be supported by the new developments which then can be extended to fully replace the former common strategies. Only known and proven technologies are accepted. So adding a completely new technology can face high barriers.

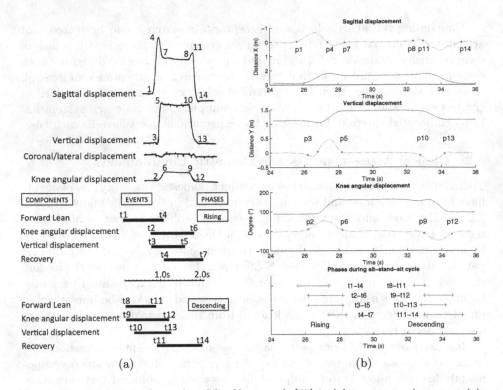

Fig. 3. Sit-stand-sit cycle analyzed by Kerr et al. [55] in laboratory environment (a) and same analysis performed by mobile robot in domestic environment (b, own work). Results seem to be comparable but how to compare such results with clinical practice?

The use of service robots in domestic environments is intensively investigated currently. Using a service robot to perform assessment test analysis is quite new. Since the development of domestic service robots is still at the early stages, questions about acceptance and usability of such a special service is highly speculative. First user tests with robot prototypes have been conducted and results are promising but still far from real world usage (see Fig. 3). This figurative example shows that state-of-the-art systems like robots are able to reproduce results that coincide with former approaches but there is still no way to actually compare both of them. Even more important - there is currently no connection to standard medical procedures that would incorporate these results.

In general an assessment analysis with either robot or other ambient technology can be regarded as feasible. However, the results of different domestic and clinical assessment systems are not comparable to each other today. The main reason for this and another open question is a missing common classification and document format for the results.

4.3   Standardization of Results

Even if technologies for performing mobility assessments in peoples' homes are available, results of such domestic assessments are not directly comparable to clinical assessment tests. Three main problems can be found:

1. Incompleteness of assessment results: Assessments in domestic environments will have to be performed as part of every-day activities without creating a test situation in order to be accepted by patients. Often, not all aspects of clinical assessment tests can be tested during every-day activities.
2. Contextual dependency on assessment results: While clinical assessment results are obtained under standardized conditions during a test, domestic assessment data is gathered in peoples' homes which may contain unclear influence factors even if people have to perform a test at home. Such unknown contextual influences factors may have an unclear influence on the assessment results.
3. Uncertainty of assessment results: Assessments in domestic environments will have to be performed unsupervised by use of sensor technologies in order to be cost-efficient. Such implementation implies that there will always remain a certain amount of uncertainty whether sensor recordings and evaluations do really reflect the abilities of a patient in a certain assessment domain.

Therefore, a common classification for aspects of clinical and domestic assessment results and for expressing contextual influence on these and their uncertainty is currently missing. Additionally, as soon as assessment information has been obtained in peoples' homes it has to be transferred to physicians and caregivers for being considered when making a medical decision. Personal Health Records (PHRs) have the ability to store and exchange this user generated data with Electronic Health Records (EHRs) of the professional domain. Mapping a classification for assessment results to an established semantically annotated document format would enable long-term storage and transfer of fine-grained assessment information on a machine interpretable level. Providing such a common classification and a mapping to standardized document-format would not only enable physicians to use domestic assessment data in their every-day decision making but maybe also enable them to gain new insights into people's daily performance.

In order to make data from clinical and domestic assessments comparable, a common classification for the results is required. Such a classification will have to solve the three described problems of incompleteness, contextual dependency, and uncertainty of assessment results. Additionally, a standardized document-format for transferring and presenting assessment results encoded by a common classification is required. Therefore, we propose three main methods for making clinical and domestic assessment results comparable by machines and medical decision makers:

1. To use component codes from the International Classification of Functioning, Disability and Health (ICF) [80] to decompose clinical and domestic assessment tests into common parts. Therefore, an assessment test will comprised

a sequence of several components from the ICF. Such break down of assessment tests solves the first described problem by enabling the standardized description of even incomplete assessments.

2. To use qualifiers from the ICF's list of activities and participation, i.e., capacity and performance, for expressing contextual influence on assessment results. Encoding assessment results as capacity values expresses low environmental influence; performance values indicate high environmental influence. Usage of aid may be encoded as well.

3. To map assessment results encoded according to our first two methods to the Clinical Document Architecture (CDA) [45] in order to enable a standardized transfer of results between PHRs/EHRs and to provide a machine-interpretable and human-readable representation of results. Additionally, to use CDA in order to annotate uncertainty of assessment results, an extension of CDA must be made.

4.4   Integration and Co-Existence of Clinical and Domestic Assessments

Even if domestic assessment results will be available to physicians in the near future in a common document format, a third open question is how recognized changes over time and differences to clinical assessment results will influence a medical decision. The explanatory power of domestic assessment results and their relationship to clinical results have to be investigated. In order to foster this process, the 3DLC model was developed [46]. 3DLC is a first step towards categorizing available assessment results and to explaining the relationship between clinical and domestic results. Within the proposed model, assessment data is categorized on three axes: relevance to clinical decision, recording frequency, and context dependence of results. Recording frequency refers to the temporal intervals in which the assessment results are obtained. While assessments in professional environments have a low frequency, i.e., once per week or twice per hospital stay, domestic assessments can be performed continuously or at least one per day. The higher frequency should provide a better insight into patients' abilities. However, domestic assessment results are more context-dependent. In a clinical setting a standardized test situation is created which makes results comparable. In a domestic setting, unclear influences, e.g., different floor covers, may results in different assessment results. Since those influences may not be clear, context dependence of results is high. These former two axes influence the third axis - the relevance to the clinical decision. The higher the result frequency and the lower the context dependence the more relevant are assessment results to a clinical decision. New technical systems for implementing both clinical and domestic (mobility) assessment tests should adhere to a common results classification and document-format in order to make their results comparable to other approaches and usable during medical decision making. In order to be accepted by patients in their homes, domestic assessment systems should be implemented unobtrusively. The question how obtained results are used during clinical decision making and how changes over time and differences between clinical and domestic assessment results have to be interpreted remains future work after more usable data was collected.

5 Future Outlook

Summarizing the current open problems and development activities, the following conclusions can be drawn (see Sect. 4 Open Questions for more detailed analysis):

1. A lot of different approaches for mobility analysis already exist. It lacks of a combined effort to bring these single-focused approaches into complete assessment systems.
2. A major factor of providing domestic technology is user acceptance - research has to put emphasis on acceptance by end-users as well as professionals for seamless integration in common work flows so that high user-acceptance is achieved. In the field of automated assessment execution there is no reliable data on user acceptance available.
3. The results of technical analysis have to be transferred into a common language which allows consistent processing. The ICF provides parts of such a tool set. This should be discussed for inclusion.
4. If data is exchanged between home and professional environments, comprehensive standards are necessary. Currently an equivalent to the PHR/EHR systems of the professional domain is missing/not sufficiently integrated in the home environment.
5. The focus should not be to completely copy common procedures but enhance them with the additional information that can be provided by technical analysis systems.
6. One future way of bringing sensors in domestic environments will be service robots. These robots usually will be designed for a different major task but they bring a set of sensors 'for free' that can clearly enhance domestic mobility analysis. Of course, robot technology itself has a lot of open research questions to be solved as well before they can be used as reliable source.

References

1. Abellanas, A., Calderón Estévez, L., Ceres Ruíz, R., Frizera Neto, A., Raya, R.: Ultrasonic time of flight estimation in assistive mobility: improvement of the model-echo fitting. In: Proceedings of Eurosensors XXII, pp. 464–467. VDI/VDE, Elsevier (2008)
2. Alwan, M., Ledoux, A., Wasson, G., Sheth, P., Huang, C.: Basic walker-assisted gait characteristics derived from forces and moments exerted on the walker's handles: results on normal subjects. Med. Eng. Phys. **29**(3), 380–389 (2007)
3. Alzheimer's Disease International. World Alzheimer Report 2009 (2009)
4. Aminian, K., Rezakhanlou, K., De Andres, E., Fritsch, C., Leyvraz, P., Robert, P.: Temporal feature estimation during walking using miniature accelerometers: an analysis of gait improvement after hip arthroplasty. Med. Biol. Eng. Comput. **37**, 686–691 (1999)

5. Auvinet, B., Berrut, G., Touzard, C., Moutel, L., Collet, N., Chaleil, D., Barrey, E.: Reference data for normal subjects obtained with an accelerometric device. Gait Posture **16**(2), 124–134 (2002)
6. Bachmann, C., Gerber, H., Stacoff, A.: Messsysteme, Messmethoden und Beispiele zur instrumentierten Ganganalyse. Schweizerische Zeitschrift für Sportmedizin und Sporttraumatologie **56**(2), 29–34 (2008)
7. Bamberg, S., Benbasat, A.Y., Scarborough, D.M., Krebs, D.E., Paradiso, J.A.: Gait analysis using a shoe-integrated wireless sensor system. IEEE Trans. Inf. Technol. Biomed. **12**(4), 413–423 (2008)
8. Beauchet, O., Allali, G., Berrut, G., Hommet, C., Dubost, V., Assal, F.: Gait analysis in demented subjects: interests and perspectives. Neuropsychiatr. Dis. Treat. **4**(1), 155–160 (2008)
9. Beer, J.M., Prakash, A., Mitzner, T.L., Rogers, W.A.: Understanding robot acceptance. Georgia Institute of Technology (2011)
10. Berg, K.: Measuring balance in the elderly: preliminary development of an instrument. Physiother. Can. **41**(6), 304–311 (1989)
11. Bergmann, J.H.M., McGregor, A.H.: Body-worn sensor design: what do patients and clinicians want? Ann. Biomed. Eng. **39**(9), 2299–2312 (2011)
12. Boonstra, M.C., van der Slikke, R.M.A., Keijsers, N.L.W., van Lummel, R.C., de Waal Malefijt, M.C., Verdonschot, N.: The accuracy of measuring the kinematics of rising from a chair with accelerometers and gyroscopes. J. Biomech. **39**(2), 354–358 (2006)
13. Bussmann, J., Damen, L., Stam, H.: Analysis and decomposition of signals obtained by thigh-fixed uni-axial accelerometry during normal walking. Med. Biol. Eng. Comput. **38**, 632–638 (2000)
14. Butler, A.A., Menant, J.C., Tiedemann, A.C., Lord, S.R.: Age and gender differences in seven tests of functional mobility. J. Neuroeng. Rehabil. **6**, 31 (2009)
15. Cameron, K., Hughes, K., Doughty, K.: Reducing fall incidence in community elders by telecare using predictive systems. In: Proceedings of the 19th Annual International Conference of the IEEE Engineering in Medicine and Biology Society, 30 October–2 November 1997, vol. 3, pp. 1036–1039 (1997)
16. Cao, E., Inoue, Y., Liu, T., Shibata, K.: A sit-to-stand trainer system in lower limb rehabilitation. In: Proceedings of the IEEE/ASME International Advanced Intelligent Mechatronics (AIM) Conference, pp. 116–121 (2011)
17. Celler, B.G., Hesketh, T., Earnshaw, W., Ilsar, E.: An instrumentation system for the remote monitoring of changes in functional health status of the elderly at home. In: Proceedings of the 16th Annual International Conference of the IEEE Engineering Advances: New Opportunities for Biomedical Engineers Engineering in Medicine and Biology Society, pp. 908–909 (1994)
18. Chan, M., Hariton, C., Ringeard, P., Campo, E.: Smart house automation system for the elderly and the disabled. In: Proceedings of the IEEE International Conference on Systems, Man and Cybernetics Intelligent Systems for the 21st Century, 22–25 October 1995, vol. 2, pp. 1586–1589 (1995)
19. Chao, E.Y.: Justification of triaxial goniometer for the measurement of joint rotation. J. Biomech. **13**(12), 989–1006 (1980)
20. Chen, C.L., Chen, H.C., Wong, M.K., Tang, F.T., Chen, R.S.: Temporal stride and force analysis of cane-assisted gait in people with hemiplegic stroke. Arch. Phys. Med. Rehabil. **82**(1), 43–48 (2001)
21. Chen, M., Huang, B., Xu, Y.: Intelligent shoes for abnormal gait detection. In: Proceedings of the IEEE International Conference on Robotics and Automation ICRA 2008, 19–23 May 2008, pp. 2019–2024 (2008)

22. Chen, Y.-C., Lin, Y.-W.: Indoor RFID gait monitoring system for fall detection. In: Proceedings of the 2nd International Aware Computing (ISAC) Symposium, pp. 207–212 (2010)

23. Chiari, L., Dozza, M., Cappello, A., Horak, F.B., Macellari, V., Giansanti, D.: Audio-biofeedback for balance improvement: an accelerometry-based system. IEEE Trans. Biomed. Eng. **52**(12), 2108–2111 (2005)

24. Cho, C.Y., Kamen, G.: Detecting balance deficits in frequent fallers using clinical and quantitative evaluation tools. J. Am. Geriatr. Soc. **46**(4), 426–430 (1998)

25. Clark, R.A., Bryant, A.L., Pua, Y., McCrory, P., Bennell, K., Hunt, M.: Validity and reliability of the nintendo wii balance board for assessment of standing balance. Gait Posture **31**(3), 307–310 (2010)

26. Currie, G., Rafferty, D., Duncan, G., Bell, F., Evans, A.: Measurement of gait by accelerometer and walkway: a comparison study. Med. Biol. Eng. Comput. **30**, 669–670 (1992)

27. Czaja, S.J., Charness, N., Fisk, A.D., Hertzog, C., Nair, S.N., Rogers, W.A., Sharit, J.: Factors predicting the use of technology: findings from the center for research and education on aging and technology enhancement (create). Psychol. Aging **21**(2), 333 (2006)

28. de Bruin, E., Najafi, B., Murer, K., Uebelhart, D., Aminian, K.: Quantification of everyday motor function in a geriatric population. J. Rehabil. Res. Dev. **44**, 417–428 (2007)

29. DeLisa, J., Scientific, U.S. Veterans Health Administration, Technical Publications Section: Gait analysis in the science of rehabilitation. Monograph (United States. Veterans Health Administration. Rehabilitation Research and Development Service). Department of Veterans Affairs, Veterans Health Administration, Rehabilitation Research and Development Service. Scientific and Technical Publications Section (1998)

30. Ezer, N., Fisk, A.D., Rogers, W.A.: Attitudinal and intentional acceptance of domestic robots by younger and older adults. In: Stephanidis, C. (ed.) UAHCI 2009, Part II. LNCS, vol. 5615, pp. 39–48. Springer, Heidelberg (2009)

31. Ezer, N., Fisk, A.D., Rogers, W.A.: More than a servant: self-reported willingness of younger and older adults to having a robot perform interactive and critical tasks in the home. In: Proceedings of the Human Factors and Ergonomics Society Annual Meeting, vol. 53, pp. 136–140. SAGE Publications (2009)

32. Fortuny-Guasch, J., Sammartino, P.F., Petit, J.: Radar techniques for human gait automatic recognition. In: Proceedings of the 43rd Annual 2009 International Security Technology Carnahan Conference, pp. 221–226 (2009)

33. Frenken, T.: Technischer Ansatz zur unaufdringlichen Mobilitätsanalyse im Rahmen geriatrischer Assessments. Ph.D. thesis. University of Oldenburg, VDI Verlag, Düsseldorf, January 2013

34. Frenken, T., Gövercin, M., Mersmann, S., Hein, A.: Precise assessment of self-selected gait velocity in domestic environments. In: Pervasive Computing Technologies for Healthcare (PervasiveHealth) (2010)

35. Frenken, T., Lipprandt, M., Brell, M., Wegel, S., Gövercin, M., Steinhagen-Thiessen, E., Hein, A.: Novel approach to unsupervised mobility assessment tests: field trial for aTUG. In: Proceedings of the 6th International Pervasive Computing Technologies for Healthcare (PervasiveHealth) Conference (2012)

36. Frenken, T., Vester, B., Brell, M., Hein, A.: aTUG: fully-automated timed up and go assessment using ambient sensor technologies. In: 2011 5th International Conference on Pervasive Computing Technologies for Healthcare (PervasiveHealth) (2011)

37. Fuerstenberg, K.C., Dietmayer, K.: Object tracking and classification for multiple active safety and comfort applications using a multilayer laser scanner. In: Proceedings of IEEE Intelligent Vehicles Symposium, pp. 802–807 (2004)
38. Gabel, M., Gilad-Bachrach, R., Renshaw, E., Schuster, A.: Full body gait analysis with kinect. In: 2012 Annual International Conference of the IEEE Engineering in Medicine and Biology Society (EMBC), pp. 1964–1967. IEEE (2012)
39. Geisheimer, J.L., Marshall, W.S., Greneker, E.: A continuous-wave (CW) radar for gait analysis. In: Proceedings of the Conference on Signals, Systems and Computers Record of the Thirty-Fifth Asilomar Conference, vol. 1, pp. 834–838 (2001)
40. Gill, T.M., Williams, C.S., Tinetti, M.E.: Assessing risk for the onset of functional dependence among older adults: the role of physical performance. J. Am. Geriatr. Soc. 43(6), 603–609 (1995)
41. Goffredo, M., Carter, J.N., Nixon, M.S.: Front-view gait recognition. In: Proceedings of the 2nd IEEE International Conference on Biometrics: Theory, Applications and Systems BTAS 2008, pp. 1–6 (2008)
42. Greene, B.R., Donovan, A.O., Romero-Ortuno, R., Cogan, L., Ni Scanaill, C., Kenny, R.A.: Quantitative falls risk assessment using the timed up and go test. IEEE Trans. Biomed. Eng. 57(12), 2918–2926 (2010)
43. Hagler, S., Austin, D., Hayes, T.L., Kaye, J., Pavel, M.: Unobtrusive and ubiquitous in-home monitoring: a methodology for continuous assessment of gait velocity in elders. IEEE Trans. Biomed. Eng. 57(4), 813–820 (2010)
44. Hausdorff, J.M., Ladin, Z., Wei, J.Y.: Footswitch system for measurement of the temporal parameters of gait. J. Biomech. 28(3), 347–351 (1995)
45. Health Level Seven International. CDA Release 2. Technical report (2005)
46. Helmer, A., Lipprandt, M., Frenken, T., Eichelberg, M., Hein, A.: 3DLC: a comprehensive model for personal health records supporting new types of medical applications. J. Healthc. Eng. 2(3), 321–336 (2011)
47. Henriksen, M., Lund, H., Moe-Nilssen, R., Bliddal, H., Danneskiod-Samsøe, B.: Test-retest reliability of trunk accelerometric gait analysis. Gait Posture 19(3), 288–297 (2004)
48. Holzinger, A., Searle, G., Wernbacher, M.: The effect of previous exposure to technology on acceptance and its importance in usability and accessibility engineering. Univ. Access Inf. Soc. 10(3), 245–260 (2011)
49. Hornsteiner, C., Detlefsen, J.: Characterisation of human gait using a continuous-wave radar at 24 GHz. Adv. Radio Sci. 6, 67–70 (2008)
50. Huang, B., Chen, M., Shi, X., Xu, Y.: Gait event detection with intelligent shoes. In: Proceedings of International Conference on Information Acquisition ICIA 2007, 8–11 July 2007, pp. 579–584 (2007)
51. Huitema, R.B., Hof, A.L., Postema, K.: Ultrasonic motion analysis system-measurement of temporal and spatial gait parameters. J. Biomech. 35(6), 837–842 (2002)
52. Imms, F.J., Edholm, O.G.: Studies of gait and mobility in the elderly. Age Ageing 10(3), 147–156 (1981)
53. Jang, Y., Shin, S., Lee, J.W., Kim, S.: A preliminary study for portable walking distance measurement system using ultrasonic sensors. In: Proceedings of 29th Annual International Conference of the IEEE Engineering in Medicine and Biology Society EMBS 2007, pp. 5290–5293 (2007)
54. Kamen, G., Patten, C., Du, C.D., Sison, S.: An accelerometry-based system for the assessment of balance and postural sway. Gerontology 44(1), 40–45 (1998)
55. Kerr, K., White, J., Barr, D., Mollan, R.: Standardization and definitions of the sit-stand-sit movement cycle. Gait Posture 2(3), 182–190 (1994)

56. Kiselev, J., Gövercin, M., Frenken, T., Hein, A., Steinhagen-Thiessen, E., Wegel, S.: A new device for the assessment of gait and mobility with an automated timed up & go (atug): study protocol of an initial validation study. Contemporary Clinical Trials (2012, submitted)

57. Kiss, R.: Comparison between kinematic and ground reaction force techniques for determining gait events during treadmill walking at different walking speeds. Med. Eng. Phys. **32**(6), 662–667 (2010)

58. Knight, H., Lee, J.-K., Ma, H.: Chair Alarm for patient fall prevention based on Gesture Recognition and Interactivity. In: Proceedings of 30th Annual International Conference of the IEEE Engineering in Medicine and Biology Society EMBS 2008, 20–25 August 2008, pp. 3698–3701 (2008)

59. Kong, K., Tomizuka, M.: A gait monitoring system based on air pressure sensors embedded in a shoe. IEEE/ASME Trans. Mechatron. **14**(3), 358–370 (2009)

60. Lai, D.T.H., Wrigley, T.V., Palaniswami, M.: Ultrasound monitoring of inter-knee distances during gait. In: Proceedings of the Annual International Conference of the IEEE Engineering in Medicine and Biology Society EMBC 2009, pp. 725–728 (2009)

61. Leu, A., Ristic-Durrant, D., Graser, A.: A robust markerless vision-based human gait analysis system. In: Proceedings of 6th IEEE International Symposium on Applied Computational Intelligence and Informatics (SACI), pp. 415–420 (2011)

62. Liao, H.-F., Mao, P.-J., Hwang, A.-W.: Test-retest reliability of balance tests in children with cerebral palsy. Dev. Med. Child Neurol. **43**(3), 180–186 (2001)

63. Liao, T.-Y., Miaou, S.-G., Li, Y.-R.: A vision-based walking posture analysis system without markers. In: Proceedings of the 2nd International Conference on Signal Processing Systems (ICSPS), vol. 3, pp. 254–258 (2010)

64. Lim, D.-W., Kim, D.-H., Shen, L., Kim, H.-M., Kim, S., Yu, H.K.: Stride rate estimation using UWB impulse radar. In: Proceedings of the 3rd Asia-Pacific International Conference on Synthetic Aperture Radar (APSAR), pp. 1–3 (2011)

65. Liu, J., Lockhart, T.E., Jones, M., Martin, T.: Local dynamic stability assessment of motion impaired elderly using electronic textile pants. IEEE Trans. Autom. Sci. Eng. **5**(4), 696–702 (2008)

66. Lombardi, R., Buizza, A., Gandolfi, R., Vignarelli, C., Guaita, A., Panella, L.: Measurement on tinetti test: instrumentation and procedures. Technol. Health Care J. Eur. Soc. Eng. Med. **9**(5), 403–416 (2001)

67. Mancini, M., Salarian, A., Carlson-Kuhta, P., Zampieri, C., King, L., Chiari, L., Horak, F.B., et al.: Isway: a sensitive, valid and reliable measure of postural control. J. Neuroengineering Rehabil. **9**(1), 59 (2012)

68. Mancini, M., Zampieri, C., Carlson-Kuhta, P., Chiari, L., Horak, F.B.: Anticipatory postural adjustments prior to step initiation are hypometric in untreated parkinsons disease: an accelerometer-based approach. Eur. J. Neurol. **16**(9), 1028–1034 (2009)

69. Marschollek, M., Goevercin, M., Wolf, K.-H., Song, B., Gietzelt, M., Haux, R., Steinhagen-Thiessen, E.: A performance comparison of accelerometry-based step detection algorithms on a large, non-laboratory sample of healthy and mobility-impaired persons. In: Proceedings of the 30th Annual International Conference of the IEEE Engineering in Medicine and Biology Society EMBS 2008, pp. 1319–1322 (2008)

70. Marschollek, M., Nemitz, G., Gietzelt, M., Wolf, K., Meyer zu Schwabedissen, H., Haux, R.: Predicting in-patient falls in a geriatric clinic. Zeitschrift fr Gerontologie und Geriatrie **42**, 317–322 (2009)

71. Mathie, M.J., Coster, A.C.F., Lovell, N.H., Celler, B.G.: Accelerometry: providing an integrated, practical method for long-term, ambulatory monitoring of human movement. Physiol. Meas. **25**(2), R1 (2004)

72. Mayagoitia, R.E., Lotters, J.C., Veltink, P.H.: Standing stability evaluation using a triaxial accelerometer. In: Proceedings of 18th Annual International Conference of the IEEE Bridging Disciplines for Biomedicine Engineering in Medicine and Biology Society, October 31–November 3 1996, vol. 2, pp. 573–574 (1996)

73. Melenhorst, A.-S., Rogers, W.A., Bouwhuis, D.G.: Older adults' motivated choice for technological innovation: evidence for benefit-driven selectivity. Psychol. Aging **21**(1), 190 (2006)

74. Menz, H.B., Lord, S.R., Fitzpatrick, R.C.: Age-related differences in walking stability. Age Ageing **32**(2), 137–142 (2003)

75. Montero-Odasso, M., Schapira, M., Soriano, E.R., Varela, M., Kaplan, R., Camera, L.A., Mayorga, L.M.: Gait velocity as a single predictor of adverse events in healthy seniors aged 75 years and older. J. Gerontol. A Biol. Sci. Med. Sci. **60**(10), 1304–1309 (2005)

76. Muras, J.: SMOOTH - a system for mobility training at home for people with Parkinson's disease. Ph.D. thesis, Trinity College Dublin (2010)

77. Najafi, B., Aminian, K., Loew, F., Blanc, Y., Robert, P.A.: Measurement of stand-sit and sit-stand transitions using a miniature gyroscope and its application in fall risk evaluation in the elderly. IEEE Trans. Biomed. Eng. **49**(8), 843–851 (2002)

78. Narayanan, M.R., Redmond, S.J., Scalzi, M.E., Lord, S.R., Celler, B.G., Ast, N.H.L.: Longitudinal falls-risk estimation using triaxial accelerometry. IEEE Trans. Biomed. Eng. **57**(3), 534–541 (2010)

79. Nester, C., Jones, R.K., Liu, A., Howard, D., Lundberg, A., Arndt, A., Lundgren, P., Stacoff, A., Wolf, P.: Foot kinematics during walking measured using bone and surface mounted markers. J. Biomech. **40**(15), 3412–3423 (2007)

80. Organization, W.H., et al.: International classification of functioning disability and health (ICF). resolution WHA 54.21 (2001)

81. Otero, M.: Application of a continuous wave radar for human gait recognition. In: Kadar, I. (ed.) Society of Photo-Optical Instrumentation Engineers (SPIE) Conference Series, vol. 5809, pp. 538–548, May 2005

82. Pallejà, T., Teixidó, M., Tresanchez, M., Palacín, J.: Measuring gait using a ground laser range sensor. Sensors **9**(11), 9133–9146 (2009)

83. Pappas, I.P.I., Keller, T., Mangold, S., Popovic, M.R., Dietz, V., Morari, M.: A reliable gyroscope-based gait-phase detection sensor embedded in a shoe insole. IEEE Sens. J. **4**(2), 268–274 (2004)

84. Pavel, M., Hayes, T., Tsay, I., Erdogmus, D., Paul, A., Larimer, N., Jimison, H., Nutt, J.: Continuous assessment of gait velocity in Parkinson's disease from unobtrusive measurements. In: Proceedings of the 3rd International IEEE/EMBS Conference on Neural Engineering CNE 2007, 2–5 May 2007, pp. 700–703 (2007)

85. Pavel, M., Hayes, T.L., Adami, A., Jimison, H., Kaye, J.: Unobtrusive assessment of mobility. In: Proceedings of the 28th Annual International Conference of the IEEE Engineering in Medicine and Biology Society EMBS 2006, pp. 6277–6280, August 2006

86. Perez, C., Oates, A., Hughey, L., Fung, J.: Development of a force-sensing cane instrumented within a treadmill-based virtual reality locomotor system. In: Proceedings of the International Conference on Virtual Rehabilitation, pp. 154–159 (2009)

87. Perry, M., Dowdall, A., Lines, L., Hone, K.: Multimodal and ubiquitous computing systems: supporting independent-living older users. IEEE Trans. Inf. Technol. Biomed. **8**(3), 258–270 (2004)
88. Podsiadlo, D., Richardson, S.: The timed "Up & Go": a test of basic functional mobility for frail elderly persons. J. Am. Geriatr. Soc. **39**(2), 142–148 (1991)
89. Poppe, R.: Vision-based human motion analysis: an overview. Comput. Vis. Image Underst. **108**, 4–18 (2007)
90. Ram, S.S., Li, Y., Lin, A., Ling, H.: Doppler-based detection and tracking of humans in indoor environments. J. Franklin Inst. **345**(6), 679–699 (2008)
91. Salarian, A., Horak, F.B., Zampieri, C., Carlson-Kuhta, P., Nutt, J.G., Aminian, K.: iTUG, a sensitive and reliable measure of mobility. IEEE Trans. Neural Syst. Rehabil. Eng. **18**(3), 303–310 (2010)
92. Scanaill, C.N., Carew, S., Barralon, P., Noury, N., Lyons, D., Lyons, G.M.: A review of approaches to mobility telemonitoring of the elderly in their living environment. Ann. Biomed. Eng. **34**(4), 547–563 (2006)
93. Shao, X., Zhao, H., Nakamura, K., Katabira, K., Shibasaki, R., Nakagawa, Y.: Detection and tracking of multiple pedestrians by using laser range scanners. In: IEEE/RSJ International Conference on Intelligent Robots and Systems, 2007, IROS 2007, pp. 2174–2179 (2007)
94. Sixsmith, A.J.: An evaluation of an intelligent home monitoring system. J. Telemedicine Telecare **6**(2), 63–72 (2000)
95. Skelly, M.M., Chizeck, H.J.: Real-time gait event detection for paraplegic FES walking. IEEE Trans. Neural Syst. Rehabil. Eng. **9**(1), 59–68 (2001)
96. Smarr, C.-A., Fausset, C.B., Rogers, W.A.: Understanding the potential for robot assistance for older adults in the home environment. Georgia Institute of Technology (2011)
97. Smith, G.E., Ahmad, F., Amin, M.G.: Micro-Doppler processing for ultra-wideband radar data. In: SPIE Defense, Security, and Sensing, pp. 83610L–83610L. International Society for Optics and Photonics (2012)
98. Spehr, J., Gietzelt, M., Wegel, S., Költzsch, Y., Winkelbach, S., Marschollek, M., Gövercin, M., Wahl, F., Haux, R., Steinhagen-Thiessen, E.: Vermessung von Gangparametern zur Sturzprädikation durch Vision- und Beschleunigungssensorik. In: Demographischer Wandel - Assistenzsysteme aus der Forschung in den Markt (AAL 2011), p. 5 (2011)
99. Steen, E.-E., Eichelberg, M., Nebel, W., Hein, A.: A novel indoor localization approach using dynamic changes in ultrasonic echoes. In: Wichert, R., Eberhardt, B. (eds.) Ambient Assisted Living. Advanced Technologies and Societal Change, pp. 61–76. Springer, Heidelberg (2012)
100. Stolze, H., Klebe, S., Baecker, C., Zechlin, C., Friege, L., Pohle, S., Deuschl, G.: Prevalence of gait disorders in hospitalized neurological patients. Mov. Disord. **20**(1), 89–94 (2005)
101. Stone, E., Skubic, M.: Mapping kinect-based in-home gait speed to tug time: a methodology to facilitate clinical interpretation. In: 2013 7th International Conference on Pervasive Computing Technologies for Healthcare (PervasiveHealth), pp. 57–64 (2013)
102. Stone, E.E., Skubic, M.: Evaluation of an inexpensive depth camera for passive in-home fall risk assessment. In: Proceedings of 5th International Conference on Pervasive Computing Technologies for Healthcare (PervasiveHealth), pp. 71–77 (2011)

103. Stone, E.E., Skubic, M.: Passive in-home measurement of stride-to-stride gait variability comparing vision and kinect sensing. In: 2011 Annual International Conference of the IEEE Engineering in Medicine and Biology Society, EMBC, pp. 6491–6494. IEEE (2011)

104. Stone, E.-E., Skubic, M.: Passive, in-home gait measurement using an inexpensive depth camera: initial results. In: Proceedings of the 6th International Conference on Pervasive Computing Technologies for Healthcare (PervasiveHealth), pp. 183–186 (2012)

105. Sutherland, D.H.: The evolution of clinical gait analysis part l: kinesiological EMG. Gait Posture **14**(1), 61–70 (2001)

106. Sutherland, D.H.: The evolution of clinical gait analysis: Part II Kinematics. Gait Posture **16**(2), 159–179 (2002)

107. Sutherland, D.H.: The evolution of clinical gait analysis part III - kinetics and energy assessment. Gait Posture **21**(4), 447–461 (2005)

108. Tinetti, M.E.: Performance-oriented assessment of mobility problems in elderly patients. J. Am. Geriatr. Soc. **34**(2), 119–126 (1986)

109. Tung, J., Gage, W., Zabjek, K., Brooks, D., Maki, D., Mihailidis, A., Fernie, G.R., McIlroy, W.E.: iWalker: a 'real-world' mobility assessment tool. In: 30th Canadian Medical and Biological Engineering Society. Canadian Medical & Biological Engineering Society (2007)

110. van Doorn, C., Gruber-Baldini, A.L., Zimmerman, S., Hebel, J.R., Port, C.L., Baumgarten, M., Quinn, C.C., Taler, G., May, C., Magaziner, J., Epidemiology of Dementia in Nursing Homes Research Group: Dementia as a risk factor for falls and fall injuries among nursing home residents. J. Am. Geriatr. Soc. **51**(9), 1213–1218 (2003)

111. Verghese, J., Lipton, R.B., Hall, C.B., Kuslansky, G., Katz, M.J., Buschke, H.: Abnormality of gait as a predictor of non-Alzheimer's dementia. N. Engl. J. Med. **347**(22), 1761–1768 (2002)

112. Vignaud, L., Ghaleb, A., Le Kernec, J., Nicolas, J.-M.: Radar high resolution range & micro-Doppler analysis of human motions. In: Proceedings of the International RADAR Conference-Surveillance for a Safer World, pp. 1–6 (2009)

113. Virone, G., Noury, N., Demongeot, J.: A system for automatic measurement of circadian activity deviations in telemedicine. IEEE Trans. Biomed. Eng. **49**(12), 1463–1469 (2002)

114. Wahab, Y., Bakar, N.A.: Microsystem based portable shoe integrated instrumentation using ultrasonic for gait analysis measurement. In: Proceedings of the 4th International Conference on Mechatronics (ICOM), pp. 1–4 (2011)

115. Wall, J.C., Bell, C., Campbell, S., Davis, J.: The timed Get-up-and-Go test revisited: measurement of the component tasks. J. Rehabil. Res. Dev. **37**(1), 109–113 (2000)

116. Wang, F., Skubic, M., Abbott, C., Keller, J.M.: Body sway measurement for fall risk assessment using inexpensive webcams. In: Proceedings of the Annual International Conference of the IEEE Engineering in Medicine and Biology Society (EMBC), pp. 2225–2229 (2010)

117. Wang, Y., Fathy, A.E.: Range-time-frequency representation of a pulse Doppler radar imaging system for indoor localization and classification. In: 2013 IEEE Topical Conference on Wireless Sensors and Sensor Networks (WiSNet), pp. 34–36. IEEE (2013)

118. Weir, R.F., Childress, D.S.: Portable devices for the clinical measurement of gait performance and outcomes. In: Proceedings of the 22nd Annual International Conference of the IEEE Engineering in Medicine and Biology Society, vol. 3, pp. 1873–1875 (2000)
119. Weiss, A., Herman, T., Plotnik, M., Brozgol, M., Giladi, N., Hausdorff, J.M.: An instrumented timed up and go: the added value of an accelerometer for identifying fall risk in idiopathic fallers. Physiol. Meas. **32**(12), 2003 (2011)
120. Whitney, J.C., Lord, S.R., Close, J.C.T.: Streamlining assessment and intervention in a falls clinic using the Timed Up and Go Test and Physiological Profile Assessments. Age Ageing **34**(6), 567–571 (2005)
121. Williamson, R., Andrews, B.J.: Gait event detection for FES using accelerometers and supervised machine learning. IEEE Trans. Rehabil. Eng. **8**(3), 312–319 (2000)
122. Yack, H.J., Berger, R.C.: Dynamic stability in the elderly: identifying a possible measure. J. Gerontol. **48**(5), M225–M230 (1993)
123. Yamada, M., Kamiya, K., Kudo, M., Nonaka, H., Toyama, J.: Soft authentication and behavior analysis using a chair with sensors attached: hipprint authentication. Pattern Anal. Appl. **12**, 251–260 (2009)
124. Yardibi, T., Cuddihy, P., Genc, S., Bufi, C., Skubic, M., Rantz, M., Liu, L., Phillips, C.: Gait characterization via pulse-Doppler radar. In: Proceedings of the IEEE International Conference on Pervasive Computing and Communications Workshops (PERCOM Workshops), pp. 662–667 (2011)
125. Zampieri, C., Salarian, A., Carlson-Kuhta, P., Aminian, K., Nutt, J.G., Horak, F.B.: The instrumented timed up and go test: potential outcome measure for disease modifying therapies in Parkinson's disease. J. Neurol. Neurosurg. Psychiatry **81**(2), 171–176 (2010)
126. Zampieri, C., Salarian, A., Carlson-Kuhta, P., Nutt, J.G., Horak, F.B.: Assessing mobility at home in people with early Parkinson's disease using an instrumented Timed Up and Go test. Parkinsonism Relat. Disord. **17**(4), 277–280 (2011).http://dx.doi.org/10.1016/j.parkreldis.2010.08.001
127. Zhu, H.S., Wertsch, J.J., Harris, G.F., Loftsgaarden, J.D., Price, M.B.: Foot pressure distribution during walking and shuffling. Arch. Phys. Med. Rehabil. **72**(6), 390–397 (1991)
128. Zijlstra, W.: Assessment of spatio-temporal parameters during unconstrained walking. Eur. J. Appl. Physiol. **92**, 39–44 (2004)
129. Zijlstra, W., Hof, A.L.: Assessment of spatio-temporal gait parameters from trunk accelerations during human walking. Gait Posture **18**(2), 1–10 (2003)
130. Zubeyde Gurbtiz, S., Melvin, W.L., Williams, D.B.: Comparison of radar-based human detection techniques. In: Proceedings of the Conference Record of the Forty-First Asilomar Conference on Signals, Systems and Computers ACSSC 2007, pp. 2199–2203 (2007)

Reading

Instead of providing even more references than already done, we want to provide a short list of further sources that continuously offer new information in this and relevant research areas (sorted alphabetically).

- International Conference on Intelligent Environments, IE, http://www.intenv. org
- International Conference on Pervasive Computing and Communications, IEEE PerCom, http://www.percom.org/
- International Conference on Pervasive Computing Technologies for Health-care, http://pervasivehealth.org
- International Conference on PErvasive Technologies Related to Assistive Envi-ronments, PETRA, http://www.petrae.org
- Journal of Ambient Intelligence and Smart Environments (JAISE), http:// www.jaise-journal.org/
- Journal IEEE Pervasive Computing, http://www.computer.org/portal/web/ computingnow/pervasivecomputing
- Journal Pervasive and Mobile Computing, Elsevier, http://www.ees.elsevier. com/pmc

Personalized Physical Activity Monitoring Using Wearable Sensors

Gabriele Bleser[1]($\boxtimes$), Daniel Steffen[1], Attila Reiss[2], Markus Weber[1],
Gustaf Hendeby[3,4], and Laetitia Fradet[5]

[1] German Research Center for Artificial Intelligence, 67663 Kaiserslautern, Germany
{gabriele.bleser,daniel.steffen,markus.weber}@dfki.de
[2] ACTLab, University of Passau, 94032 Passau, Germany
attila.reiss@uni-passau.de
[3] Department of Electrical Engineering, Linköping University,
SE-581 83 Linköping, Sweden
hendeby@isy.liu.se
[4] Department of Sensor and EW Systems, Swedish Defence Research Agency (FOI),
SE-581 11 Linköping, Sweden
[5] Université de Poitiers, 86000 Poitiers, France
laetitia.fradet@univ-poitiers.fr

Abstract. It is a well-known fact that exercising helps people improve their overall well-being; both physiological and psychological health. Regular moderate physical activity improves the risk of disease progression, improves the chances for successful rehabilitation, and lowers the levels of stress hormones. Physical fitness can be categorized in cardiovascular fitness, and muscular strength and endurance. A proper balance between aerobic activities and strength exercises are important to maximize the positive effects. This balance is not always easily obtained, so assistance tools are important. Hence, *ambient assisted living* (AAL) systems that support and motivate balanced training are desirable. This chapter presents methods to provide this, focusing on the methodologies and concepts implemented by the authors in the *physical activity monitoring for aging people* (PAMAP) platform. The chapter sets the stage for an architecture to provide personalized activity monitoring using a network of wearable sensors, mainly *inertial measurement units* (IMU). The main focus is then to describe how to do this in a personalizable way: (1) monitoring to provide an estimate of aerobic activities performed, for which a boosting based method to determine activity type, intensity, frequency, and duration is given; (2) supervise and coach strength activities. Here, methodologies are described for obtaining the parameters needed to provide real-time useful feedback to the user about how to exercise safely using the right technique.

Keywords: Physical activity monitoring · ADL · Strength exercises · Personalization · Wearable sensors · Inertial sensors · HCI · Ambient assisted living

© Springer International Publishing Switzerland 2015
A. Holzinger et al. (Eds.): Smart Health, LNCS 8700, pp. 99–124, 2015.
DOI: 10.1007/978-3-319-16226-3_5

1   Introduction

Regular physical activity is highly recommended and is known to improve both physiological and psychological health [41]. Physical exercise can be divided into two categories, aerobic activity (promoting mainly cardiovascular health) and strength training (beneficial for the whole musculoskeletal system [45], not only muscle strength). These are all good arguments to exercise [13], but it is especially important for frail populations to help them maintain functional independence [20,41]. However, improperly executed, physical activity may cause injury [9,16]; hence, tools to allow for exercising efficiently and at minimal risk are desirable, still no general purpose systems are yet available for purchase.

In this chapter, this lack is addressed by describing the PAMAP system. The system's modular design allows for efficient customization, which could enable support tools as described above. Two use cases are studied in more detail: (1) monitoring of aerobic activities and (2) monitoring of strength exercises. For the former, a state-of-the-art boosting algorithm is provided. For the latter, different methodologies necessary for supervising exercises are outlined. In both cases, personalization is emphasized and the described methods are evaluated using data from field trials.

This chapter is intended to be interesting for both generally knowledgeable readers with a general interest for current advances in (AAL) solutions to *activities of daily living* ADL monitoring and support for strength activities using inertial sensing. Specialists in the field with interest in machine learning and multivariate signal pattern recognition looking for detailed algorithm descriptions to solve the aforementioned exercise monitoring problems.

This book chapter is organized as follows: Sect. 2 provides a short overview and the definitions of the most important terms that will be used throughout this chapter. Section 3 starts by presenting a generic platform concept for (AAL) systems. It describes the important components as well as the modular and flexible architecture for a physical activity monitoring using wearable sensors. Following, Sect. 3.2 showcases the implementation of the generic platform concept for the aerobic activity monitoring use case. Then, Sect. 3.3 illustrates the implementation for the strength exercise monitoring use case. Both use cases focus on the objectives, the initial requirements as well as the personalization of the (AAL) system. Section 4 briefly outlines the problems of the current setup, its implementations and the research challenges that should be addressed in future. Finally, for the general reader, a recommended reading list is presented in Sect. 4.

2   Glossary

ADL. The term activities of daily living summarizes daily activities within an individual's place or in outdoor environments. The term is mainly related to health care.

EHR. An electronic health record is a computerized record of a person or patient. Generally, it includes the history of illnesses, diagnosis, medical treatments, etc.

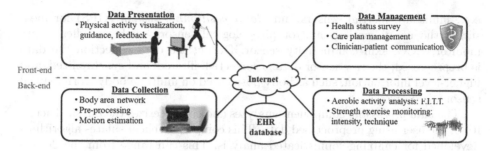

Fig. 1. The proposed modular monitoring platform architecture.

FITT. The frequency, intensity, time, type principle can be considered as a set of rules in order to benefit from any form of fitness training and is applicable to individual exercise training.

IMU. An inertial measurement unit usually combines multiple accelerometers, gyroscopes, and magnetometers providing measurements of linear acceleration, angular rate, and magnetic field.

GPS. A global positioning system determines the position (latitude and longitude) of a receiver on earth by calculating the time difference for signals from different satellites to reach the receiver.

MET. The metabolic equivalent of task is a unit to measure the energy cost of physical activities. It is used to estimate the amount of oxygen used by the body during physical activity and is defined as the ratio of metabolic rate during a specific physical activity to a reference metabolic rate.

PSD. The power spectral density describes how the power of a signal or time series is distributed over the different frequencies.

3   A State-of-the-Art System Example

This section first proposes an AAL system architecture for physical activity monitoring using wearable sensors. It then details the two use cases, monitoring of aerobic activities and supporting strength activities, in terms of requirements, hardware platform, and monitoring methodology. The discussion is supported with experimental results.

3.1   System Overview

The proposed system is modular and flexible. As illustrated in Fig. 1, it comprises four major components that communicate with each other over network using efficient protocols. The individual components (data collection, data processing, data presentation, and data management) are outlined in the following.

The *data collection* component is based on a network of sensors and possibly a mobile processing unit worn by the user. The sensor network can include, *e.g.,* miniature inertial sensors and *global positioning system* (GPS) for measuring the users' motions and/or physiological sensors, such as a heart rate monitor, ECG, skin conductivity sensor. During the data collection the data is preprocessed; the raw sensor data is corrected, filtered, and synchronized, and higher-level information, such as body pose based on multiple body-worn inertial sensors, is derived.

The *data processing* component analyzes and characterizes the physical activity of the user using preprocessed data. This component encapsulates algorithms developed for enabling sophisticated analysis. This can range from the derivation of the general *frequency, intensity, time, type principle* (FITT) parameters to the accurate evaluation of strength exercises. One of the key points in this context is to provide easy means for personalization in order to be able to target individuals or groups with specific needs.

The *data presentation* component provides reminders and physical activity visualization, guidance, and feedback to the user while training. Online user interfaces can range from a simplistic mobile device interface (a smartphone app), that provides alerts and just-in-time information about the current activity or daily profile. While being on the move, to a complete digital exercise trainer shown on a stationary display at home or in the gym, that guides a user through an exercise session whilst providing feedback on the way the exercises are performed.

The *data management* component connects the monitoring system to a private or public cloud. In a medical context, this could include uploading activity data to an *electronic health record* EHR enabling reviewing of this data by health care professionals. In a private context, activity data could be uploaded to social communities and shared with informal carers, such as family or friends. This sharing could promote friendly competition and motivate users to improve their performance.

By providing standards for the system components described above, the different components can easily be exchanged. This way the functionality of the system can be easily extended and specialized to create various target applications based on the same generic architecture.

The following sections showcase the implementation for the use case of aerobic activity monitoring Sect. 3.2 and strength exercise monitoring Sect. 3.3. The topics data collection and data processing will be described in detail.

3.2   Aerobic Activity Monitoring

In the field of physical activity monitoring, the recognition of basic aerobic activities (such as walking, running or cycling) and basic postures (lying, sitting, standing) is well researched and is possible with just one 3D-accelerometer [11,18]. However, since these approaches only consider a limited set of similar activities, they only apply to specific scenarios. Therefore, current research focuses among others on increasing the number of activities to recognize, with the goal to give a more accurate and more detailed description of an individual's daily routine [3].

Another challenge in this research field is the monitoring of physical activities in real life scenarios, which is usually neglected or even completely ignored. Moreover, recent benchmark results on physical activity monitoring datasets show that the difficulty of the more complex classification problems appearing in real life situations exceeds the potential of existing classifiers [32, 33].

This section addresses these shortcomings by describing a robust activity monitoring system for everyday life, as instantiation of the above described overall system architecture for the aerobic activity monitoring use case. The focus lies thereby on the presentation and evaluation of algorithms for monitoring a large and extensible set of activities of daily living based on a system for longterm and everyday use. Furthermore, the personalization of activity recognition algorithms — a new topic of interest in this field [19, 23] — will also be addressed, considering its feasibility in mobile applications and its applicability in everyday life situations.

Objectives and Requirements. The aerobic activity monitoring use case has two main objectives: to estimate the intensity of performed activities and to identify the aerobic activities traditionally recommended. The former objective is motivated by the goal to tell how far individuals meet physical activity recommendations, such as given in [13]. For this purpose, the system should distinguish activities of light, moderate, and vigorous effort. The ground truth for this rough intensity estimation is based on the *metabolic equivalent* (MET) of physical activities, provided by [1]. Moreover, to give a more detailed description of an individual's daily routine, an activity recognition task is defined. The goal thereby is the recognition of a few (recommended) activities and postures of interest, but as part of a classification problem where a large amount of other activities are included as well. This simulates the common behavior of how activity monitoring systems are used in real life scenarios.

Due to the special characteristics of classification problems defined on aerobic activity monitoring tasks, the evaluation methodology of such systems deserves a few remarks. The commonly used standard k-fold *cross-validation* (CV) only simulates the scenario in which a classifier was trained. The evaluation this way is limited to the known set of users and activities, thus delivering "optimistic" results for real life scenarios. The simulation of subject independence can be achieved with *leave-one-subject-out* (LOSO) CV. Moreover, to simulate when unknown activities are performed, *leave-one-activity-out* (LOAO) CV is recommended. The combination of LOSO and LOAO evaluation gives the best simulation of how developed methods would behave in everyday life scenarios, as described in [30]. Finally, it should be noted that traditional performance measures are used in this section to quantify the classification performance: precision, recall, F-measure, and accuracy.

Data Collection. Since aerobic activities are monitored over a long period in daily life, the hardware system for this use case has important constraints to adhere: only a limited number of sensors can be used and only relaxed requirements can be defined for calibration and fixation of the sensors. Therefore, a mobile and unobtrusive system is proposed, consisting of the following components: three wireless inertial sensors (attached on the chest, over the wrist on the dominant arm and on the dominant side's ankle, respectively), a wireless heart rate monitor, and a mobile unit for data collection, processing, and online feedback. An analysis of the necessity of the different sensors showed that this proposed sensor setup is the minimum required to achieve an accurate monitoring and assessment of the user's aerobic activities in daily life [31].

Due to the lack of commonly used, standard datasets in the field of physical activity monitoring the described hardware system was used to record a new dataset [32,33]. The created PAMAP2 dataset includes inertial and heart rate data from 9 subjects performing 18 different physical activities. The categorization of the latter into intensity classes is given in Table 1. The dataset not only includes basic activities and postures (lying, sitting/standing, walking, running, cycling and Nordic walking) traditionally used in the activity monitoring field, but also a wide range of everyday, household and fitness activities (*e.g.,* car driving, vacuum cleaning or playing soccer). Therefore, it is suitable for defining complex classification tasks and to simulate developed methods under realistic conditions. The dataset has been made publicly available in the UCI machine learning repository [27] and will be used in the rest of this section for evaluation purposes.

Data Processing. The PAMAP2 dataset provides raw sensory data. Therefore, a common *data processing chain* (DPC) is applied to obtain the aimed intensity and activity class. The DPC consists of preprocessing, segmentation, feature extraction, and classification steps, as depicted in Fig. 2. The preprocessing step provides synchronized, timestamped, and labeled acceleration and heart rate data. This data is then segmented using a sliding window. Previous work shows (*e.g.,* [15]) that for segmentation there is no single best window length for all activities.

Table 1. Definition of the intensity estimation task: mapping of physical activities included in the PAMAP2 dataset to the three intensity classes.

Light effort (< 3.0 METs)	Moderate effort (3.0–6.0 METs)	Vigorous effort (> 6.0 METs)
lie	walk	run
sit	cycle	ascend stairs
stand	descend stairs	rope jump
drive car	vacuum clean	play soccer
iron	Nordic walk	
fold laundry		
clean house		
watch TV		
computer work		

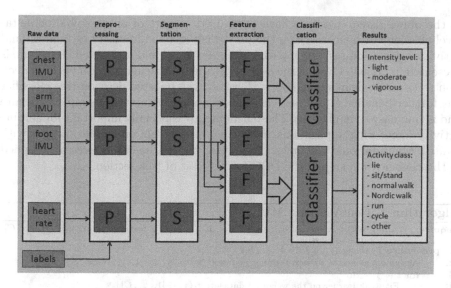

Fig. 2. The data processing chain applied in the aerobic activity monitoring use case.

To obtain at least two or three periods of all different periodic movements, a window length of about 3 to 5 s is reasonable. Furthermore, to assure an effective discrete Fourier transform computation for the frequency domain features, a window size of 512 samples was selected. Since the sampling rate of the raw sensory data was 100 Hz in the recorded PAMAP2 dataset, the segmentation step results in signal windows of 5.12 s length. Thus, the preprocessed data is segmented using a sliding window with the defined 5.12 s of window size, shifted by 1 s between consecutive windows. On each of these segments, various signal features are computed in both time (*e.g.,* mean, standard deviation) and frequency domain (*e.g.,* energy, entropy). In total, 137 features are extracted, which then serve as input to the classification step. The entire DPC is described in more detail in [32].

To deal with the *other* activities in the activity recognition task different models have been proposed. Common approaches include regarding all background activities as separate activity classes ('allSeparate' model), introducing a single background activity class ('bgClass' model, basically a null-class approach) or separating the basic and background activities in a classification step before or after the actual differentiation of the activities of interest ('preReject' or 'postReject' model, respectively). With the application of the above described LOSO and LOAO evaluation techniques the model with best generalization characteristics can be identified. As shown in [30], the 'bgClass' model behaves the most robust in real life scenarios and will thus be used hereafter.

A wide range of classification methods has been proposed and applied in the literature of physical activity monitoring. Most common choices are supervised learning approaches such as decision trees, Bayesian or instance based classifiers, support vector machines, neural networks, *etc.* A comparison of different methods applied for activity recognition can be found, *e.g.,* in [2, 24]. Moreover, some of the above listed classifiers have been used as part of an ensemble or meta-level classifier. A benchmark on the previously defined intensity estimation and activity recognition tasks, comparing different base- and meta-level classifiers, is presented in [32,33]. Overall, the best performance is achieved with boosted decision trees and k-nearest neighbors. However, the boosted decision tree classifier has further benefits: it is a fast classification algorithm with a simple structure and is thus easy to implement. These benefits are especially important for aerobic activity monitoring applications, since they usually run on mobile systems with limited computational resources. Therefore, boosted decision trees are applied in the classification step of the DPC for the rest of this section.

Algorithm 1. ConfAdaBoost.M1

Require: Training set of N instances: $(\underline{x}_i, y_i)$ $i = 1, \ldots, N$ ($\underline{x}_i$: feature vector, $y_i \in [1, \ldots, C]$)
      New instance to classify: $\underline{x}_n$
 1: **procedure** TRAINING($(\underline{x}_i, y_i)$ $i = 1, \ldots, N$)
 2:    Assign equal weight to each training instance: $w_i = \frac{1}{N}$, $i = 1, \ldots, N$
 3:    **for** $t \leftarrow 1, T$ **do**
 4:        Fit weak learner on the weighted dataset: $f_t(\underline{x}) \in [1, \ldots, C]$
 5:        Compute the confidence of the prediction that instance $\underline{x}_i$ belongs to the
            predicted class: p_{ti}, $i = 1, \ldots, N$
 6:        Compute error e_t of model on weighted dataset: $e_t = \sum_{i: y_i \neq f_t(\underline{x}_i)} p_{ti} w_i$
 7:        **if** $e_t = 0$ or $e_t \geq 0.5$ **then**
 8:            Delete last $f_t(\underline{x})$ and terminate model generation.
 9:        **end if**
10:        Compute $\alpha_t = \frac{1}{2} \log \frac{1 - e_t}{e_t}$
11:        **for** $i \leftarrow 1, N$ **do**
12:            $w_i \leftarrow w_i e^{\left(\frac{1}{2} - \mathrm{I}(y_i = f_t(\underline{x}_i)) \right) p_{ti} \alpha_t}$
13:        **end for**
14:        Renormalize the weight of all instances so that $\sum_i w_i = 1$
15:    **end for**
16: **end procedure**

17: **procedure** PREDICTION($\underline{x}_n$)
18:    Set zero weight to all classes: $\mu_j = 0$, $j = 1, \ldots, C$
19:    **for** $t \leftarrow 1, T$ **do**
20:        Predict class with current model: $[c, p_t(\underline{x}_n)] = f_t(\underline{x}_n)$, where $p_t(\underline{x}_n)$ is the
          confidence of the prediction that instance $\underline{x}_n$ belongs to the predicted class c
21:        $\mu_c \leftarrow \mu_c + p_t(\underline{x}_n) \alpha_t$
22:    **end for**
23:    The output class is $arg\,max_j \mu_j$ $j = 1, \ldots, C$
24: **end procedure**

One of the key challenges identified by the benchmark is the necessity to improve existing algorithms to achieve good performance results on complex activity monitoring classification problems. Therefore, a novel boosting method called ConfAdaBoost.M1 is presented here. ConfAdaBoost.M1 (*cf.* Algorithm 1) is a confidence-based extension of the well-known AdaBoost.M1 algorithm. It is a direct multiclass classification technique, keeping the algorithmic structure of AdaBoost.M1. The main idea of ConfAdaBoost.M1 can be described as follows. In the training part of the algorithm, the confidence of the classification estimation is returned for each instance by the weak learner (line 5). These p_{ti} confidence values are used when computing the error rate of the weak learner (line 6): the more confident the model is in the misclassification the more that instance's weight counts in the overall error rate. Moreover, the p_{ti} confidence values are used to recompute the weights of the instances. The more confident the weak learner is in an instance's correct classification or misclassification, the more that instance's weight is reduced or increased, respectively (line 12). Finally, the confidence values are used in the prediction part of the algorithm: the more confident the weak learner is in a new instance's prediction the more it counts in the output of the combined classifier (line 21).

The ConfAdaBoost.M1 algorithm has been evaluated on various benchmark datasets, comparing it to the most commonly used boosting techniques. Results achieved on the defined activity recognition (PAMAP2_AR) and intensity estimation (PAMAP2_IE) classification problems are shown in Table 2. It is clear that ConfAdaBoost.M1 performed significantly best among the compared algorithms. For example, on the activity recognition task the test error rate was reduced by nearly 20 % compared to the second best performing classifier. A more detailed description of ConfAdaBoost.M1 and further results of its thorough evaluation can be found in [29].

Personalization of Physical Activity Recognition. The benchmark results on the PAMAP2 dataset show that although good overall performance is achieved on various activity monitoring tasks, the individual performance of the included subjects varies a lot [32, 33]. Therefore, personalization approaches are highly encouraged, thus to adapt a general activity monitoring model to a new user. This has become a topic of interest recently, suggesting personalization either in the feature extraction or classification step of the DPC. Drawbacks of existing approaches are that either the general model is simple (allowing only low performance on complex classification tasks) or too complex for mobile applications, resulting in unfeasible computational costs.

This section presents a novel general concept of personalization, applying it in the decision fusion step of the DPC. In this concept the general model consists of a set of S classifiers (experts), all weighted the same ($w_i = 1$, $i = 1, \ldots, S$). Using new labeled data from a previously unknown subject, only the weights of the experts are retrained, the classifiers themselves remain the same. To show that this concept is a valid approach for personalization, different methods based on the idea of weighted majority voting are applied to increase the performance of the general model for new individuals. The baseline performance is given by

Table 2. Comparison of ConfAdaBoost.M1 to common boosting algorithms: test error rates [%] on the PAMAP2 activity recognition and intensity estimation tasks.

Task	AdaBoost.M1	Quinlan-AdaBoost.M1	Conf-AdaBoost.M1	SAMME
PAMAP2_AR	29.28 ± 1.4	27.9 ± 1.06	$\mathbf{22.22 \pm 0.77}$	27.98 ± 1.34
PAMAP2_IE	7.98 ± 1.04	7.73 ± 0.66	$\mathbf{5.60 \pm 0.31}$	7.81 ± 0.6

majority voting (MV), thus when no retraining is performed. Using a set of N labeled samples from the new subject, three existing approaches are applied to retrain the general model: *weighted majority algorithm* (WMA), *randomized weighted majority algorithm* (RWMA) and *weighted majority voting* (WMV). Moreover, based on the proposed general concept, a novel algorithm called *dependent experts* (DE, *cf.* Algorithm 2) is introduced. The main idea of the DE algorithm is that the confidence of an expert's prediction depends on the decision of all other experts. Therefore, the result of training the weights is a matrix of size SC (**W**, line 13), where $w_{i,c}$ stands for the weight of the ith expert when the majority vote of all other experts is the class c (defined as the performance rate of the ith expert on this subset of samples, *cf.* line 8–10). This way, DE is more flexible compared to existing algorithms: it supports the case when an expert is performing good on some classes, but poorly on others.

The described general concept of personalization and the novel DE algorithm have been thoroughly evaluated on the PAMAP2 activity recognition task, using the LOSO evaluation technique [34]. The results show the validity of the proposed methods: compared to MV, the overall performance measures and especially the lowest individual performance increases significantly. Moreover, the new DE algorithm clearly outperforms all other methods and is thus a very promising approach for personalization. Since the presented algorithms are computationally not intensive, they are feasible for mobile activity monitoring systems. Finally, the proposed personalization approach requires less interaction from a new user than existing solutions and has a short response time [34].

Algorithm 2. Dependent Experts

Require: **S** is the set of S different experts (classifiers): s_i, $i = 1, \ldots, S$
      C is the set of C classes the classification task is composed of: c_i, $i = 1, \ldots, C$
      N is the set of N new labeled samples: $\underline{n}_i = (\underline{x}_i, y_i)$, $i = 1, \ldots, N$
          ($\underline{x}_i$: feature vector, $y_i \in [1, \ldots, C]$)
      New instance to classify: $\underline{x}_{new}$
1: **procedure** TRAINING_WEIGHT(**S,C,N**)
2:     **for** $i \leftarrow 1, S$ **do**
3:         **for** $j \leftarrow 1, N$ **do**
4:             Predict label of $\underline{x}_j$ with expert s_i: $\hat{y}_j$
5:             Predict label of $\underline{x}_j$ with the ensemble $\mathbf{S} \cap s_i$, using majority voting: $\hat{\tilde{y}}_j$
6:         **end for**
7:         **for** $c \leftarrow 1, C$ **do**
8:             $\mathbf{P}_c = \{\forall \underline{n} \in \mathbf{N} \,|\, \hat{\tilde{y}} = c\}$
9:             $\mathbf{P}_{c\_good} = \{\forall \underline{n} \in \mathbf{P}_c \,|\, \hat{y} = y\}$
10:            $w_{i,c} = |\mathbf{P}_{c\_good}| / |\mathbf{P}_c|$
11:        **end for**
12:    **end for**
13:    **W** is the return weight matrix, composed of $w_{i,c}$ $i = 1, \ldots, S$ and $c = 1, \ldots, C$
14: **end procedure**
15: **procedure** PREDICTION(**S,C,W**,$\underline{x}_{new}$)
16:    $\mu_c = 0$, $c = 1, \ldots, C$
17:    **for** $i \leftarrow 1, S$ **do**
18:        Predict label of $\underline{x}_{new}$ with expert s_i: class $\hat{c}$
19:        Predict label of $\underline{x}_{new}$ with the ensemble $\mathbf{S} \cap s_i$: class $\hat{\tilde{c}}$
20:        $\mu_{\hat{c}} \leftarrow \mu_{\hat{c}} + w_{i,\hat{\tilde{c}}}$
21:    **end for**
22:    The output class is $arg\,max_c \mu_c$ $c = 1, \ldots, C$
23: **end procedure**

3.3 Strength Exercise Monitoring

Different systems and methodologies for monitoring and supervising home-based motor retraining and coordination exercises have been proposed during the past years. See [25] for a thorough review of wearable sensors and systems for rehabilitation applications. Examples of rehabilitation solutions that have entered into the market are Hocoma's ValedoMotion [14] and CoRehab's Riablo [8]. Using few wearable IMUs, both system monitor specific body parts, such as back, knee, or elbow, with respect to range of motion and use gamification techniques to motivate the user.

Current video games include feedback based on wearable motion or external vision sensors in order for users to follow fitness exercises of general interest. While such gaming systems are motivating and can have a positive effect on strength, balance, and overall fitness, the considered parameters are undocumented leading to a lack of proper monitoring and helpful feedback. Moreover, the available systems cannot be personalized for users with specific needs and individual limitations and their use in frail populations has led to injuries as reported in a recent survey [38]. Finally, external vision sensors suffer from the line-of-sight problem and therefore restrict the set of available exercises to those which allow full visibility of the user in the relevant plane.

To summarize, previous work has mostly focused on a single body joint rather than providing a flexible solution for the whole body. Moreover, it has concentrated on the motivational aspect of the system rather than on developing sophisticated monitoring methodology. Therefore, this section focuses on a recently developed methodology, which takes both exercise load and technique into account and stands out due to the complexity of evaluation parameters, the inclusion of the complete body, and its generic concept with inherent personalization.

Objectives and Requirements. The aim of the strength exercise use case is to guide a user through a training session and to provide valuable online feedback in order to ensure positive training effects and prevent injuries through correct exercise execution. For this, the exercise load, as well as, the performed movement have to be monitored and evaluated. The latter includes verifying that the muscles loaded during the exercise are the targeted ones and that the range of motion and the assumed postures are correct. Monitoring these parameters requires, in contrast to the aerobic activity use case, short-term, but accurate tracking of relevant body segments.

The following paragraphs describe the technical realization of these requirements in terms of the back-end components depicted in Fig. 1. Data collection addresses the hardware platform, as well as, full-body motion tracking, while data processing encapsulates methods for: (1) to learn and then recognize motion patterns (single exercise repetitions) in continuous motion data streams; and (2) to compare segmented patterns to previously learnt reference motions and to evaluate their execution in terms of the above mentioned parameters.

Data Collection. Strength exercises are monitored over a short period of time, typically during training indoors and require accurate tracking of all involved body segments. Therefore, the hardware system for this use case is based on a stationary processing and display infrastructure (*e.g.*, a laptop and a television) and a comparably complex wearable inertial sensor setup.

Any commercially available IMU, providing sufficient measurement quality can be in the system. While the latest generation wireless sensors, such as [39, 46], are rather costly and obtrusive due to their form factor, recent developments in sensor miniaturization enable low-cost and light-weight solutions [36].

The number of sensors, the sensor positioning, fixation, and calibration, is a trade-off between ease of use and data accuracy. The latter receives more emphasis here compared to the aerobic monitoring use case. To precisely capture the user's movements, it is typically assumed to have one IMU on each major body segment that should be monitored. Moreover, sensors should be placed on bones, ligaments, and between muscles in order to be unobtrusive and limit the skin and muscle motion artifacts. Furthermore, an easy, fast and repeatable fixation method is required that neither allows for too many degrees of freedom nor is too size-dependent.

While previous systems emphasize flexibility and are mostly based on Velcro straps on top of the normal cloths [8, 14], the system in focus here, the solution proposed in [6], uses a modified sports suit with pre-defined sensor fixation points in order to reduce the burden on the user to remember the correct positioning. Moreover, an interactive, but easy-to-perform calibration procedure is used to improve data accuracy. Recent developments in the direction of smart garment with highly integrated miniaturized sensors provide a promising future platform for the considered application [36].

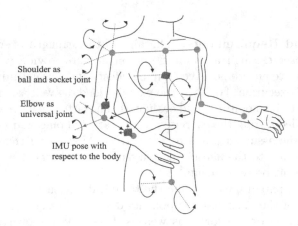

Fig. 3. Functional upper body model with indicated IMU placement (red cubes) (Color figure online).

A conventional approach to body motion tracking is to determine the joint angles and angle kinematics by comparing the IMU measurements (accelerations, angular velocities, and magnetic fields) to predictions based on a biomechanical body model using model based sensor fusion. This biomechanical model is typically a functional model consisting of rigid bodies and joints, such as the upper-body model illustrated in Fig. 3 in relation to the sensor positions. To capture more detailed motions or additional body parts, the model complexity can be increased by including additional segments and respective IMUs. While commercially available inertial motion capturing systems based on the aforementioned type of IMUs [40, 47] provide rather closed solutions, dedicated implementations of the underlying method as described in e.g., [10, 21, 28] provide more flexibility. In particular, [21] describes a generic method for tracking arbitrary kinematic chains based on IMUs.

The inertial motion capturing system used in this section is based on the model illustrated in Fig. 3, while assuming the same structure also for the lower body. The full-body model consists of ten rigid bodies (torso, pelvis, upper-arms, forearms, upper-legs, and lower-legs) connected by anatomically motivated restricted joints. The orientations of torso and pelvis, as well as, the shoulder and hip joints are modeled with three degrees of freedom, while elbow and knee joints are modeled as pivot joints with two degrees of freedom. Hence, in total, 26 angles are available for data processing.

Due to a lack of commonly available datasets for the type of application described here, a new dataset has been created using this setup. This dataset is particularly interesting, since it has been generated in the context of a clinical study with an extremely relevant target group of elderly people between the ages of 55 and 86. The dataset contains motion tracking data (26 joint angles at 100 Hz) from 30 participants performing 10 to 13 different upper and lower body exercises. These exercises were performed once under the supervision of a physical activity teacher and once autonomously. Labels indicate the start and end of each exercise repetition. From the 30 participants, ten were fit and healthy, ten were cardiac patients and ten suffered from upper or lower body functional disabilities. Hence, this dataset is suitable for evaluating personalized monitoring methodologies and will be used in the rest of this section for evaluation purposes[1].

Data Processing. From a technical point of view, monitoring both exercise load and performed movement requires to automatically detect single exercise repetitions and to accurately evaluate each repetition with respect to certain parameters. A promising concept for achieving personalized monitoring is to learn personalized exercise models from example executions of individual users. This is illustrated in Fig. 4: During a teach-in phase, training data is collected from a user, while he/she performs a certain number of exercise repetitions (per exercise), e.g., under supervision of a physical activity specialist. The training data is then used to automatically construct a personalized exercise model, which

---

[1] The dataset is publicly available at http://www.pamap.org/PAMAP_trials.tar.gz.

serves as gold standard during the trainer mode, *i.e.*, during online exercise monitoring. This generic reference model concept not only enables personalization, but it also provides independence of a fixed exercise selection with pre-defined parameters for each exercise.

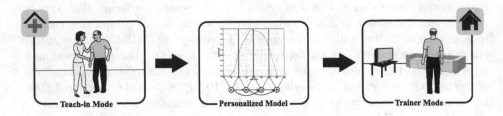

Fig. 4. Concept for personalized strength exercise monitoring.

Subsequently, the technique to automatically generate a personalized exercise model from training data is described. This includes finding all repetitions of the performed exercise in the recorded sequence and then creating a statistical model from the detected repetitions. Afterwards, it is explained, how this model is used to detect and evaluate motion cycles during online monitoring.

Teach-in Mode. The following paragraphs describe a fully automated method for reliably extracting known numbers of exercise repetitions within continuous motion sequences. Technically, this corresponds to the problem of detecting motifs in multivariate training sequences, which is also referred to as unsupervised motif discovery. A motif is here a recurring motion segment, representing one repetition of strength exercise execution. The detected segments can then be used to generate a personalized statistical model, which can serve as reference for both online motion cycle detection and evaluation.

In the following, the different steps of motif discovery will be described. First, the dimensionality of the motion data is reduced. Figure 5a shows an example recording of the 26 angles for the full body. Based on the assumption that the most moving joints contain the most relevant information, the angles with highest variances are extracted (see Fig. 5b). Let

$$C_i = \{c_{i,1}, c_{i,2}, \cdots, c_{i,n}\},$$

with $0 \leq i < b$, be a time series of angle values for joint angle i, where b is the number of tracked angles and n the length of the sequence. Then, each channel with $\mathrm{var}(C_i) > \mu_{var}$ is considered to be relevant, with

$$\mu_{\mathrm{var}} = \frac{1}{b} \cdot \sum_{i=0}^{b} \mathrm{var}(C_i).$$

Since, in this case, the length of the pattern (one exercise repetition) is unknown, the second step is to estimate a suitable window size w_{est}, *i.e.*, the length of one motion cycle. This is an extension to most previous approaches, which are based on a predefined window size [22]. Here, the windows size depends on the sampling rate of the system and is measured in number of samples.

Based on the assumption that the repetitions in the training sequence are performed consecutively with roughly the same speed, a dominant frequency should be present in the signal. This can be extracted using the combined *power spectral density* (PSD) [44] (*cf.* Fig. 5b). The window length w_{est} is then initialized as the wavelength of the dominant frequency, $w_{est} = \lambda = \frac{v}{f_{dominant}}$, with v being the sampling rate; *i.e.*, here 100 Hz.

The next step detects the motif candidates. For this, an extended version of Minnen's method [22] parametrized with w_{est} is used. The method collects overlapping sub-sequences, S_i, of length w_{est} from the training signal, S, and determines the k-nearest neighbors for each subsequence as $\text{kNN}(S_i) = S_{i,1...k}$. Here, k is the predefined number of repetitions. In order to reduce the sensitivity to local time shift and slightly varying execution speed, *dynamic time warping* (DTW) is used as distance measure. A real motif should have at least k similar sub-sequences. Hence, in order to find good motif candidates, for each subsequence, S_i, the distance density is estimated as the reciprocal of the distance to the least similar neighbor k: $\text{den}(S_i) \propto \frac{1}{\text{dist}(S_i, S_{i,k})}$. The motif candidates, $cand_i$, are then identified as the local maxima of the densities among their k nearest neighbors:

$$\text{maxima}(S_i) = \{S_i : \forall\ S_{i,j}\ \text{den}(S_i) > \text{den}(S_{i,j})\},$$

where $j = [1, k]$. Motif candidates are highlighted in Fig. 5c.

In the next step of the algorithm, a model for each candidate is generated and used to segment the signal. As most of the learning approaches fail, if there are only few training samples available, either constructed models [42] or template-based approaches are feasible. Here, a template approach, based on the *online dynamic time warping* (ODTW) [17] is described. The motif candidate is chosen as the template for the DTW and its k-neighbors are used for defining the cost threshold.

Finally, the candidate, which model provides the best signal segmentation, is chosen as the motion motif. As criteria, the difference between the number of segmented patterns and the known number of executions in the training sequence, as well as, the average normalized DTW costs are used. In Fig. 5c, the selected candidate is marked red.

The chosen motif and its nearest neighbors can now be either used to generate a class template from a set of the best templates, *e.g.*, extract the templates from the nearest neighbors that have the best minimum inter-class DTW distances [17], or they can be used to generate a *hidden Markov model* (HMM) as proposed in [42]. Both approaches are suitable for an online real-time segmentation.

The proposed motif discovery method was evaluated on the previously mentioned dataset in terms of precision, recall, and overlap. Precision is defined as the fraction of segmented exercise executions that are relevant, while recall is defined as the fraction of correctly retrieved executions. A segment, *i.e.*, a motion cycle, is considered as correctly retrieved, if it overlaps with the ground truth segment exceeds 30 %.

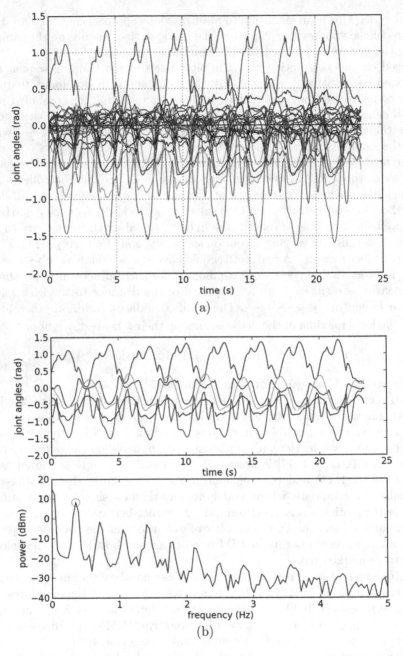

Fig. 5. Consecutive steps of the motif discovery on a sample teach-in sequence: (a) plots 26 joint angles recorded during a teach-in session for one exercise; (b) illustrates the reduced motion tracking signal, *i.e.,* the most moving joint channels (top) and the PSD (bottom), where the dominant frequency is marked with a red circle (estimation of w_{est}); in (c), the annotated area shows the result of the motif candidate (green) selection, as well as the finally selected motif (red) (Color figure online).

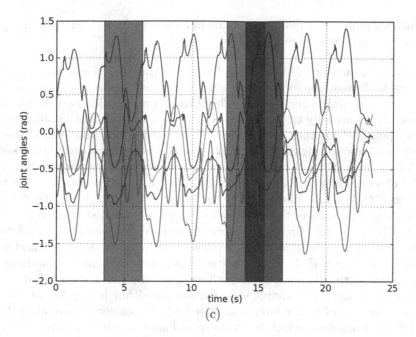

Fig. 5. (*Continued*)

Table 3. Exemplary motif discovery results averaged over all performed exercises in terms of precision, recall, and percental overlap.

#	Precision $\mu \pm$ var	Recall $\mu \pm$ var	Overlap $\mu \pm$ var
1	0.77 ± 0.10	0.80 ± 0.10	0.59 ± 0.06
2	0.85 ± 0.08	0.86 ± 0.08	0.71 ± 0.08
3	0.98 ± 0.00	0.97 ± 0.01	0.75 ± 0.03
4	0.93 ± 0.02	0.95 ± 0.02	0.76 ± 0.02
5	0.98 ± 0.00	0.90 ± 0.01	0.73 ± 0.03
⋮	⋮	⋮	⋮
30	0.95 ± 0.01	0.88 ± 0.01	0.59 ± 0.04
∅	0.93 ± 0.00	0.91 ± 0.00	0.72 ± 0.00

Table 3 exemplifies the experimental results for selected participants represented in the dataset, averaged over all performed exercises. A more detailed analysis of the results is given in [43]. In the following the methods for generating personalized models for real-time, online motion cycle detection, as well as, for motion cycle evaluation are introduced.

Model Construction and Motion Cycle Detection. Based on the motion segments extracted in the teach-in mode, a method for constructing an HMM for a motion pattern, is discussed in this section. The HMM representation is chosen for two reasons: (1) it naturally takes variations in motion into account by allowing for time-warping and has thus been successfully applied in domains such as speech, gesture, and handwriting recognition; (2) standard algorithms, such as the short-time Viterbi algorithm [7] can be applied for online, real-time monitoring.

The observation probabilities of the HMM are modeled using *Gaussian mixture models* (GMM), as illustrated in the left plot in Fig. 6. Here, the different joint angle components of the multivariate signal are handled separately.

Let RM be the set of reference motions recorded for one exercise performed by one individual, during the teach-in phase. Now, a model M_{RM} is learnt from the reference motion RM. Since traditional parameter estimation methods for HMMs, such as the Baum-Welch algorithm, typically fail when applied to too few training examples, a simple construction algorithm is applied to capture the characteristics of each reference motion RM_i. This algorithm builds a HMM with left-right topology, which is a wide-spread approach to model time-varying sequential data [26]. Self-transitions and skip-transitions are added to allow for a faster and slower execution of the pattern. The number of states, N, is chosen as half the average sample length l_{avg}: $N = \lceil \frac{l_{avg}}{2} \rceil$ of the reference motion patterns RM. For each state, ST_i, a GMM is then trained using an expectation-maximization algorithm on all respective elements of $RM_i[j : j + l_{avg}]$. Thus, each segment is described by one normal distribution $\mathcal{N}(\mu_j, \sigma_j)$.

The HMMs obtained during the personalized model creation enable online detection of the represented reference motion within continuous motion data by utilizing the short-time Viterbi algorithm [7]. In general, the Viterbi algorithm computes the most likely path of states given a sequence of observations. Here, the observations are given by the continuous joint angles as streamed by the data collection component. Thus, the algorithm can determine, to which state, respectively frame, of the reference motion the current motion matches. If the probability of the Viterbi algorithm is below a defined threshold, the current observation is considered represent an incorrect motion. The motion cycle detection immediately allows for counting exercise repetitions and deducing their duration. Whenever a complete motion cycle has been detected, the detailed evaluation starts as will be detailed below.

Motion Cycle Evaluation. According to the system requirements, it is fundamental to evaluate the load of the exercise, the muscles that work, as well as, the posture assumed during the exercise in order to ensure effectiveness and safety. Translating these constraints into objective data that can be derived from the measured motion data resulted in the following criteria: For movement load, the exercise intensity is quantified by the number of repetitions, the movement speed, the movement amplitude, and the movement smoothness. Whether the

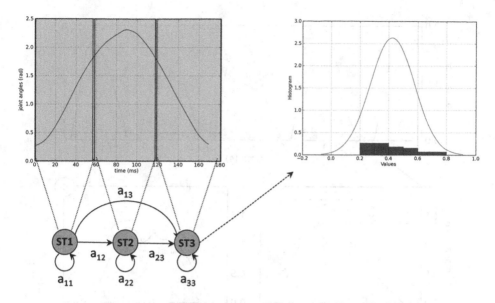

Fig. 6. HMM for one angle of the motion signal.

muscles that work are the correct ones is evaluated based on the axes of rotation during motion. Finally, for safety issues, the posture is evaluated based on a number of fixed distances or angles to be kept when performing the movement. This could, for instance, be the distance between the feet during squat exercises, or the angle at the pelvis during push-ups.

The number of repetitions and their duration are given by the motion cycle detection step described above. For the other criteria, an algorithm has been proposed in [6], which evaluates each detected motion cycle using the model constructed during the teach-in mode as reference. The different steps of the algorithms are the following. First, different angles and distances that must be respected during the movement in order to avoid injuries are computed and compared with those obtained during the reference movement. Afterwards, the principal rotation axis is computed for the current cycle at each joint. The principal rotation axes are then compared to the ones obtained during the reference movement. Using the same formalism, the rotation amplitudes are also compared. Finally, the number of local extrema of the time derivative of the joint trajectory (*i.e.*, its velocity) that has the greatest range of motion during the movement is evaluated and compared in order to determine movement smoothness. The procedure is illustrated in Fig. 7. The movement duration used to evaluate velocity, the pose (fixed angles and distances), and the rotation amplitudes of the movement to evaluate should not differ by more than a certain threshold from the reference model. The principal rotation axes should not deviate more than a certain threshold from those obtained from the reference. For the smoothness, the same number of extrema has to be found, since any other number of extrema indicates a deviation from the prescribed movement,

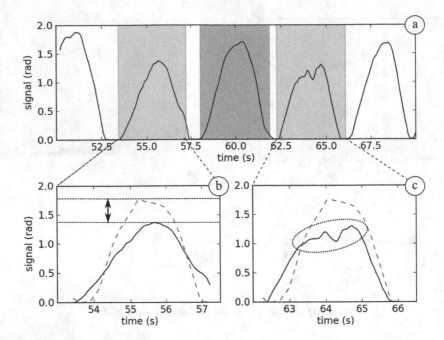

Fig. 7. Motion cycle evaluation: Detected motion cycles are evaluated separately by comparing them to a reference motion. The cycles overlaid with a red area show a significant deviation from the reference movement (illustrated as dashed red lines) (a), either in amplitude (b) or in the number of extrema (c). The green area indicates a correctly performed cycle (Color figure online).

e.g., in the form of a parasite movement or a break in motion flow during the execution of the exercise. For providing online user feedback, if any of these above mentioned criteria are not met, an alert can be generated and sent to the user interface, which translates this into explanatory feedback. The motion cycle evaluation concept is summarized in Table 4. Moreover, a technical evaluation of the proposed algorithm in terms of a confusion matrix for the considered parameters within a small-scale study can be found in [6].

4   Open Problems and Future Outlook

This chapter has outlined a platform for personalized physical activity monitoring by means of wearable sensors and has showcased different possible use cases. Even though promising results have been shown that indicate the potential of the technology, there are still open problems and challenges to be solved before this technology can be widely applied.

In the aerobic exercise monitoring use case, it should be investigated how well the developed methods and algorithms perform with different user groups. The evaluation on a publicly available physical activity monitoring dataset — including only young, healthy adult subjects — indicate good performance results. However, the ability to generalize the developed approaches with significantly different user groups (*e.g.,* elderly) remains an open question. Moreover, it is also planned to investigate the effect of increasing the number of known (thus in the training included) other activities, with the goal to improve even more the robustness with respect to unknown other activities while sustaining the high performance regarding the basic activity classes of interest. Furthermore, although the mobile aerobic activity monitoring system in its current form (using small wireless sensor units and a smartphone as mobile control unit) is as unobtrusive as possible with today's technology, its acceptance amongst different user groups needs to be evaluated in a user study.

Table 4. Motion cycle evaluation concept: The fixed angles and distances are provided by physical activity experts. The other measures are directly deduced from the movement of reference. The values x and θ are parameters of the algorithm.

Constraints	Parameters	Measures	Thresholds
Safety	Posture	Fixed angles and distances at/between joints	$\pm x\%$ of reference value
Load of exercise	Number of repetitions	Number of cycles	Same as reference
	Movement velocity	Movement duration	$\pm x\%$ of reference value
	Movement amplitude	Range of motion from quaternions at moving joints	$\pm x\%$ of reference value
	Movement smoothness	Number of extrema in velocity of most moving joint	Same as reference
Muscles to work	Joint rotation axes	Quaternion axes at moving joints	Angle deviation, θ, from reference axis

In the strength exercise use case, for instance, the detailed motion capturing needs to be more robust and the wearable sensory equipment even less obtrusive to be reliably deployed in the users' homes. Current developments in miniaturized sensors and smart clothes are fully in line with the latter requirement and open up for new possibilities. Moreover, stationary vision and depth sensors used in current gaming consoles could be fused with wearable motion sensors in order to create synergies and increase precision and robustness or reduce the number of required wearable sensors. A purely vision-based approach, however, is not feasible for the type of motions performed, due to the line-of-sight problem.

Another challenge is posed by the machine learning algorithms used to learn, segment, and evaluate motion cycles of arbitrary exercise motions. Today, these algorithms require engineering know-how to some extend to tune various parameters and thresholds. Here, further experiments and the development of data-driven parameter selection methods are crucial in order to improve the usability of such technologies for *e.g.,* health care professionals.

A last aspect to mention for the strength exercise use case is the fact that recognition algorithms sometimes fail. This raises the question how this should be handled by both the monitoring system and the user interface. Here, in particular false negative motion cycle detections or false positive incorrect motion detections could decrease the motivation of the user rather than providing support. Furthermore, a system accepting incorrect motions could be even more dangerous and could encourage the user to hurt himself. A forgiving user interface and the possibility for online learning based on some type of feedback from the user could be subject of future research.

Even though open problems still exist, monitoring technologies, such as the ones presented in this chapter, have taken a big step forward and in view of today's societal challenges, the aging society and the aging workforce, it is to be expected that mobile health technologies will gain even more importance and enter various application fields from personal health and fitness over work-life-balance support to human factor research.

References

1. Ainsworth, B.E., Haskell, W.L., Whitt, M.C., Irwin, M.L., Swartz, A.M., Strath, S.J., O'Brien, W.L., Bassett, D.R., Schmitz, K.H., Emplaincourt, P.O., Jacobs, D.R., Leon, A.S.: Compendium of physical activities: an update of activity codes and MET intensities. Med. Sci. Sports Exerc. **32**(9), 498–516 (2000)
2. Altun, K., Barshan, B., Tunçel, O.: Comparative study on classifying human activities with miniature inertial and magnetic sensors. Pattern Recogn. **43**(10), 3605–3620 (2010)
3. Bao, L., Intille, S.S.: Activity recognition from user-annotated acceleration data. In: Ferscha, A., Mattern, F. (eds.) PERVASIVE 2004. LNCS, vol. 3001, pp. 1–17. Springer, Heidelberg (2004)
4. Berger, K.: The Developing Person: Through the Life Span. Worth Publishers, New York (2008)
5. Bishop, C.: Pattern Recognition and Machine Learning. Information Science and Statistics. Springer, New York (2006)
6. Bleser, G., Steffen, D., Weber, M., Hendeby, G., Stricker, D., Fradet, L., Marin, F., Ville, N., Carré, F.: A personalized exercise trainer for the elderly. J. Ambient Intell. Smart Environ. **5**, 547–562 (2013)
7. Bloit, J., Rodet, X.: Short-time Viterbi for online HMM decoding: evaluation on a real-time phone recognition task. In: IEEE International Conference on Acoustics, Speech and Signal Processing, pp. 2121–2124 (2008)
8. Costa, C., Tacconi, D., Tomasi, R., Calva, F., Terreri, V.: RIABLO: a game system for supporting orthopedic rehabilitation. In: Conference of the Italian SIGCHI Chapter (CHItaly 2013), September 2013
9. Dick, F.W.: Sports Training Principles. A. & C. Black, London (1997)
10. El-Gohary, M., McNames, J.: Shoulder and elbow joint angle tracking with inertial sensors. IEEE Trans. Biomed. Eng. **59**(9), 2635–2641 (2012)
11. Ermes, M., Pärkkä, J., Cluitmans, L.: Advancing from offline to online activity recognition with wearable sensors. In: Proceedings of 30th Annual International IEEE EMBS Conference, Vancouver, Canada, pp. 4451–4454, August 2008
12. Fisk, A.D., Rogers, W.A., Charness, N., Czaja, S.J., Sharit, J.: Designing for Older Adults: Principles and Creative Human Factors Approaches. CRC Press, Boca Raton (2009)

13. Haskell, W.L., Lee, I.-M., Pate, R.R., Powell, K.E., Blair, S.N., Franklin, B.A., Macera, C.A., Heath, G.W., Thompson, P.D., Bauman, A.: Physical activity and public health: updated recommendation for adults from the American College of Sports Medicine and the American Heart Association. Med. Sci. Sports Exerc. **39**(8), 34–1423 (2007)

14. Hocoma.   VALEDO®MOTION.   http://www.hocoma.com/de/produkte/valedo-konzept/valedomotion/. Accessed June 2014

15. Huynh, T., Schiele, B.: Analyzing features for activity recognition. In: Proceedings of Joint Conference on Smart Objects and Ambient Intelligence (sOc-EuSAI), pp. 159–163 (2005)

16. Kirkendall, D.: Exercise prescription for the healthy adult. Prim. Care **11**(1), 23–31 (1984)

17. Ko, M.H., West, G., Venkatesh, S., Kumar, M.: Using dynamic time warping for online temporal fusion in multisensor systems. Inf. Fusion **9**(3), 370–388 (2008)

18. Long, X., Yin, B., Aarts, R.M.: Single-accelerometer based daily physical activity classification. In: Proceedings of 31st Annual International IEEE EMBS Conference, Minneapolis, MN, USA, pp. 6107–6110, September 2009

19. Maekawa, T., Watanabe, S.: Unsupervised activity recognition with user's physical characteristics data. In: Proceedings of IEEE 15th International Symposium on Wearable Computers (ISWC), San Francisco, CA, USA, pp. 89–96, June 2011

20. Mazzeo, R., Tanaka, H.: Exercise prescription for the elderly: current recommendations. Sports Med. **31**, 809–818 (2001)

21. Miezal, M., Bleser, G., Schmitz, N., Stricker, D.: A generic approach to inertial tracking of arbitrary kinematic chains. In: International Conference on Body Area Networks, Bosten, US, September 2013

22. Minnen, D., Isbell, C., Essa, I., Starner, T.: Discovering multivariate motifs using subsequence density estimation and greedy mixture learning. In: Proceedings of the 22nd National Conference on Artificial Intelligence (AAAI), vol. 1, pp. 615–620 (2007)

23. Pärkkä, J., Cluitmans, L., Ermes, M.: Personalization algorithm for real-time activity recognition using PDA, wireless motion bands, and binary decision tree. IEEE Trans. Inf. Technol. Biomed. **14**(5), 1211–1215 (2010)

24. Patel, S., Mancinelli, C., Healey, J., Moy, M., Bonato, P.: Using wearable sensors to monitor physical activities of patients with COPD: a comparison of classifier performance. In: Proceedings of 6th International Workshop on Wearable and Implantable Body Sensor Networks (BSN), Berkeley, CA, USA, pp. 234–239, June 2009

25. Patel, S., Park, H., Bonato, P., Chan, L., Rodgers, M.: A review of wearable sensors and systems with application in rehabilitation. J. Neuroeng. Rehabil. **9**(21), 1–17 (2012)

26. Rabiner, L.: A tutorial on Hidden Markov Models and selected applications in speech recognition. Proc. IEEE **77**(2), 257–286 (1989)

27. Reiss, A.: PAMAP2 Physical Activity Monitoring Data Set. http://archive.ics.uci.edu/ml/datasets/PAMAP2+Physical+Activity+Monitoring, 22 November 2013

28. Reiss, A., Hendeby, G., Bleser, G., Stricker, D.: Activity recognition using biomechanical model based pose estimation. In: Lukowicz, P., Kunze, K., Kortuem, G. (eds.) EuroSSC 2010. LNCS, vol. 6446, pp. 42–55. Springer, Heidelberg (2010)

29. Reiss, A., Hendeby, G., Stricker, D.: Confidence-based multiclass AdaBoost for physical activity monitoring. In: Proceedings of IEEE 17th International Symposium on Wearable Computers (ISWC), Zurich, Switzerland, September 2013

30. Reiss, A., Hendeby, G., Stricker, D.: Towards robust activity recognition for everyday life: methods and evaluation. In: Proceedings of 7th International Conference on Pervasive Computing Technologies for Healthcare (PervasiveHealth), Venice, Italy, May 2013

31. Reiss, A., Stricker, D.: Introducing a modular activity monitoring system. In: Proceedings of 33rd Annual International IEEE EMBS Conference, Boston, MA, USA, pp. 5621–5624, August–September 2011

32. Reiss, A., Stricker, D.: Creating and benchmarking a new dataset for physical activity monitoring. In: Proceedings of 5th Workshop on Affect and Behaviour Related Assistance (ABRA), Crete, Greece, June 2012

33. Reiss, A., Stricker, D.: Introducing a new benchmarked dataset for activity monitoring. In: Proceedings of IEEE 16th International Symposium on Wearable Computers (ISWC), Newcastle, UK, pp. 108–109, June 2012

34. Reiss, A., Stricker, D.: Personalized mobile physical activity recognition. In: Proceedings of IEEE 17th International Symposium on Wearable Computers (ISWC), Zurich, Switzerland, September 2013

35. Russell, S., Norvig, P.: Artificial Intelligence: A Modern Approach. Prentice Hall Series in Artificial Intelligence. Prentice Hall, Englewood Cliffs (2010)

36. Salehi, S., Bleser, G., Schmitz, N., Stricker, D.: A low-cost and light-weight motion tracking suit. In: IEEE International Conference on Ubiquitous Intelligence and Computing, Vietri sul Mare, Italy, December 2013

37. Sears, A., Jacko, J.A.: The Human-Computer Interaction Handbook: Fundamentals, Evolving Technologies and Emerging Applications. CRC Press, Baco Raton (2007)

38. Taylor, M., McCormick, D., Impson, R., Shawis, T., Griffin, M.: Activity promoting gaming systems in exercise and rehabilitation. J. Rehabil. Res. Dev. **48**, 1171–1186 (2011)

39. Trivisio. Colibri Wireless - Inertial Motion Tracker. http://www.trivisio.com/trivisio-products/colibri-wireless-inertial-motion-tracker-3/. Last Accessed June 2014

40. Trivisio. MotionVizard. http://www.trivisio.com/trivisio-products/motionvizard-4/. Accessed June 2014

41. Warburton, D., Nicol, C., Bredin, S.: Health benefits of physical activity: the evidence. Can. Med. Assoc. J. **174**(6), 801–809 (2006)

42. Weber, M., Bleser, G., Hendeby, G., Reiss, A., Stricker, D.: Unsupervised model generation for motion monitoring. In: IEEE International Conference on Systems, Man and Cybernetics - Workshop on Robust Machine Learning Techniques for Human Activity Recognition, Anchorage, pp. 51–54. IEEE (2011)

43. Weber, M., Liwicki, M., Bleser, G., Stricker, D.: Unsupervised motion pattern learning for motion segmentation. In: International Conference on Pattern Recognition (ICPR), Tsukuba Science City, Japan (2012)

44. Welch, P.: The use of fast Fourier transform for the estimation of power spectra: a method based on time averaging over short, modified periodograms. IEEE Trans. Audio Electroacoust. **15**(2), 70–73 (1967)

45. Winnett, R.A., Carpinelli, R.N.: Potential health-related benefits of resistance training. Prev. Med. **33**, 503–513 (2001)

46. Xsens. MTx. http://www.xsens.com/products/mtx/. Accessed June 2014

47. Xsens. MVN - Inertial Motion Capture. http://www.xsens.com/products/xsens-mvn/. Accessed June 2014

Reading

The generic platform concept for physical activity monitoring using wearable sensors, as well as the two implemented use cases have been presented in the previous Sect. 3. Especially the technical requirements in terms of the hardware platform and monitoring methodology have been addressed. However, in order to design such a system it is inevitable to consider end user requirements and to evaluate its overall usability. Particularly, when designing for diversity (*e.g.*, elderly population) additional requirements have to be considered.

Targeting the elderly population various aspects and effects of aging on mental and physical health and fitness have to be considered. Among others the book

> K. Berger. *The developing person: Through the life span.* Worth Publishers, 2008

describes the cognitive changes with aging (decreased ability to perceive a high amount of information at the same time, decrease of memory), the physiological changes (decrease of sensory abilities, *e.g.*, vision and hearing, decrease of movement accuracy and coordination) and the ability to deal with recent technology. The cognitive and the physiological changes should be taken into account during the conception of the user interface and the conception of the wearable sensors. Regarding the user interface, the quantity of information presented to the user should be reduced to the most useful and simplest form and should be presented by different sensory means (visual, auditive). The interaction with the system, as well as the manipulation and the fixation of the wearable sensors, should not require any fine movements. Finally, the user interface should be integrated into a system familiar to the user in order to limit the required learning of unknown technology. For a detailed description regarding the above mentioned requirements the interested reader is referred also to the following books

> A. D. Fisk, W. A. Rogers, N. Charness, S. J. Czaja, and J. Sharit. *Designing for older adults: Principles and creative human factors approaches.* CRC press, 2009

and

> A. Sears and J. A. Jacko. *The Human-Computer Interaction Handbook: Fundamentals, Evolving Technologies and Emerging Applications.* CRC Press, 2007

Moreover, recent advances in the miniaturization of sensors have made it possible to realize a great variety of new applications and open up new possibilities. However, this vast amount of sensor data has to be captured, stored and analyzed. Finding patterns and trends in this data is a challenging task. Witten *et al.* presents in

> I. Witten and E. Frank. *Data Mining: Practical Machine Learning Tools and Techniques, Second Edition.* The Morgan Kaufmann Series in Data Management Systems. Elsevier Science, 2005

a description of the Weka toolkit, along with a thorough foundation for the machine learning concepts the toolkit uses, and practical advice for using the different tools and algorithms. Weka is a collection of machine learning algorithms for data mining tasks. It includes tools for data pre-processing, classification, regression, clustering, association rules, and visualization. It is also well-suited for developing new machine learning systems.

A comprehensive and up-to-date introduction to the theory and practice of artificial intelligence is given by Russell and Norvig in

S. Russell and P. Norvig. *Artificial Intelligence: A Modern Approach.* Prentice Hall series in artificial intelligence. Prentice Hall, 2010

A great introduction to ubiquitous computing is given by Krumm in

J. Krumm. *Ubiquitous Computing Fundamentals.* Taylor & Francis, 2009

This book covers the contributions of 11 of the most prominent researchers in the field of ubiquitous computing. Based on the categories systems, experience, and sensors the authors describe various research topics in the field of ubiquitous computing.

Finally, pattern recognition from the Bayesian viewpoint is addressed in the book

C. Bishop. *Pattern Recognition and Machine Learning.* Information Science and Statistics. Springer, 2006

This book does not require any previous knowledge of pattern recognition or machine learning concepts. Furthermore, it includes a self-contained introduction to basic probability theory.

Energy Harvesting on Human Bodies

Gregor Rebel[1]([envelope]), Francisco Estevez[1], Peter Gloesekoetter[1],
and Jose M. Castillo-Secilla[2]

[1] Fachhochschule Muenster, Stegerweldstr. 39, 48565 Münster, Germany
gregor@fh-muenster.de
[2] Computer Architecture, Electronics and Electronics Technology,
University of Cordoba, CU Rabanales, 14071 Cordoba, Spain

Abstract. Human body has an interesting potential to provide energy
to micro-electronic systems. There are several techniques that can harvest energy from human body and convert it in energy to be used by
electronic systems. Usually this energy cannot be used immediately and
needs to be conditioned. This chapter summarizes about current trends
of energy storage systems. Techniques for extracting energy from human
body, estimations and experimental results based on previous works are
discussed. The merge of all the above mentioned concepts, providing a
general idea to the reader about the state of the art in energy harvesting
from human bodies.

Keywords: Energy harvesting · Energy storage · Human body systems

1 Introduction

Based on techniques and analysis of recent research results, this chapter gives
a detailed overview of the different energy flows on human bodies and how to
scavenge energy from them. Several experimental results and estimations are
presented and discussed, providing an easy to grasp approach to this topic.
At the same time this chapter presents a sketchy approach to energy storage
systems. Also, a special section focused on energy harvesting and energy usage
on human body, can be read.

Several flows of energy can be found on the human body. Each flow is presented
in a separate section focusing on the particular scavenging technique. Following
an intuitively classification makes it for the reader easy to follow. This chapter
is specially recommended to people who are interested in an introduction to this
topic, people with a good level of knowledge on this topic and researchers. Readers
can find a lot of summarized information with helpful suggestions and representations.

2 Glossary

Following, the main concepts used in this chapter are explained in order to help
the reader in the comprenhension of this work.

A. Holzinger et al. (Eds.): Smart Health, LNCS 8700, pp. 125–159, 2015.
DOI: 10.1007/978-3-319-16226-3_6

ATP: Adenosine triphosphate is a nucleoside triphosphate used in cells as a coenzyme. It is called the molecular unit of currency of intracellular energy transfer.

ADP: Adenosine diphosphate is an organic compound used in the flow of energy to living cells.

DVB-T: Digital video broadcasting – terrestrial is the European-based consortium standard for the broadcast transmission of digital terrestrial television.

DSP: Digital signal processing is the mathematical manipulation of an information signal to modify or improve it in some way.

Exoskeletons: It is an external skeleton that supports and protects an animal's body. It is used in several purposes with humans.

Gravimetric energy density: Battery capacity in weight (Wh/Kg).

MEMS: Microelectromechanical system is the technology of very small devices. It merges at the nano-scale into nanoelectromechanical systems (NEMS).

mmHg: Unit used to measure the blood pressure. It is usually expressed in terms of the systolic pressure over diastolic pressure and is measured in millimeters of mercury.

Mole: It is an unit of measurement used in chemistry to express amounts of a chemical substance. It is defined as the amount of any substance that contains as many elementary entities as there are atoms in $12\,g$ of pure $carbon^{-12}$.

MPPT: It is a technique that grid connected inverters, solar battery chargers and similar devices use to get the maximum possible power from one or more photovoltaic devices, typically solar panels.

Peltier Element: It is an electronic device consisting of metal strips between which alternate strips of n-type and p-type semiconductors are connected. Passage of a current causes heat to be absorbed from one set of metallic strips and emitted from the other by the Peltier effect.

PVDF: Polyvinylidene fluoride (or difluoride) is a highly non-reactive and pure thermoplastic fluoropolymer. It is used in applications requiring the highest purity, strength and resistance to solvents, acid, bases and heat.

RF: Radio frequency is a rate of oscillation in the range of about 3 kHz to 300 GHz, which corresponds to the frequency of radio waves.

RFID: Radio frequency identification is the wireless non-contact use of radio-frequency electromagnetic fields to transfer data. The purposes of automatically identifying and tracking tags attached to objects, animals or people.

TEG: Thermoelectric generator is a device that converts heat directly into electrical energy, using a phenomenon called the Seebeck effect.

Thermopile: It is an electronic device that converts thermal energy into electrical energy. It is composed of several thermocouples connected usually in series.

Wi-Fi: Wireless Fidelity is a technology that allows an electronic device to exchange data or connect to the internet wirelessly using radio waves.

3 State of the Art

The human body comprises quite a few potential power sources. Figure 1 shows an overview of the different available power sources which can be found on human bodies. In the above mentioned figure, brackets show the total amount of generated power. The figure above gives the amount of harvestable energy by use of state of the art harvesting technology. The amount of power available for energy harvesting must be much less than the total amount to avoid negative physical effects on the user [3]. Also, an up to date overview of energy storage concepts available for storing energy in human body applications, is presented.

3.1 Chemical Energy

Food is the energy source of human bodies. It has nearly the same gravimetric energy density as gasoline and 100 times greater than batteries [1]. Human bodies store energy in fat cells distributed in various regions. Each gram of fat stores and equivalent of 37.7 kJ. An average person of 68 kg (150 lbs) with 15 % body fat stores an approximate equivalent of 384 mega joule [3]. Fat cannot

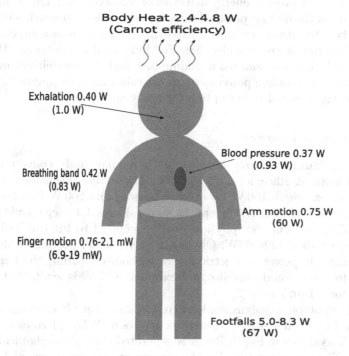

Fig. 1. Energy sources on human body [3]

be directly consumed by body cells. Fat molecules are long chains of glucose molecules (C6H12O6). These are cut into single molecules and injected into the bloodstream. Glucose is the main source of energy for the brain and a basis for smaller molecules like ATP. One glucose molecule stores an energy equivalent of 16 kilo joules. In the human body, it can be converted into two ATP molecules (C10H16N5O13P3) in anaerobic respiration and into 32 ATP molecules in aerobic respiration. The ATP is then usable for muscle contraction. Both enzymatic breakdown processes require two ATP molecules for processing. In aerobic respiration, a glucose molecule is much more profitable than in its anaerobic form [5]. The total quantity of ATP in the human body is about 0.2 mol, providing roughly the same amount of energy as a AA battery [8]. At any given time, the total amount of ATP and ADP (a similar type of energy molecule) is fairly constant and recycled continuously. Within 24 h, all cells in the human body consume about 100–150 mol of ATP which is around 50–75 kg [7]. A human will typically use up his or her body weight of ATP over the course of the day.

3.2   Energy from Liquid Fuels

Common liquid fuels are formic acid, ammonia or methanol. They show energy densities of 1.6, 5.2, and 5.6 kWh/Kg. Liquid hydrocarbon fuels have gravimetric energy densities around 13 kWh/Kg. Typical electric generators based on these fuels provide a conversion efficiency of 25 %. Electric energy generators powered from liquid fuel can provide energy densities of 3.25 kWh/Kg. This value is near the upper end of the desired personal power range. This high gravimetric energy density is the often stated reason for exploring combustion as a superior power source to batteries at small scales [58]. For individual applications, the entire power system has to be evaluated including fuel, fuel storage delivery and power conversion. When complete power systems are taken into the equation, batteries remain a strong personal power option for many applications.

3.3   Mechanical Energy

Power from Human Gait: Muscles in the human body convert food into mechanical work at efficiencies up to 25 %. The usable mechanical output of human bodies can reach 100 W for average persons and 200 W for elite athletes [1]. A 68 kg man walking at 3.5 mph (2 steps/s) uses 1.1 mega joule per hour or 324 W of power. The raw physical energy required to lift the heel through 5 cm during a walk is only 67W. Obviously only a small portion of these 67 W can be detoured to power an electric device without disturbing the human gait. According to Starner and Paradiso, a maximum of 13 W is available for energy harvesting for a 1 cm stroke [3].

Several prototyping designs implemented in shoes have been designed by the MIT Media Lab team leaded by Paradiso. It uses a PVDF piezo electric foil as a shoe insole as shown in Fig. 2. Power is generated through mechanical bending of the sole. Their prototype is able to generate an average power of 1.3 mW at

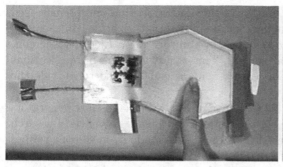

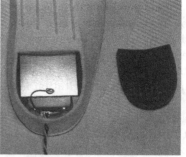

Fig. 2. Prototype PVDF bimorph generator

Fig. 3. Prototype piezoceramic composite on spring steel

an optimum load resistance of 100 kOhm per shoe. The user weighted 52 kg and was walking at 1 Hz per leg.

The team also produced another prototype that inserts a generator into the heel of a shoe. The generator was built of a flexible piezo-ceramic composite laminated on a curved piece of spring steel. The spring steel placed flat when the heel came down. The power generated by this design was measured as 60 mW peak and 1.8 mW on average [3, 20]. An improved design from Shenck and Paradiso uses two generators placed back-to-back (see Fig. 3). It generates power by the user's heel striking and flattening of the clamshell.

To this prototype, the material used is an EAP [35], which is similar to piezoelectrics. In that material, mechanical stress produces a voltage which one is stored in capacitors. The latest studies confirm that polymers have more strains and are more versatile than piezoelectric. This design generates 8.4 mW of power in average [3, 21].

Continuing with EAPs, these are similar to electrostatic generators, it is necessary to maintain a constant voltage to change on the electrodes. For a dielectric elastomer generator is necessary a relatively high voltage, between 1 and 6 KV for operation [36]. Those ones give us more energy per compression and, for extension, more power generation.

In this class, we have dielectric elastomers, these are basically electrostrictive elements. Usually they are made of silicone rubber or soft acrylics, trying always to have flexible materials, and they are extremely compliant. They have a similar performance as piezoelectric materials when they accumulate enough strain, but in these devices it is easy to drive a 50–100 % area strain. Like electrostatic mechanisms, these designs require a very high potential to be applied across the dielectric. Current is produced as the material is compressed and its capacitance changes, this is the same process that variable capacitor follows. However, they can produce higher voltage and are more versatile, thus they have excellent properties allowing much strain energy to be stored for power generation.

One important note is energy density of the generator, that can be increased by decreasing the capacitor spacing, increasing miniaturization, but energy density decreases when we reduce the capacitor surface area. Electrostatic generators also require also an initial voltage. This is not an issue in applications that use the generator to charge a battery, as this can be used to provide the necessary initial excitation level.

Pelrine, Kornbluh and others [24,37], have developed electrostatic generators around materials called dielectric elastomers for the Defense Advanced Research Projects Agency (DARPA). Dielectric elastomers are made from silicone rubber or soft acrylic. A displacement of 2–6 mm can drive these materials to 50–100 % area strain. This makes them ideal to be built into the elastic heel of a shoe as shown in Fig. 4. The prototype generated an energy output of 0.8 J per step for a heel compression of only 3 mm. The generated power was 800 mW per shoe at 2 Hz. For higher compressions up to 9 mm, up to 1 W of output power has been anticipated [19,24].

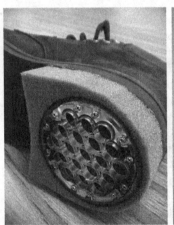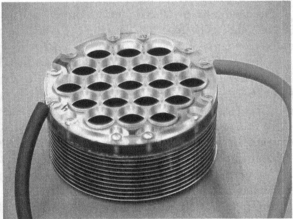

Fig. 4. Dielectric elastomers built into heel of a shoe [3]

3.4   Power from General Movement

Inertial Systems: These kind of systems generate power when moved cyclically. Despesse et al. [30] research analyses a structure for electrostatic transduction with high electrical damping. This electrostatic transduction is designed to operate with low frequencies, typically less than 100 Hz. The structure used, was an in-plane gap with a charge constrained cycle. In the proposed scenario, the electrostatic force is linearly proportional to the inertial mass displacement in the same way. This allows two forces to be balanced for all displacements of the inertial mass. If the electrical stiffness is close to mechanical stiffness is achieved a high electrical damping. Beeby et al. [31] explain how an 18 cm^2 1 cm volume device with a 0.104 kg inertial mass was electro discharge machined from tungsten and produced a scavenged power of $1052\,\mu W$ for a vibration amplitude of $90\,\mu m$ at $50\,Hz$. This represents a scavenged efficiency of $60\,\%$ with the losses being accounted for by charge/discharge losses and transduction losses. A similar geometry silicon micro structure of volume $81\,mm^2$ $0.4\,mm$ with a $2 \cdot 10^3 Kg$ inertial mass excited by a vibration amplitude of $95\,\mu m$ at $50\,Hz$ is predicted to produce a scavenged power of $70\,\mu W$. Pelrine et al. [19] presented a design of an electrostatic generator for linear movement as shown in Fig. 5.

There are other experiments using electrostatic generators that show how to use this technology on inertial systems. Meninger et al. [28] simulated an in-plane overlap varying electrostatic generator based on a comb-driven structure and generated $8\,\mu W$ from $2.5\,kHz$ input motion. The limit to operate on the electrostatic generator is the high voltage produced. An integrated circuit was used and limited to the voltage of $8\,V$ in this structure. It was necessary to charge and discharge the electrostatic generator at several points. In order to do this, Meninger et al. used several feedback algorithms in addition to a measurement technique to take threshold and to choose the specific points to charge and discharge.

Ma et al. [29] predict $1\,\mu W$ load for a $5\,\mu m$ displacement at $4.3\,kHz$. The inertial mass is $2107\,kg$ and the device is operated at resonance with a damping coefficient of $0.002\,kg\,s^1$. The floating gate is charged by electron tunneling and power is generated by a variable capacitor of which one plate is a moving gold proof mass and the other is the fixed floating gate.

Experiments at the ETH in Zrich showed a theoretical harvest of $200\,\mu W$ during normal walking using a mass of $1\,g$ [13]. Another study showed that the available power output from walking is over $0.5\,mW/cm$ for most body locations and over $10\,mW/cm$ when running. The ankle and knee locations showed an up to 20 times larger amount of available power [15].

Inertial microsystems can be attached at various positions on the human body. Positions exposed to higher accelerations will generate more power.

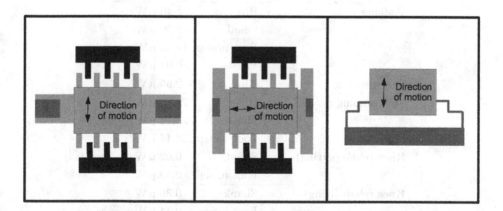

Fig. 5. Left: In-plane overlap varying type. Center: In-plane gap closing type. Right: Out-of plane gap closing type

The best mounting position is at the wrist. Todays self-winding wrist watches use a 2 g mass mounted off-center on a spindle. As the user walks around, the mass swings around the spindle and winds up the watch. Several electro-mechanical generators exist that fit into a watch [3]. The ETA Autoquartz Self-Winding Electric Watch generates 16 V at 6 mA in 50 ms pulses [11]. Another watch size generator is the Seiko AGS that creates 5 μW on average and 1 mW if shaken hard [12].

A study from 2010 build a 50 g mass on a piezo electric bender attached to an AC-DV converter electronics and tested it on various body positions. The measures of generated average power are shown in Table 1.

Electromagnetic Generators: Compared with electrostatic generators, electromagnetic generators (see Fig. 6) are heavier and more difficult to tailor and require rotary movements. But magnetic machines running at sufficient speed can provide much higher efficiencies.

Some motions of human body are rotary, though not fully 360°, and the speed of motions is cyclic and relatively slow. Other motions, such as heel strike, are distinctly linear requiring a linear machine or some mechanical converter to use a rotary machine. The best position to harvest power from cyclic movement on the human body is the wrist. The wrist moves faster than any other part of the human body. Power can be harvested whenever the user is walking.

Though this seems unpromising for magnetic machines, the rotation speed can be increased by using flywheel arrangements in rotary motions. For linear motions, a mechanical spring can give high bursts of speed by releasing stored energy. The machine speed is not limited by the 1 Hz walking as some have proposed [38]. Better than 90 % efficiency is routinely obtained in good machines

Table 1. Average generated power at different body positions [26]

Activity	Position	Average power
Walking	Hip	1.40 μW
	Shank	10.30 μW
	Foot instep	11.52 μW
	Wrist	0.04 μW
Slow running	Hip	9.65 μW
Fast running	Hip	22.89 μW
	Shank	28.74 μW
	Foot instep	28.44 μW
Knee rehab (sitting)	Shank	0.02 μW
	Foot instep	0.39 μW
Knee rehab (lying)	Shank	0.36 μW
	Foot instep	0.44 μW
Arm swinging	Wrist	3.08 μW
Arm trembling simulation	Wrist	0.62 μW

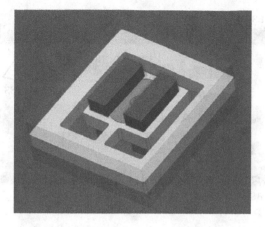

Fig. 6. A silicon electromagnetic generator [39]

with sufficiently high speed. An important disadvantage of magnetic methods is that the material is relatively heavy compared to other methods. Several problems exist with such energy systems. They tend to be big and heavy. Their power output is proportional to the scale of coils or length of stroke. Rotary magnetic power generators have a long tradition in the history of electrical generators. A wide variety of spring/mass configurations can be used with various types of material that are well suited and proven in cyclically stressed applications. Comparatively high output current levels are achievable at the expense of low voltages. These systems, however, are quite difficult to build because the number of turns on planar coils are limited and because the magnet/coil velocity is restricted.

Linear Motors: This kind of design is able to convert linear motion directly into electrical energy. A linear motor consists of sets of coils and magnets arranged on a line [40]. Induction is based on Faradays law about the variation in magnetic flux. When the magnetic flux changes, a current is induced in the inductor. Traditionally, conductors are shaped like a coil. An output current is generated when either the relative movement of the magnet and coil, or when the magnetic field changes.

Low transduction efficiency yet high power output due to cumbersome mounting and bulk scale has been described in many applications [41]. Their power generation ability is characterized by direct proportion to the scale of coils or length of stroke. However, new designs outperform their predecessors several times.

In a scenario with permanent magnet generators, it is clear that they are most efficient at higher speeds and in a rotary arrangement, like wrist movements. Kulah and Najafi [42] focused on low frequency resonant structures but only measured 4 nW from a millimeter-scale mock-up with an efficiency less than 2 %. For an excitation level provided, for example by finger typing, a device can generate 0.16 μW like Huang et al. have demonstrated [43]. On a larger scale,

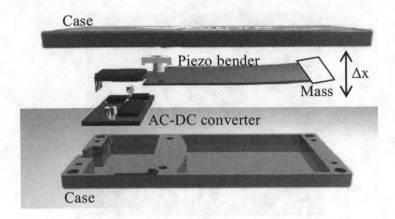

Fig. 7. PEH20W piezo electric generator from Midé Technologies [26]

Amirtharajah et al. [44] described a moving coil electromagnetic generator contained in a low-power DSP application. The resonant frequency of the generator was 94 Hz, but the model of its performance predicted that an average of 400 μW could be generated from a 2 cm movement at 2 Hz in human-powered applications.

Magnetostrictive Materials: These kind of systems, are often used in combination with piezoelectric generators (see Figs. 7, 8, and 9). These materials possess suitable characteristics to be used on human energy scavenging. They deform when placed in a magnetic field and conversely if strained can induce changes in a magnetic field (see Fig. 10). Magnetostrictive materials can be used independently but usually have been employed in piezoelectric-magnetostrictive composites. Staley and Flatau generated a maximum DC output voltage of less than 0.35 V with Terfeno-D. Piezoelectric-magnetostrictive composites were originally intended for use in magnetic field sensors [55].

Ferromagnetic Materials: Exhibit only low energy conversion. As a result, Metglas 2605SC [56] outperforms its predecessors, with a maximum output power and power density of 200 μW/cm^3 and 900 μW/cm^3, respectively, in low frequency. Huang et al. [43] report that the frequency of the rotary resonance depends upon the spring constant of the springs that control the motion of the disc and the size of the eccentric proof mass used to achieve rotary motion. This device achieved 1.2 mW of power at 30 Hz at 5 ms^2 and claims were made that more than 10 mW could be harvested from a volume of 1 cm^3 at 5 m s^2.

Power from Respiration: Breath pressure is 2 % above atmospheric pressure. The power consumption of human breathing ranges from 0.1 to 40 W. Because of physiological effects, only exhalation can be used as an energy source. The maximum available power from exhalation is 1.0 W. Use of an aircraft-style pressure mask can increase available power 2.5 times, but also puts the user under

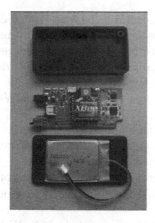

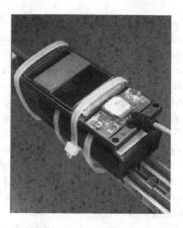

Fig. 8. WAGYRO energy harvesting device [26]

Fig. 9. WAGYRO with mounted PEH20W [26]

significant stress. These devices are already in use but combinations of turbine and generator only achieve a total efficiency of 40 % [3].

Another approach to harvest energy from breathing applies a tight band around the chest of the user. Empirical measurements show a 2.5 cm change in chest circumference (5 cm for heavy breathing). Given an average breathing rate of 10/s and an ambitious 100 N force over 5 cm distance calculates as 0.83 W. Due to friction losses, the effectively harvested power reduces to less than 0.42 W [3].

Power from Blood Pressure: Typical physical measures of human blood flow show a blood pressure of 100 mm Hg, a resting heart rate of 60 beats per minute and a heart stroke volume of 70 ml passing through the aorta at every heart beat. The power generated from blood stream is 0.93 W. Harvesting only 2 % of this power would be enough to run a microprocessor [3].

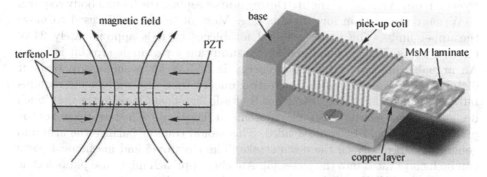

Fig. 10. Magnetostrictive effect-based vibration harvester [10]

An out-of-plane gap closing electrostatic generator type was depicted by Miyazaki [32], this kind of generators is very interesting for blood pressure energy scavenging systems. Miyazaki presented an out-of-plane cantilever based generator with a base capacitance of 1 nF and a variable capacitance in the range of 30 and 350 pF. The device resonated at 45 Hz with a Q factor of 30. The device was tested on a wall with a 1 μm displacement up to 100 Hz. 120 nW was harvested for the wall acceleration of $0.08\,ms^2$.

Tashiro et al. [33] described a honeycomb structure made up by folding a strip of a polyester film with aluminium evaporated on one surface. This structure has a variable capacitor was suspended between acrylic boards using 12 springs and an inertial mass attached to one of the acrylic boards. The spring constant of the resonator was $1100\,Nm^{-1}$ with a total mass of 0.78 Kg resulting in a resonant frequency of 6 Hz.

Experiments performed by Tashiro [34] report the generation of 58 μW from the simulated heart movements of a goat after an initial charging voltage of 24 V. They used a similar structure honeycomb generator which had an initial capacitance of 32 nF varying to 200 nF and was resonant at 4.76 Hz. In this study the inertial mass was 1.2 kg and the resonator spring constant was $570\,Nm^1$. Newer designs can harvest up to $4.15\,\mu W/cm^3$ at 1.5 Hz and tens of micro watts per cubic centimeter of blood are predicted [10].

Power from Finger Press: Though not directly connected to the human body, keyboards can be used to generate power from key presses, e.g., a user could wear a device that shows a keyboard for interaction. The keyboard could also be used for energy harvesting. A design from Paradiso and Feldmeier uses a piezoelectric element with resonantly-matched transformer and electronics that generates 0.5 mJ at 3 V for each 15 N push. This amount of energy allows to transmit a digital RF code after a single push [14]. The german company EnOcean sells a magnetic energy converter called ECO 200 for linear movements. The ECO 200 is less than 30207 mm in size and outputs 120–210 μJ at 2 V for each finger press at <3.9 N in 1.2 mm [23].

Power from Arm Movement: During housekeeping, the human body requires 35 W more power than for still standing. Most of this power is used to move the upper limbs. The power required for biceps curls is approximately 24 W for both arms. The maximum power consumption for a single arm lift is 30 W. An arguable amount of harvested energy is 0.75 W for a single arm without disturbing the user too much. Harvesting energy from arm movements requires bulky and uncomfortable exoskeletons that add significant mass to the user. Such designs may use jackets with pulley systems in the elbows. The take-up reel of the pulley system could be spring-loaded. This would counter balance the arm and generate energy only on the down stroke. The electronic and mechanical parts can be incorporated into the jacket [3]. Another approach might use piezoelectric polymers like PVDF or dielectric elastomers because they do not require complex mechanical parts like reels. If piezoelectric foils are stretched along their most sensitive axis, their maximum extension is limited to 1 %–2 %. This makes them

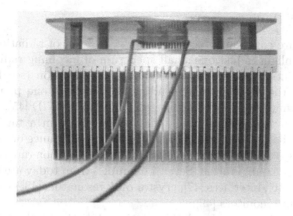

Fig. 11. TEG with attached heat sink

incompatible to human movements. Dielectric elastomers on the other hand are soft and rubbery materials providing 50 %–100 % of area strain. The elastomers are placed between capacitor plates. When the plates of a charged capacitor are stretched, the voltage increases as energy is put into the electrical field. Power scales with the square of capacitor voltage. Typical operating voltages for elastomers are 1–6 kV. A full compression/expansion cycle can produce more than 1 J of energy [3,19].

3.5   Thermal Energy

The human body produces waste heat in the range from 81 W (sleeping) up to 1630 W (sprinting). Table 2 shows the individual energy consumption of a typical human in various situations. During sitting, a mere of 116 W is available [3].

Carnot efficiency limits the amount of power that can be harvested. Harvesting thermal energy always requires a temperature difference. The bigger the difference the more energy can be harvested. Assuming normal body temperature of 37 °C, the Carnot efficiency is 5.5 % for 20 °C (difference of 17 °K) and 3.2 % for 27 °C (difference of 10 °K) room temperature. Using a Carnot heat engine to model the recoverable energy yields 3.7–6.4 W of power. Carnot efficiency defines a theoretical upper limit to the efficiency of every thermoelectric generator. Todays standard thermo piles provide 0.2 %–0.8 % for temperature differences of 5–20 °K [17]. A design of a micro machined thermopile from 2007 shows output voltage of 13 mV/K/cm^2. Simulations showed an output power around 1.5 μW at 1 V for a watch sized TEG placed on a human body. For a temperature difference of 10 °K, an output voltage of 130 mV was measured [18]. Another kind of design uses the commercially available Peltier element PKE 128 A 1030 with an attached heat sink as shown in Fig. 11. The TEG setup generated 2.05 mW at 334 mV for 6.71 °K temperature difference and 4.97 mW at 530 mV for 11.36 °K [23].

3.6 Incoming Radiation

Human bodies are constantly receiving energy in form of radiation of different wavelengths. Sunlight is just one small spectrum of incoming radiation. One of the available solutions uses a wireless energy transmission (see Fig. 12). This technique offers the possibility for sending energy from one point to another one. A well known technology which uses this design is RFID [45], which derives their energy inductively, capacitively, or radiatively from a tag reader. Most RFID chips talk back to the reader changing their impedance or reflection coefficient. These chips are low power devices on the consumption range of $1–100\,\mu W$, depending of their configuration. Several examples from today are keyless access systems, sensors [46], interfaces [47], crystal bulk resonators [48] or new proposals like blood pressure monitors [49].

It is also possible to use the above mentioned method for wireless transmission for systems based on IEEE 802.15.4. To scavenge enough energy a dipole antenna and an impedance are required on the receiver side. The received signal is rectified and mixed down to a lower frequency.

Signals in a frequency range between 500 MHz and 10 GHz from different electromagnetic sources have been led in practice and failed to produce any useful results, because the signal strength of DVB-T, WiFi or mobile network is very high and disturb other smaller signals for that hereby energy harvesting could operate. A different situation exists when a transmission signal whose energy is to be used for the comparison supply of an embedded system, is itself produced. One example is a wireless system from PowerCast company. The wireless sensor

Table 2. Human energy consumption [3]

Activity	Power (W)
Sleeping	81
Lying quietly	93
Sitting	116
Standing at ease	128
Conversation	128
Eating meal	128
Strolling	163
Driving a car	163
Playing a violin or piano	163
Housekeeping	175
Carpentry	268
Swimming	582
Mountain climbing	698
Long distance run	1048
Sprinting	1630

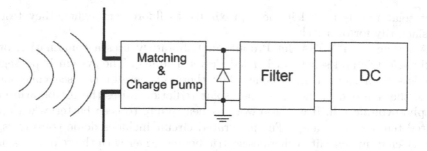

Fig. 12. A proposal of RF energy harvesting schema

nodes work at 915 MHz frequency and they are put to the power harvester boards that work with a P2110 receiver, which supplies them with energy. The chip constitutes P2110 received RF energy into a DC voltage, which is stored in a capacitor on the board, so that the supply of the sensor node is made possible [59]. The required energy is self-generated, but this approach actually does not comply with the principle of energy harvesting. The P2110 Receiver converts signals in 850–950 MHz at a DC voltage.

On the other hand, the use of solar cells could be another possibility on radiation systems. This system involves several factors such as chemistry of the batteries, power management features of the system and the own characteristics from solar cells. Solar energy harvesting through photo-voltaic conversion technique provides up to $15 \, \mathrm{mW/cm^3}$ of power [50]. Solar cells make use of photons, which come from sunlight radiations and hit the solar panel to be absorbed by semi conducting materials, such as silicon. Electrons are energized and flow through the material to produce electricity. Due to the special composition of solar cells, the electrons are only allowed to move in a single direction. This energy includes the electromagnetic spectrum between infrared and ultraviolet light. Indoor power density typically ranges from $100 \, \mathrm{\mu W/cm^2}$ to $1000 \, \mathrm{\mu W/cm^2}$, and outdoors can be up to $100 \, \mathrm{mW/cm^2}$. Solar cells efficiency can be up to more than 30 % [51]. Power densities are similar for indoor solar cells, around $0.017 \, \mathrm{mW/cm^2}$, and batteries. On the other hand, outdoor solar cells provide around $1.42 \, \mathrm{mW/cm^2}$, this is more than 80 times more power [52].

There is a very interesting case that Hande et al. [53] have presented. Indoor application for solar cells using fluorescent lights. This indoor light harvesting is aimed to power wireless sensor networks for biomedical sensing applications. A testbed using indoor lighting was presented for hospital use employing mono-crystalline solar panels. Mono-crystalline solar cells with typical efficiencies of less than 3 % under indoor lighting conditions have a power density between 0.5 and $1 \, \mathrm{mW/cm^2}$, under light conditions of $1–5 \, \mathrm{W/m^2}$, which still surpasses other energy scavenger devices. Hande et al. employed commercial mono-crystalline solar panels placed at 1 cm distance from overhead 34 W fluorescent lights. Two crossbow MICAz router nodes operating at a 50 % duty cycle were powered by eight solar panels placed in close proximity to fluorescent lights, they tested satisfactorily for over 24 h.

A design from NASA Jet Propulsion Laboratory uses a combination of a thermo-electric and solar panel called Power Tile [54]. The system is packaged in a less than 2 mm thick volume. The thermo-generator can scavenge some of the thermal energy incurred when solar radiation raises the temperature on the photovoltaic cell. It can also work as heat pump to keep batteries within a desired temperature range. The integrated circuit includes dc-dc converters, a battery-charging circuit, a thermo-electric heater driver with the required sense, and control circuits. In full sunlight, the photo voltaic cell produces 125 mA at 2.1 V and the thermo-generator generates 20 mA at 0.8 V, when a temperature difference of 35 °C is present.

3.7   Conversion

Energy harvesting on the human body is a tough job. The different generator designs described in the previous chapter deliver minimal quantities of energy. The energy flows are neither constant nor can they be directly consumed by micro controllers. Some generators provide voltages of just a few hundred milli-volts while others output several kilovolts in short spikes. Efficient voltage converters and energy storages are required to operate sensors, micro controllers and transmitters.

DC/DC Step-Up Converters: A step-up (boost) converter basically consists of an inductor, a diode and a switch as shown in Fig. 13. When the switch is activated, the power supply causes an increasing current through the inductor. When the switch is deactivated, the current through the inductor cannot stop immediately because of its established magnetic field. The energy in the magnetic field causes the current to continue and thus increasing the voltage at the diode. Once the voltage at the diode is higher than $U_{Flow} + U_{Load}$ then the current will flow through the diode and increase U_{Load} too. If the switch is alternating at high frequency, U_{Load} will see a nearly constant voltage that is flattened by the capacitor and is higher than U_{Supply}. In practical circuits, the switch is controlled by a feedback network that constantly compares U_{Load} to a configured voltage reference and adapts on and off time of the switch automatically [72].

Commercial step-up converters start at input voltages of 0.7 V due to the minimum threshold value of their switching transistors. This is too high for the output of TEGs which output typically less than 300 mV for temperature differences less than 10 K.

For input voltages lower than 0.7 V a charge pump (see Fig. 15) with special low-threshold transistors has to be used. Loreto Mateu et al. [27] presented a design especially for TEGs as shown in Fig. 10. His charge pump started switching at 150 mV and provided an output of 3.7 V at an efficiency of 63 %–40 % [22]. Measures of input voltage and current are shown in Table 3.

A more advanced step–up DC–DC converter has been presented by Pollack, Mateu and Spies provides up to 70 % efficiency in the range of 200–500 mV for

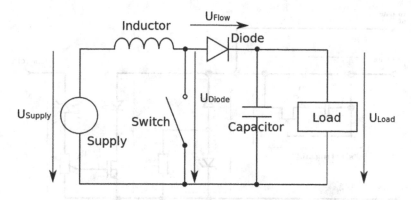

Fig. 13. Simplified circuit of a boost converter [72]

Table 3. Input voltage and charge pump current consumption [22]

V_N	300 mV	250 mV	200 mV	150 mV	130 mV
I_N	0.35 mA	1.5 mA	3.5 mA	2.6 mA	6.4 mA

a minimum startup at 70 mV. Schematics of this boost converter are shown in Figs. 14 and 16. The converter can turn a 300–500 mV input to 2 V output at an efficiency greater than 70 % [27].

DC/DC Step-Down Converters: A Step-Down (Buck) converter converts an input voltage into a lower output voltage. In contrast to a linear regulator, a Buck converter is more efficient and the output current can be higher than the input current. In an idealized converter, all of its components are considered to be perfect. Especially the switch, the inductor and the diode have zero voltage drop when on and no current when off.

A simplified circuit of a Buck converter is shown in Fig. 17. At start, when the switch is off, no current flows through the circuit. When the switch is turned on, current cannot start immediately because the inductor needs time to build up its magnetic field. So the inductor causes a voltage drop UInductor. This voltage drop will constantly decrease while the magnetic field builds up until only the internal resistance of the inductor is limiting the current. As the voltage drop decreases, U_{Load} will increase. When the switch is turned off before the inductor has completely build up its field, then U_{Load} will stay lower than U_{Supply}. In practical circuits, the switch is controlled by a feedback network that constantly compares U_{Load} to a configured voltage reference and adapts on and off time of the switch automatically.

In the area of human body applications step-down converters are mostly used to convert the high output voltages of piezoelectric foils and dielectric elastomers which can provide several kilovolts, down to a value that is suitable to run electronics in the range of 1.8 V–5 V.

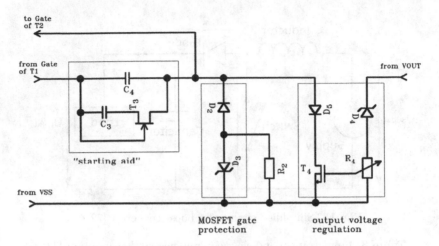

Fig. 14. Simplified schematic of boost converter [27]

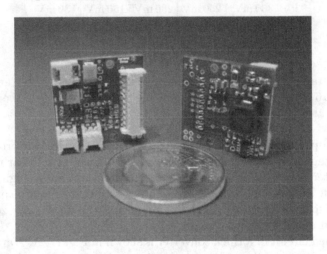

Fig. 15. DC-DC charge pump

A design from Ottman, Hofmann and Lesieutre in 2002 uses a step-down converter build up around an NE555 timer device to convert the output of a piezoelectric generator down to 3.3 V to charge a battery. Through of a converter, the amount of energy stored in the battery increased by 325 % compared to connecting the battery directly to the rectified output of the generator. Their control circuit theoretically consumed 5.74 mW. Experiments showed a conversion efficiency of 60–70 % for input voltages in the range of 35–70 V [74].

Maximum Power Point Circuits: The previous chapter provided a variety of energy harvesting generators for using it on the human body. Each generator can act as a power supply for an application circuit. For a given power supply, only an

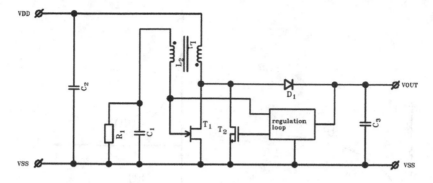

Fig. 16. Regulation loop circuit of boost converter [27]

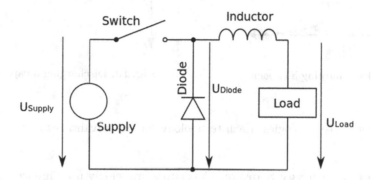

Fig. 17. Simplified step-down converter

optimal matched load resistance will extract the maximum available power. This resistance varies for many energy harvesting generators when the energy flow of its energy source (amplitude/ frequency of vibrations, temperature difference) changes. A maximum power point tracking circuit can adapt its input resistance dynamically to the actual internal resistance of the power supply to always operate in the optimum setting. Mateu, Pollack and Spies provided the design of a Maximum Power Point Tracker (MPPT) circuit that uses only for low power operational amplifiers. The circuit automatically adapts its duty cycle to achieve the MPP whenever the input voltage increases or decreases. Due to their tracking nature, MPPTs cannot stay at the ideal maximum power point. Simulations show that this MPPT will not deviate more than 5 % of the theoretical maximum power point of a selected, state of the art TEG [28].

3.8   Energy Storage

The amount of harvestable power shows great variation over time for all types of power harvesting. If an electronic device should be powered constantly, the harvested energy must be stored somewhere. This chapter lists various avadilable

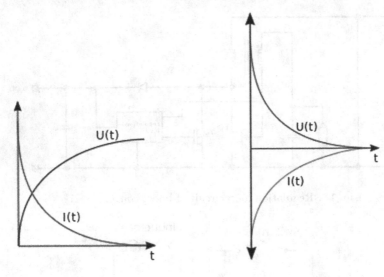

Fig. 18. Charging a capacitor   **Fig. 19.** Discharging a capacitor

energy storage technologies. Each technology has its advantages and disadvantages.

Capacitors as Energy Storage: Capacitors are widely used in electronics to stabilize supply voltages directly at each chip. But they can also be used to stabilize the fluctuating output of harvesting generators. The main unit for capacitors is Capacitance, C, which is given in Farad (F). 1 F = 1 As/V. Energy is stored in the electric field between two plates. When a capacitor is charged at a constant voltage, the charge current starts like a shortcut with the maximum current. While the electric field is built up, the voltage at the capacitor poles increases. When this voltage increases, automatically decreases the current charge exponentially as shown in Fig. 18. When the power supply is disconnected and a load resistance is connected, discharging starts at high negative current. While the electric field diminishes, voltage at the capacitor poles reduces exponentially as shown in Fig. 19.

The classical capacitor uses two parallel plates in a fixed distance. The space between the plates is filled with air or special material. The capacity of a classical capacitor is calculated as shown in Eq. (1). The effective electrode surface is denoted by A, d is the thickness of the dielectric. ε_0 is the dielectric constant of the vacuum with $8.85 \cdot 10^{12}$ As/Vm. Usually, it is necessary as an indication of the relative dielectric constant (ϵ_r), which is referred to as permittivity, $\epsilon = \epsilon_0 \cdot \epsilon_r$. This value is used to indicate the increment of dielectric constant when another dielectric, different to air, is used.

$$C = \varepsilon_0 \cdot \varepsilon_r \cdot \frac{A}{d} \quad \textit{Capacity of classic Capacitor} \tag{1}$$

Capacitors and elastic elements have high power densities because they can release all their stored energy in a short time, but these devices do not have a good storage capabilities on a mass basis. Chang et al. [61] reported that the energy density of hybrid capacitors was in the range from 0.074 to 0.233 J/g and the power density was in the range from 19 to 259 W/g. Both energy density and power density increased when increasing the maximum operational voltage. But exceeding the maximum allowed operating voltage will decrease the lifetime dramatically. Hoffman et al. analyzed hybrid capacitors response to over voltages. Lifetime of the tested supercharge capacitors reduced from 5023 days at 2 V to 13 days at 2.3 V, at constant temperature [60].

Li-Ion Capacitors: A lithium-ion capacitor (LIC) is a hybrid type of capacitor. Activated carbon is used as a cathode. The anode of the LIC consists of carbon material which is pre-doped with lithium ion. This pre-doping process lowers the potential of the anode and allows a high output voltage. The positive electrode (cathode) employs activated carbon material in which charges are stored in an electric double layer which is developed at the interface between the carbon and the electrolyte similar to electric double-layer capacitors (EDLC). The pre-doping process of the anode lowers the anode potential and results in a high cell output voltage. Typically, output voltages for LICs are in the range of 3.8–4.0 V. As a consequence, LICs have a higher energy density than EDLC. Furthermore, the capacity of the anode is several orders of magnitude larger than the capacity of the cathode. As a result, the change of the anode potential during charge and discharge is much smaller than the change in the cathode potential. The electrolyte used in an LIC is a lithium-ion salt solution. In order to avoid direct electrical contact between anode and cathode, a separator material is used.

Lithium-ion capacitors have a higher power density as compared to batteries, and LICs are safer in use than lithium ion batteries, in which thermal runaway reactions may occur. Compared to the electric double-layer capacitor (EDLC), the LIC has a higher output voltage. They have similar power densities, but energy density of an LIC is much higher.

Figure 20 shows that the lithium-ion capacitor combines the high energy of lithium-ion batteries with the high power density of EDLCs [70, 71]. They provide a superb cycle life compared to other technologies, but lifetime highly depends on operating voltage [65]. Lithium-ion capacitors possess very high power densities of over 3,000 Wh/kg (see Fig. 20). The charging efficiency reaches more than 95 %. Short charging times of below 1 min are attainable. Charging an LIC is simple, because no full-charge detection is needed thus avoiding the danger of overcharging. When used in conjunction with rechargeable batteries, in some applications the LIC can supply energy for a short time, reducing battery cycling duty and extending life. LIC experience almost no degradation when completely discharged [65].

Batteries as Energy Storage: Batteries are an electrochemical energy storage that consist of one or more voltaic cells. Each cell consists of two half-cells that

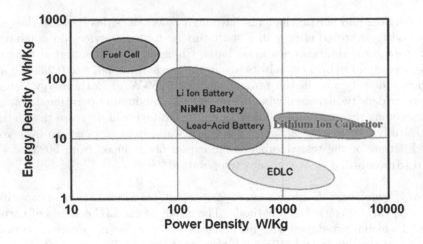

Fig. 20. Power density VS energy density for different storage technologies

are connected in series by a conductive electrolyte. Conductivity of the electrolite is given by containing anions (negatively charged ions) and cations (positive charged ions). One half-cell contains the electrode that attracts anions and the electrode in the other half-cell attracts cations. The battery is powered by a redox-reaction. Cathions are reduced at the cathode (electrons are added) and anions are oxidized (electrons are removed) at the anode [63].

A cell provides a certain voltage that is typical for the active chemical elements in it. Batteries are divided into primary and secondary cells. Most primary cells cannot be recharged (except Alkali-Mangan cells). Secondary cells can be recharged for different times. Typical examples of secondary cells are Nickel-Cadmium (NiCd), Lead-Acid, Nickel-Metal Hydride, Nickel-Zinn (NiZn), Silver-Oxide (AgZn) and Lithium-Ion (LiIon).

Nickel Metal Hydride (NiMH) Batteries: Nickel-metal-hydride batteries are related to sealed nickel-cadmium batteries and only differ from them in that instead of cadmium, hydrogen is used as the active element at a hydrogen-absorbing negative electrode (anode). This electrode is made from a metal hydride usually alloys of Lanthanum and rare earths that serve as a solid source of reduced hydrogen that can be oxidized to form protons. The electrolyte is alkaline potassium hydroxide. Cell voltage is 1.2 V. The low self-discharge nickel-metal hydride battery (LSD NiMH) was introduced in November 2005. These batteries were developed by Sanyo, who called them "eneloop". Subsequently, other manufacturers also offered LSD NiMH.

Low Self-discharge (LSD) NiMH Batteries: This kind of battery reduces self-discharge and, therefore lengthens shelf life compared to normal NiMH batteries. By using an improved electrode separator and improved positive electrode the batteries retain 70–85 % of their charged capacity after one year when stored at room temperature. Standard NiMH batteries may lose half their charge in the same time period (see Fig. 21) [64]. Retention of charge depends a lot on the battery's impedance or internal resistance and on the size of the battery. High quality separators are very important for battery performance. Thick separators take up space and reduce capacity, while providing a low-tech way of reducing self discharge, while thin separators tend to raise the self discharge rate. Some batteries may have overcome this obstacle with more precise manufacturing techniques and by using a more advanced sulfonated polyolefin separator [64]. Specifications for the self discharge rate are not always clear or widely published, and virtually any LSD may claim to maintain some level of charge after 12 months. A non-LSD battery typically self discharges at a rate of about 20 % within the first 24 h, then from 1 %–4 % per day thereafter. In devices not accurately calibrated to closely predict battery level, run-times for LSD NiMH batteries can be as well or even better than normal cells with higher rated capacity, because the slightly higher operating voltage doesn't trip a device's under-voltage shut off circuit [66, 67]. Figure 21 reveals exemplary different discharge curves with invariant cell potential and, Fig. 22 sloped cell potential. LSD NiMH batteries were introduced in November 2005 by Sanyo [64].

Rechargeable Lithium Batteries: Lithium is the lightest of metals and it floats on water. It also has the greatest electrochemical potential which makes it one of the most reactive of metals. These properties give Lithium the potential to achieve very high energy and power densities in high power battery applications such as automotive and standby power.

Many variations of the basic Lithium chemistry have been developed to optimize the cells for specific applications or perhaps in some cases to get around the patents on the original technology. Lithium metal reacts violently with water and can ignite into flame. Early commercial cells with metallic lithium cathodes were considered unsafe in certain circumstances. However, modern cells don't use

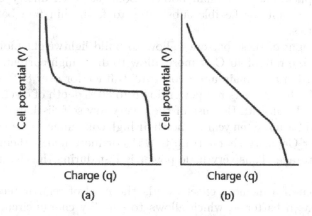

Fig. 21. Discharge characteristics LSD VS Standard NiMH batteries [64]

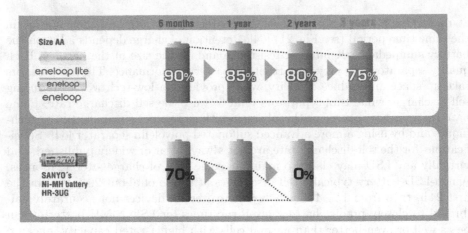

Fig. 22. Discharge characteristics LSD vs. Standard NiMH batteries [64]

free Lithium but instead the Lithium is combined with other elements into more benign compounds which do not react with water. The typical Lithium-ion cells use Carbon for their anode and Lithium Cobalt dioxide or a Lithium Manganese compound as the cathode. The electrolyte is usually based on a Lithium salt in an organic solvent. Lithium batteries have now taken their place as the rechargeable battery of choice for portable consumer electronics equipment. Though they were expensive when introduced, volume production has brought the prices down.

The high cell voltage of 3.6 V allows the use fewer cells to supply electronics. Thus reducing the amount of associated connections and electronics. One Lithium cell can replace three NiMH cells which have a cell voltage of only 1.2 V. The lack of liquid electrolyte means that Li-Ion batteries are immune from leaking. Their energy density is about 4 times greater than Lead acid.

The availability of extra small Li-Ion batteries make them ideally suited for mobile applications on human bodies. Solid state chemistry can even be printed on to ceramic or flexible substrates to form thin film batteries with unique properties.

The low weight of these batteries allow to build lightweight mobile applications. A discharge rate of 40°C or more allow to drive high currents of accumulated energy.Li-Ion cells maintain a constant voltage for over 80 % of their discharge curve. It thus delivers full power down to 80 % depth of discharge (DOD) versus 50 % for Lead acid. Because of their very low self discharge rate, charge can be retained for up to ten years. And their high coulombic efficiency (Capacity discharged over Capacity charged) up to 95 % or more makes them a very efficient energy storage. Thus very little power is lost during the charge/discharge cycles.

The absence of a memory effect avoids the need of regular reconditioning, as do nickel based batteries, which allows to simplify charge circuits. As these batteries tolerate microcycles, they can be charged with very low currents from energy harvesters over a long period of time. A long cycle life possible. The cycle life can be extended significantly by using protective circuits to limit the permissible DOD of the battery.

This mitigates against the high initial costs of the battery.

They are available in a wide range of cell constructions with capacities from less than 500 mAh–1000 Ah from a large number (over 100) of suppliers worldwide.

Stability of the chemicals has been a concern in the past. Because Lithium is more chemically reactive special safety precautions are needed to prevent physical or electrical abuse and to maintain the cell within its design operating limits. Lithium polymer cells with a solid electrolyte overcome some of these problems. Though stricter regulations on shipping methods exists than for other cell chemistries.

Some of the negative aspects of Li-Ion batteries are:

- Degrades at high temperatures.
- Capacity loss or thermal runaway when overcharged.
- Degradation when discharged below 2 V.
- Venting and possible thermal runaway when crushed.
- Need for protective circuitry.

Measurement of the state of charge of the cell is more complex than for most common cell chemistries. The state of charge is normally extrapolated from a simple measurement of the cell voltage, but the flat discharge characteristic of lithium cells, that is so desirable for applications, renders it unsuitable as a measure of the state of charge and other more costly techniques such as coulomb counting have to be employed.

Although Lithium cell technology has been used in low power applications for some time now, there is still not a lot of field data available about long term performance in high power applications. Reliability predictions based on accelerated life testing show that the cycle life matches or exceeds that of the most common technologies currently in use [68]. These drawbacks are far outweighed by the advantages of Lithium cells and several variations of Li-Ion batteries have been developed which overcome some of them.

Charging Lithium Batteries: Lithium batteries should be charged regularly. The cell voltage is typically 4.2 V. A battery lasts longer with partial charges rather than full charges. Charging to 4.1 V increases the lifecycle but reduces the effective cell capacity by about 10 % [69]. These kind of batteries can not tolerate overcharging and hence should not be trickle charged.

Charging method (Constant Current - Constant Voltage): Fast chargers typically operate during the constant current charging phase only when the charging current is at a maximum. They switch off at the point when the constant voltage, reducing current phase starts. At this point the battery will only be charged to about 70 % of its capacity.

Lithium's unique properties have been used as a basis of numerous battery chemistries both for primary and secondary cells. Using nano - electrode materials provides a bigger active surface area and hence a higher current carrying capacity. This technology allows current rates of 10 °C or more making the cells even suitable for hybrid electric vehicles (HEV) applications.

Lithium-Ion: Lithium-ion batteries were designed to overcome the safety problems associated with the highly reactive properties of Lithium metal. The essential feature of the Lithium ion battery is that at no stage in the charge-discharge cycle should there be any Lithium metal present. Rather, Lithium ions are intercalated into the positive electrode in the discharged state and into the negative electrode in the charged state and move from one to the other across the electrolyte.

Lithium-ion batteries therefore operate based on what is sometimes called the "rocking chair" or "swing" effect. This involves the transfer of Lithium ions back and forth between the two electrodes. The anode of a Lithium-ion battery is composed of Lithium, dissolved as ions, into a carbon or in some cases metallic Lithium. The cathode material is made up from Lithium liberating compounds, typically the three electro-active oxide materials, Lithium Cobalt-oxide $LiCoO2$, Lithium Manganese-oxide $LiMn2 O4$ and Lithium Nickel-oxide $LiNiO2$. Lithium salt constitutes the electrolyte.

The origin of the cell voltage is then the difference in free energy between $Li +$ ions in the crystal structures of the two electrode materials. Lithium-ion cells have no memory effect and have long life-cycles and excellent discharge performance. For safety reasons, charge control circuitry is required for virtually all Lithium-ion applications.

Lithium-ion technology uses a liquid or gel type electrolyte. This cell chemistry and construction permits very thin separators between the electrodes which can consequently be made with very high surface areas. This in turn enables the cells to handle very high current rates making them ideal for use in high power applications. Some early cells used flammable active ingredients which required substantial secondary packaging to safely contain these potentially hazardous chemicals. This additional packaging not only increased the weight and cost, but it also limited the size flexibility. Modern cell chemistries and additives have essentially eliminated these problems.

Lithium-Ion Polymer: Lithium-ion polymer batteries use liquid Lithium-ion electrochemistry in a matrix of ion conductive polymers that eliminate free electrolytes within the cell. The electrolyte thus plasticises the polymer, producing a solid electrolyte that is safe and leak resistant. Lithium polymer cells are often called Solid State cells [69].

Because there's no liquid, the solid polymer cell does not require the heavy protective cases of conventional batteries. The cells can be formed into flat sheets or prismatic/rectangular packages or they can be made in odd shapes to fit whatever space is available. As a result, manufacturing is simplified and batteries can be packaged in a foil. This provides added cost and weight benefits and design flexibility. Additionally, the absence of free liquid makes Lithium-ion polymer batteries more stable and less vulnerable to problems caused by overcharge, damage or abuse. Solid electrolyte cells have long storage lives, but low discharge rates.

There are some limitations on the cell construction imposed by the thicker solid electrolyte separator which limits the effective surface area of the electrodes and hence the current carrying capacity of the cell, but at the same time the added volume of electrolyte provides increased energy storage. This makes them ideal for use in high-capacity low-power applications [69].

Despite of the above comments, there are some manufacturers who make cells designated as Lithium polymer which actually contain a liquid or a gel. Such cells are more prone to swelling than genuine solid polymer cells.

Other Lithium Cathode Chemistry Variants: Numerous variants of the basic Lithium-ion cell chemistry have been developed. Lithium Cobalt and Lithium Manganese were the first to be produced in commercial quantities, but Lithium Iron Phosphate (LiFePO4) is taking over for high power applications because of its improved safety performance. The rest are either at various stages of development or they are awaiting investment decisions to launch volume production.

While the basic technology is well known, there used to be a lack of operating experience and hence system design data with some of the newer developments which also hampered their adoption.

Lithium Cobalt LiCoO2: Lithium Cobalt is a mature, proven, industry-standard battery technology that provides long cycle life and very high energy density. The polymer design makes the cells inherently safer than "canned" construction cells that can leak acidic electrolyte fluid under abusive conditions. The cell voltage is typically 3.7 V. Cells using this chemistry are available from a wide range of manufacturers [69]. Unfortunately, the use of Cobalt is associated with environmental and toxic hazards.

Lithium Manganese LiMn2O4: Lithium Manganese provides a higher cell voltage than Cobalt based chemistries at 3.8–4 V but the energy density is about 20 % less. It also provides additional benefits to Lithium-ion chemistry, including lower cost and higher temperature performance. This chemistry is more stable than Lithium Cobalt technology and thus inherently safer but the trade off is lower potential energy densities. Lithium Manganese cells are also widely available but they are not yet as common as Lithium Cobalt cells [69]. Manganese, unlike Cobalt, is a safe and more environmentally benign cathode material. Manganese is also much cheaper than Cobalt, and is more abundant.

Lithium Nickel LiNiO2: Lithium Nickel based cells provide up to 30 % higher energy density than Cobalt but the cell voltage is lower at 3.6 V. They also have the highest exothermic reaction which could give rise to cooling problems in high power applications. Cells using this chemistry are therefore not generally available [69].

Lithium (NCM) Nickel Cobalt Manganese - Li(NiCoMn)O2: Tri-element cells combine slightly improved safety (better than Cobalt oxide) with lower cost without compromising the energy density but with slightly lower voltage. Different manufacturers may use different proportions of the three constituent elements, in this case Ni, Co and Mn [69].

Lithium (NCA) Nickel Cobalt Aluminium - Li(NiCoAl)O2: As above, another tri-element chemistry which combines slightly improved safety (better than Cobalt oxide) with lower cost without compromising the energy density but with slightly lower voltage [69].

Lithium Iron Phosphate LiFePO4: Phosphate based technology possesses superior thermal and chemical stability which provides better safety characteristics than those of Lithium-ion technology made with other cathode materials. Lithium phosphate cells are incombustible in the event of mishandling during charge or discharge, they are more stable under overcharge or short circuit conditions and they can withstand high temperatures without decomposing. When abuse does occur, the phosphate based cathode material will not burn and is not prone to thermal runaway. Phosphate chemistry also offers a longer lifecycle. Recent developments have produced a range of new environmentally friendly cathode active materials based on Lithiated transition metal phosphates for Lithium-ion applications [69].

The operating performance of the cell can also be "tuned" by changing the identity of the transition metal. This allows the voltage as well as the specific capacity of these active materials to be regulated. Cell voltages in the range 2.1–5 V are possible.

Phosphates significantly reduce the drawbacks of the Cobalt chemistry, particularly the cost, safety and environmental characteristics. Once more the trade off is a reduction of 14 % in energy density. Due to the superior safety characteristics of phosphates over current Lithium-ion Cobalt cells, batteries have been designed using larger cells and with a reduced reliance upon additional safety devices [69].

Summary of Batteries as Energy Storage: This section has provided an overview of the current state of battery technologies. A system designer can choose from a variety of battery types depending on the requirements of the actual energy source and appliance. Table 4 shows an overview of the characteristics of commonly used battery types.

4   Outstanding Issues

Researchers among the world have dealt with the problem of energy scavenging from human bodies. Nevertheless, not all the human energy-scavenging problems have been solved. Most of these problems are related to quantity, availability and reliability of the energy.

As it has been described among this book chapter, human body can be used as source of electric energy. To achieve that, a merge between hardware and

Table 4. Most commonly used batteries characteristics

	NiMH w/wo LSD	Li-Ion	Li-Ion Polymer	LiFePo_4	LIC
Commercial use since	2005/1986	1991	1999	2008	1995
Gravimetric energy Density (J/g)	210–360	430–750	360–720	320–400	36–54
Gravimetric power Density (mW/g)	250–1000	250–340	250–340	>300	>3000
Lifecycle (to 80 % of initial capacity)	500	500–1000	300–500	>1000	>10000
Coulombic efficiency (charging efficiency)	70 %	90 %	90 %	90 %	95 %
Typical fast change time	2 h/1 h	1 h	1 h	<1 h	<1 min
Overcharge tolerance	Low	Very low	Low	Moderate	High
Nominal cell Voltage	125 V	3.6 V	3.6 V	3.2 V–3.3 V	2.5 V–3.8 V
Self-discharge/month @ room tmp	<2/20 %	5–10 %	5–10 %	5–10 %	<5 %
Operating Temperature	−20°C–60°C	−20°C–60°C	0°C–60°C	−30°C–60°C	−20°C–70°C

software focused on human energy scavenging is required. Applications have to be tailored to fit to the potentially small footprint of the system and to the available energy source.

In order to obtain the best solutions, an interrelated optimization of transducer, electronics and storage elements have to be addressed. The following paragraphs are focused on explain the main solutions which can be found to solve the above mentioned issues.

4.1 Energy Limitation

Efficiency of current available scavenging approaches is far from being optimal. Most of these systems can scavenge and store between 25 %–40 % of the theoretically available electrical energy. Typical ambient energy sources (e.g. such as light, temperature gradients, motion/vibrations, etc.) need to be transformed into electrical energy. Environmental conditions on the human body will determine the choice of the necessary energy converter. Also, as another constraint, the energy converter should be very small and lightweight to be comfortable for the user. Finally, the position and system functionality will determine the power source.

4.2 Intermittent Energy Supply

The own nature of human bodies impede the continuous harvesting of energy from them. Not all the human beings movements have the same capability to harvest energy and, in consequence, the best or worse location of the harvest devices will determine the amount of energy scavenged. Locations as, e.g., wrist, feet, hit or schrank are the most interesting to obtain the best results in terms of scavenging. If the user is barely moving, the available energy from these positions is insignificant.

Generated by heat gradiants on the human body, the heat gradients are another kind of source power. These gradients harvest energy in ranges between 81 W–1630 W. Special applications may be able to profit from a high power output for a limited time.

Scavenging from radio frequencies depends on a steady level of incoming radiation. Energy transmitters have very short ranges. If the user is moving a lot. The amount of harvestable radiation will vary several orders of magnitude. Another aspect is the short band sensitivity of current radio harvesting circuits which prevents them from harvesting over multiple radio frequency bands.

In any case, an average user, can not ensure a constant and stable power supply. This situations have to be studied by the research community in order to obtain better solutions.

4.3 Limitted Experience of Reliability

Currently, most promising energy harvesting systems seem to be mechanical systems. These systems directly use the movement from the human body and convert it into electrical energy. These systems give a promising conversion rate and can be installed as practical devices, e.g., in the heel of a shoe. The main drawback on these promising systems is the limited reliability, since the used rubbery materials are exposed to high mechanical stress. The reliability of these materials is not high enough in a practical sense.

4.4 Annoying Systems

Most of the current devices are not comfortable for the user. Several studies declare that the compromise point to have an effective system is when the user is not annoyed and it is possible to scavenge enough energy to supply the device. Currently no suggested approach reaches this trade-off point. Existing devices either annoy the user or produce too less energy. More research efforts and better technologies will be required to solve this contradiction.

5 Future Directions

Future research in this area will aim the main open problems described in the previous chapter. Major efforts are needed in order to improve the amount of harvestable energy from human body.

Latest trends are focused on blood pressure, thermal and radio frequency scavenging techniques. Also, there are, advances in new materials that can be used to harvest energy more efficiently and make wearable harvester devices more comfortable for the human beings.

To sum up, the main goals to be achieved in the next decade are the improvement of energy harvesters and the reduction of energy consumption of electronic devices in order to make viable autonomous human-powered systems.

References

1. Maxwell, J., Naing, V., Li, Q.: Biomechanical Energy Harvesting. Locomotion Lab, Simon Fraser University, Burnaby (2009)
2. Khan, Q.A., Bang, S.J.: Energy Harvesting for Self Powered Wearable Health Monitoring System, pp. 11–15. Oregon State University (2009)
3. Starner, T., Paradiso, J.A.: Human Generated Power for Mobile Electronics GVU Center, College of Computing Responsive Environments Group, Media Laboratory Georgia Tech MIT Atlanta, Responsive Environments Group, Media Laboratory MIT Cambridge (2004). http://resenv.media.mit.edu/pubs/books/Starner-Paradiso-CRC.1.452.pdf
4. Kim, H.H., Mano, N., Yhang, Y., Heller, A.: A miniature membrane-less biofuel cell operating under physiological conditions at 0.5 V. J. Electrochem. Soc. **150**(2), A209–A213 (2003)
5. http://en.wikipedia.org/wiki/Glucose
6. http://en.wikipedia.org/wiki/Adenosine_triphosphate
7. Di Carlo, S.E., Coliins, H.L.: Submitting illuminations for review. Adv. Physiol. Educ. **25**(2), 70–71 (2001)
8. Nature's Batteries May Have Helped Power Early Lifeforms
9. Morton, D.: Human Locomotion and Body Form. The Williams & Wilkins Co., Baltimore (1952)
10. Deterre, M., Lefeuvre, E., Zhu, Y., Woytasik, M., Bosseboeuf, A., Boutaud, B., Dal Molin, R.: Micromachined piezoelectric spirals and ultra-compliant packaging for blood pressure energy harvesters powering medical implants. In: IEEE 26th International Conference on Micro Electro Mechanical Systems (MEMS) (2013)
11. Gilomen, B., Schmidi, P.: Mouvement a quartz dame dont lenergie est fournie par une generatrice, calibre ETA 204.911. In: Congres Europeen de Chronometrie, Geneva (2000)
12. Matsuzawa, K., Saka, M.: Seiko human powered quartz watch Space Power Institute, Auburn Univ. Prospector IX: Human-Powered Systems Technologies, pp. 359–384, Auburn (1997)
13. Bueren, T., Lukowicz, P., Troester, G.: Kinetic energy powered computing - an experimental feasibility study. In: ISWC, pp. 22–24 (2003)
14. Paradiso, J., Feldmeier, M.: A compact, wireless, self-powered pushbutton controller. In: Abowd, G.D., Brumitt, B., Shafer, S. (eds.) Ubicomp 2001: Ubiquitous Computing. LNCS, pp. 299–304. Springer, Heidelberg (2001)
15. Romero, E., Warrington, R.O., Neuman, M.R.: Powering Biomedical Devices with Body Motion. In: Conference on Proceedings of IEEE Engineering in Medicine and Biology Society (2010)
16. Stevens, J.: Optimized thermal design of small thermoelectric generators. In: Proceedings of the 34th Intersociety Energy (1999)
17. Society of Automotive Engineers: Conversion Engineering Conference Vancouver, BC, Canada, Paper 1999-01-2564, pp. 2–5 (1999)
18. Wang, Z., Leonov, V., Fiorini, P., Van Hoof, C.: Micromachined Thermopiles For Energy Scavenging On Human Body. Katholieke Universiteit Leuven, Transducers & Eurosensors, Leuven, Belgium (2007)
19. Pelrine, R., Kornbluh, R., Eckerle, J., Jeuck, P., Oh, S., Pei, Q., Stanford, S.: Dielectric elastomers: Generator mode fundamentals and applications. In: SPIE Electroactive Polymer Actuators and Devices, vol. 4329, pp. 148–156. Newport Beach (2001)

20. Hellbaum, R.F., Bryant, R.G., Fox, R.L.: Thin layer composite unimorph ferro-electric driver and sensor. US Patent, 27 May 1997

21. Shenck, N.S., Paradiso, J.A.: Energy scavenging with shoe-mounted piezoelectrics. IEEE Micro **21**(3), 30–42 (2001)

22. Mateu, L., Condrea, C., Lucas, N., Pollack, M., Spies, P.: Human Body Energy Harvesting Thermogenerator for Sensing Applications. In: Proceedings of IEEE International Conference on Sensor Technologies and Applications (2007)

23. EnOcean Corp. Oberhaching Germany: Energy Harvester ECO 200 - An energy harvester for linear motion. http://www.enocean.com/de/enocean_module/ECO_200_Data_Sheet_Sep12_03.pdf (2012)

24. Nowak, R.: DARPA Energy Harvesting Program Review, pp. 13–14, Washington, D.C., April 2000. http://www.darpa.mil/dso/trans/energy/briefing.html

25. Olivares, A., Olivares, G., Gloesekoetter, P., Gorriz, J.M., Ramirez, J.: A study of vibration based energy harvesting in activities of daily living. In: Proceedings of International Conference on Pervasive Computing Technologies for Healthcare, pp. 1–4, March 2010

26. Pollak, M., Mateu, L., Spies, P.: Step-Up DC-DC-Converter with Coupled Inductors for Low Input Voltages Thermogenerators. Power Efficient Systems Department, Fraunhofer IIS, Nuremberg

27. Mateu, L., Pollak, M., Spies, P.: Analog Maximum Power Point Circuit Applied to Thermogenerators. Power Efficient Systems Department, Fraunhofer IIS, Nuremberg

28. Meninger, S., Mur-Miranda, J., Lang, J., Chandrakasan, A., Slocum, A., Schmidt, M., Amirtharajah, R.: Vibration to electric energy conversion. IEEE Trans. Very Large Scale Integr. VLSI Syst. **9**, 64–76 (2001)

29. Ma, W., Wong, M., Ruber, L.: Dynamic simulation of an implemented electrostatic power micro-generator. In: Proceedings of Design, Test, Integration and Packaging of MEMS and MOEMS, pp. 380–385 (2005)

30. Despesse, G., Jager, T., Chaillout, J., Leger, J., Vassilev, A., Basrour, S., Chalot, B.: Fabrication and characterisation of high damping electrostatic micro devices for vibration energy scavenging.In: Proceedings of Design, Test, Integration and Packaging of MEMS and MOEMS, pp. 386–90 (2005)

31. Beeby, S.P., Tudor, M.J., White, N.M.: Energy harvesting vibration sources for microsystems applications. Meas. Sci. Technol. **17**, R175–R195 (2006)

32. Miyazaki, M., Tanaka, H., Ono, G., Nagano, T., Ohkubo, N., Kawahara, T., Yano, K.: Electric-energy generation using variable-capacitive resonator for power-free LSI: efficiency analysis and fundamental experiment ISLPED 03, pp. 193–198 (2003)

33. Tashiro, R., Kabei, N., Katayama, K., Tsuboi, F., Tsuchiya, K.: Development of an electrostatic generator for a cardiac pacemaker that harnesses the ventricular wall motion. J. Artif. Organs **5**, 239–245 (2002)

34. Tashiro, R., Kabei, N., Katayama, K., Tsuboi, F., Tsuchiya, K.: Development of an electrostatic generator that harnesses the motion of a living body. JSME Int. J. C **43**, 916–922 (2000)

35. Roundy, S., Wright, P., Pister, K.: Micro-electrostatic vibration-to-electricity converters. In: Proceedings of IMECE, pp. 1–10 (2002)

36. Niu, P., Chapman, P., Riemer, R., et al.: Evaluation of motions and actuation methods for biomechanical energy harvesting. In: 35th Annual IEEE Power Elecrronics Specialisrs Conference. Piscataway: IEEE, pp. 2100–2106 (2004)

37. Kymissis, J., Kendall, C., Paradiso, J., Gershenfeld, N.: Parasitic power harvesting in shoes. In: IEEE International Symposium on Wearable Computers, pp. 132–139, October 1998

38. Kymissis, J., Kendall, C., Paradiso, J., et al.: Parasitic power harvesting in shoes. In: Second IEEE Conference on Wearable Computing, pp. 132–139. IEEE Computer Society, Washington, DC (1998)

39. Beeby, S.P., Tudor, M.J., Koukharenko, E., White, N.M., ODonnell, T., Saha, C., Kulkarni, S., Roy, S.: Micromachined silicon generator for harvesting power from vibration. In: Proceedings of Transducers, Seoul, Korea, pp. 780–3 (2005)

40. Poulin, G., Sarraute, E., Costa, F.: Generation of electrical energy for portable devices comparative study of an electromagnetic and a piezoelectric system. Sens. Actuators, A 116(3), 461–471 (2004)

41. Saha, C.R., ODonnell, T., Wang, N., et al.: Electromagnetic generator for harvesting energy from human motion. Sens. Actuators, A 137(1), 1–7 (2008)

42. Kulah, H., Najafi, K.: An electromagnetic micro power generator for low-frequency environmental vibrations. In: 17th IEEE International Conference on MEMS. Piscataway: IEEE, pp. 237–240 (2004)

43. Huang, W.S., Tzeng, K.E., Cheng, M.C., et al.: Design and fabrication of a vibrational micro-generator for wearable MEMS. In: Proceedings of Eurosensors XVII, pp. 695–69. Eurosensors, Barcelona (2003)

44. Amirtharajah, R., Chandrakasan, A.P., Mit, C.: Self-powered signalprocessing using vibration-based powergeneration. IEEE J. Solid-State Circuits 33(5), 687–695 (1998)

45. Finkenzeller, K.: RFID Handbook: Fundamentals and Applications in Contactless Smart Cards and Identification. Wiley, New York (2003)

46. Spillman, W.B., Durkee Jr., S., Kuhns, W.W.: Remotely interrogated sensor electronics (RISE) for smart structures applications. In: Proceedings of the SPIE Second European Conference on Smart Structures and Materials, vol. 2361, pp. 282–284. SPIE, Glasgow, October 1994

47. Paradiso, J.A., Pardue, L.S., Hsiao, K.-Y., Benbasat, A.Y.: Electromagnetic tagging for electronic music interfaces. J. New Music Res. 32(4), 395–409 (2003)

48. Bartels, O.: Apparatus for wire-free transmission from moving parts. US Patent, 30 April 2002

49. Pohl, A., Steindl, R., Reindl, L.: The intelligent tire: utilizing passive SAW sensorsmeasurement of tire friction. IEEE Trans. Instrum. Meas. 48(6), 1041–1046 (1999)

50. Bhuvaneswari, P.T.V., Balakumar, R., Vaidehi, V., Balamuralidhar, P.: Solar energy harvesting. In: First International Conference on Computational Intelligence, Communications Systems and Networks (2009)

51. Green, M.A., Emery, K., Hishikawa, Y., Warta, W.: Short communication solar cell efficiency tables (version 33). Prog. Photovoltaics Res. Appl. 17, 85–94 (2009)

52. Penella, M.T., Albesa, J., Gasulla, M.: Powering wireless sensor nodes: primary batteries versus energy harvesting. In: I2MTC 2009 - International Instrumentation and Measurement (2009)

53. Hande, A., Polk, T., Walker, W., Bhatia, D.: Indoor solar energy harvesting for sensor network router nodes. Microprocess. Microsyst. 31, 420–432 (2007)

54. NASA's Jet Propulsion Laboratory: Integrated Solar-Energy-Harvesting and - Storage Device. NASA's Jet Propulsion Laboratory, Pasadena, California

55. Staley, M., Flatau, A.: Characterization of energy harvesting potential of terfenol-d and galfenol. In: Proceedings of SPIE, pp. 630–640, SPIE, Bellingham (2005)

56. Wang, L., Yuan, F.G.: Energy harvesting by magnetostrictive material (msm) for powering. Wireless sensors in SHM. In: 2007 SPIE/ ASME Best Student Paper Presentation Contest SPIE, p. 652941, SPIE, Bellingham (2007)
57. Dunn-Rankin, D., Martins Leal, E., Walther, D.C.: Personal power systems. Prog. Energy Combust. Sci. **31**, 422–465 (2005)
58. Ragone, D.: Review of battery systems for electrically powered vehicles. Mid-Year meeting of the Society of automotive engineers, pp. 20–24, Detroit, MI, May 1968
59. Dembowski, K.: Energy Harvesting fr die Mikroelektronik, pp. 41–46. VDE Verlag Gmbh, Berlin (2011). cap. 2
60. Hoffmann, F., Loechte, A., Rebel, G., Krimphove, C., Gloesekoetter, P.: Degradation aware energy storage using hybrid capacitors. In: 2nd IEEE ENERGYCON (2012)
61. Chang, T., Wang, X., Evans, D.A., Roberson, S.L., Zheng, J.P.: Characterization of tantalum oxide-ruthenium oxide hybrid capacitors. IEEE Trans. Ind. Electron. **51**(6), 1313–1317 (2004)
62. Brown, J.T., Klein, M.G.: Design Factors for a Super High Energy Density Ni-MH Battery for Military Uses. Electro Energy Inc., Danbury (1997)
63. Dingrando, L., et al.: Chemistry: Matter and Change (Chapter 21). Glencoe/McGraw-Hill, New York (2007). ISBN 978-0-07-877237-5
64. http://www.eneloop.info/home/whats-eneloop.html
65. Hoffmann, F.: Degradation aware energy storage using hybrid capacitors. In: 2nd IEEE ENERGYCON Conference & Exhibition, 9–12 September 2012, Florence, Italy (2012)
66. http://www.stefanv.com/electronics/sanyo_eneloop.html
67. Beeby, S.: Energy Harvesting for Autonomous Systems. Artech House Publishers, Norwood (2010). ISBN-13: 978-1-59693-718-5
68. http://www.jsrmicro.be/en/lic
69. http://www.mpoweruk.com/lithiumS.htm
70. Gholam-Abbas, N.: Lithium Batteries, Science and Technology. Springer, New York (2009). ISBN: 978-1-4020-7628-2
71. http://en.wikipedia.org/wiki/Lithium-ion_capacitor
72. http://en.wikipedia.org/wiki/Boost_converter
73. http://en.wikipedia.org/wiki/Buck_converter
74. Ottman, G.K., Hofinann, H.F., Lesieutre, G.A.: Optimized piezoelectric energy harvesting circuit using step-down converter in discontinuous conduction mode. IEEE Trans. Power Electron. **18**, 696–703 (2003)

Readings

75. Colomer-Farrarons, J., Miribel, P.: A CMOS Self-Powered Front-End Architecture for Subcutaneous Event-Detector Devices. Springer, Heidelberg (2011). ISBN 978-94-007-0686-6
76. Kamierski, T.J., Beeby, S.: Energy Harvesting Systems. Springer, New York (2011). ISBN 978-1-4419-7566-9
77. Du, R., Xiu, L.: The Mechanics of Mechanical Watches and Clocks. Springer, Berlin (2013). ISBN 978-3-642-29308-5
78. Bonfiglio, A., De Rossi, D.: Wearable Monitoring Systems. Springer, New York (2011). ISBN 978-1-4419-7384-9
79. Zhang, Y.T.: Wearable Medical Sensors and Systems. Springer, New York (2014). ISBN 978-3-319-01005-2

80. Lay-Ekuakille, A.: Wearable and Autonomous Biomedical Devices and Systems for Smart Environment. Springer, Heidelberg (2011). ISBN 978-3-642-15687-8
81. Marrn, P.J., Minder, D., Karnouskos, S.: The Emerging Domain of Cooperating Objects. Springer, Heidelberg (2012). ISBN 978-3-642-28469-4
82. Songjun, L., Jagdish, S., He, L., Ipsita, A.B.: Biosensor Nanomaterials. Wiley-VCH, Weinheim (2011). ISBN: 978-3-527-63517-7
83. Bhaskaran, M., Sriram, S., Iniewski, K.: Energy Harvesting with Functional Materials and Microsystems. CRC Press, Nottingham (2013). ISBN 978-1-466-58723-6

On Distant Speech Recognition for Home Automation

Michel Vacher[1]([✉]), Benjamin Lecouteux[2], and François Portet[2]

[1] LIG, CNRS, 38000 Grenoble, France
Michel.Vacher@imag.fr
[2] LIG, University Grenoble Alpes, 38000 Grenoble, France
{Benjamin.Lecouteux,Francois.portet}@imag.fr

Abstract. In the framework of Ambient Assisted Living, home automation may be a solution for helping elderly people living alone at home. This study is part of the Sweet-Home project which aims at developing a new home automation system based on voice command to improve support and well-being of people in loss of autonomy. The goal of the study is vocal order recognition with a focus on two aspects: distance speech recognition and sentence spotting. Several ASR techniques were evaluated on a realistic corpus acquired in a 4-room flat equipped with microphones set in the ceiling. This *distant speech* French corpus was recorded with 21 speakers who acted scenarios of activities of daily living. Techniques acting at the decoding stage, such as our novel approach called Driven Decoding Algorithm (DDA), gave better speech recognition results than the baseline and other approaches. This solution which uses the two best SNR channels and *a priori* knowledge (voice commands and distress sentences) has demonstrated an increase in recognition rate without introducing false alarms. Generally speaking, a short overview allows then to outline the research challenges that speech technologies must take up for Ambient Assisted Living and Augmentative and Alternative Communication, and the current reseach avenues in this domain.

Keywords: Distant speech recognition · Keyword detection · Triggered language models · Home automation · Smart home · Application of speech processing for assistive technologies · Ambient assisted living

1 Introduction

Demographic change and ageing in developed countries are challenging the society effort in improving the well being of its elderly and frail inhabitants. The evolution of the Information and Communication Technologies led to the emergence of Smart Homes equipped with ambient intelligence technology which provides high man-machine interaction capacity [1]. However, the technical solutions implemented in such Smart Homes must suit the needs and capabilities of their users in the context of *Ambient Assisted Living*. Under some circumstances, classic tactile commands (e.g., the switch of the lamplight) may not be adapted to the aged population who have some difficulties in moving or seeing. Therefore, tactile commands can be complemented by speech based solutions that would provide voice

© Springer International Publishing Switzerland 2015
A. Holzinger et al. (Eds.): Smart Health, LNCS 8700, pp. 161–188, 2015.
DOI: 10.1007/978-3-319-16226-3_7

command and would make it easier for the person to interact with her relatives or with professional carers (notably in case of distress situations) [2]. Moreover, analysis of sounds emitted in a person's habitation may be useful for activity monitoring and context awareness.

The SWEET-HOME project was set up to integrate sound based technology within smart homes to provide natural interaction with the home automation system at any time and from anywhere in the house. As emphasized by Vacher et al. [3], major issues still need to be overcome. For instance, the presence of uncontrolled noise is a real obstacle for distant speech recognition and identification of voice commands in continuous audio recording conditions when the person is moving and acting in the flat. Indeed, it is not always possible to force the user to take up a position at a short distance and in front of a microphone when he has to manage a specific device, such as a remote control device. Therefore, some microphones are set in the ceiling to be available without any action of the user.

This paper presents preliminary results of speech recognition techniques evaluated on data recorded in a flat by several persons in a daily living context. A glossary is given in Sect. 2 in order to define all specific terms used in this chapter. The background, the state of the art and the challenges to tackle are given in Sect. 3. The data recording and the corpus are presented in Sect. 4. In Sect. 6, several techniques of multisource speech recognition are detailed and evaluated. Section 6.5 is devoted to word spotting needed to recognize voice commands in sentences. The chapter finishes with Sect. 7 which makes a review of the open problems with regard to the application of speech processing for Assistive Technologies and with Sect. 8 which emphasizes the future work and studies necessary to design a usable system in the real world.

2   Glossary

Activities of daily living (ADL) are, as defined by the medical community, the things we normally do in daily living, including any daily activity we perform for self-care (such as feeding ourselves, bathing, dressing, grooming), work, and leisure. Health professionals routinely refer to the ability or inability to perform ADLs as a measurement of the functional status of a person, particularly in regard to people with disabilities and the elderly. A well known scale for ADL was defined by Katz and Akporn [4].

Ambient Assisted Living (AAL) aims to help seniors to continue to manage their daily activities at home thanks to ICT solutions for active and healthy ageing.

Automatic Speech Recognition (ASR) is the translation of spoken words into text by an automatic analysis system.

Blind Source separation (BSS) is the separation of a set of source signals from a set of mixed signals, without the aid of additional information (or with very little information) about the source signals or the mixing process.

Driven Decoding Algorithm (DDA) is a method that allows to drive a primary system search by using the one-best hypotheses and the word posteriors gathered from a secondary system in order to improve the recognition performances.

Distant Speech Recognition is a particular case of Automatic Speech Recognition when the microphone is moved away from the mouth of the speaker. A broad variety of effects such as background noise, overlapping speech from other speakers, and reverberation are responsible of the high degradation of performances of the conventional ASR in this configuration.

Hidden Markov Model (HMM) is a statistical Markov model in which the system being modelled is assumed to be a Markov process with unobserved (hidden) states.

Home Automation is the residential extension of building automation. Home automation may include centralized control of lighting, appliances and other systems, to provide improved convenience, comfort, energy efficiency and security.

Home Automation Network is a network specially designed to ensure the link between sensors, actuators and services.

KNX (KoNneX) is a worldwide ISO standard (ISO/IEC 14543) for home and building control.

Maximum A Posteriori (MAP) estimator, as the maximum likelihood method, is a method that can be used to estimate a number of unknown parameters, such as parameters of a probability density, connected to a given sample. This method is related to maximum likelihood however, it differs in the ability to take into account a non-uniform a priori on the parameters to be estimated.

Maximum Likelihood Linear Regression (MLLR) is an adaptation technique that uses small amounts of data to train a linear transform which, in case of Gaussian distribution, warps the Gaussian means so as to maximize the likelihood of the data.

Recognizer Output Voting Error Reduction (ROVER) is based on a 'voting' or re-scoring process to reconcile differences in ASR system outputs. It is a post-recognition process which models the output generated by multiple ASR systems as independent knowledge sources that can be combined and used to generate an output with reduced error rate.

Smart Home is a house that is specially equipped with devices giving it the ability to anticipate the needs of their inhabitants while maintaining their safety and comfort.

Signal to Noise Ratio (SNR) it is a measure that compares the level of a desired signal to the level of a reference or to background noise: $SNR = \frac{P_{signal}}{P_{reference}}$ The signal and the noise are usually measured across the same impedance and the SNR is generally expressed in dB scale: $SNR_{dB} = 10.\log_{10}\left(\frac{P_{signal}}{P_{reference}}\right) = 20.\log_{10}\left(\frac{A_{signal}}{A_{reference}}\right)$, where P and A denote respectively the power and amplitude of signal or reference.

Wizard of Oz It is an interaction method in which the user is not informed that the reaction of a device is actually controlled by a human (the 'wizard'). This is a reference to the 1939 American musical fantasy film "The Wizard of Oz".

Word Error Rate (WER) is a common metric of the performance of a speech recognition or machine translation system. $WER = \frac{S+D+I}{N}$, where S is the number of substitutions, D the number of deletions, I the number of insertions, N the number of words in the reference.

Word Spotting is related to search and retrieval of a word in an audio stream.

3   Background and State of the Art

As reported in Sect. 1, Smart Homes have been designed with the aim of allowing seniors to keep control of their environment and to improve their autonomy. Despite the fact that audio technology has a great potential to become one of the major interaction modalities in Smart Home, this modality is seldom taken into consideration [5–8]. The most important reason is that audio technology as not reached a sufficient stage of maturity and that there is still some challenges to overcome [3]. The SWEET-HOMEproject presented in Sect. 3.1 aims at designing an audio analysis system running in real-time for voice commands recognition in a realistic home automation context. The state of the art and the challenges to tackle are developed in Sect. 3.2 while Sect. 3.3 focuses on keyword spotting.

3.1   The SWEET-HOMEproject

Main Goals. The SWEET-HOME project is a French national supported research project (http://sweet-home.imag.fr/). It aims at designing a new smart home system by focusing on three main aspects: to provide assistance via *natural man-machine interaction* (voice and tactile command), to ease *social inclusion* and to provide *security reassurance* by detecting situations of distress. If these aims are achieved, then the person will be able to pilot his environment at any time in the most natural way possible [9].

Acceptance of the system is definitely a big issue in our approach therefore, a qualitative user evaluation was performed to assess the acceptance of vocal technology in smart homes [10] at the beginning of the project and before the study presented in Sect. 4. Height healthy persons between 71 and 88 years old, seven relatives (child, grand-child or friend) and three professional carers were questioned in co-discovery in a fully equipped smart home alternating between interview and Wizard of Oz periods. Important aspects of the project have been evaluated: voice command, communication with the outside world, domotic system interrupting a person's activity, and electronic agenda. In each case, the voice based solution was far better accepted than more intrusive solutions. Thus, in accordance with other user studies [11,12], audio technology seems to have a great potential to ease daily living for elderly and frail persons. To respect privacy, it must be emphasized that the adopted solution will analyse the audio information on the fly and is not designed to store the raw audio signal. Moreover, the speech recognizer must be made to recognize only a limited set of predefined sentences in order to prevents recognition of intimate conversations.

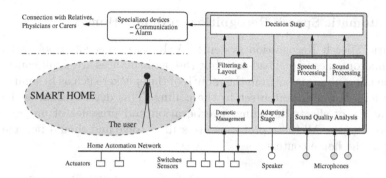

Fig. 1. The general organisation of the SWEET-HOME system

SWEET-HOME **Technical Framework.** The SWEET-HOME system is depicted in Fig. 1. The input of the system is composed of the information from the domotic system transmitted via a local network and information from the microphones transmitted through radio frequency channels. While the domotic system provides symbolic information, raw audio signals must be processed to extract information from speech and sound. This extraction is based on our experience in developing the AUDITHIS system [13], a real-time multi-threaded audio processing system for ubiquitous environments. The extracted information is analysed and either the system reacts to an order given by the user or the system acts pro-actively by modifying the environment without an order (e.g., turns off the light when nobody is in the room). Output of the system thus includes domotic orders, but also interaction with the user when a vocal order has not been understood for instance, or in case of alert messages (e.g., turn off the gas, remind the person of an appointment). The system can also make it easier for the user to connect with her relative, physician or caregiver by using the e-lio[1] or Visage[2] systems. In order for the user to be in full control of the system and also in order to adapt to the users' preferences, three ways of commanding the system are possible: voice order, PDA or classic tactile interface (e.g., switch).

The project does not include the definition of new communication protocols between devices. Rather than building communication buses and purpose

---

[1] www.technosens.fr.

[2] camera-contact.com.

designed material from scratch, the project tries to make use of already stan-dardised technologies and applications. As emphasized in [14], standards ensure compatibility between devices and ease the maintenance as well as orient the smart home design toward cheaper solutions. The interoperability of ubiquitous computing elements is a well known challenge to address [15]. Another exam-ple of this approach is that SWEET-HOME includes systems which are already specialised to handle the social inclusion part. We believe this strategy is the most realistic one given the large spectrum of skills that are required to build a complete smart home system.

3.2   Automatic Speech Recognition in Smart Homes

Automatic Speech Recognition systems (ASR) are especially good with close talking microphones (e.g., head-set), but the performances are significantly lower when the microphone is far from the mouth of the speaker such as in smart homes where microphones are often set in the ceiling. This deterioration is due to a broad variety of effects including reverberation and presence of undetermined background noise. All these problems are still to solve and should be taken into account in the home context.

Reverberation. Distorted signals can be treated in ASR either at the acoustic model level or at the input (feature) level [16]. Deng et al. [17] showed that feature adaptation methods provide better performances than those obtained with systems trained with data with the same distortion as the ones coming from the target environment (e.g., acoustic model learned with distorted data) for both stationary and non stationary noise conditions. Moreover, when the reverberation time is above 500 ms, ASR performances are not significantly improved when the acoustic models are trained on distorted data [18]. In the home involved in the study, the only glazed areas that are not on the same wall are right-angled, thus the reverberation is minimal. Given this and the small dimensions of the flat we can assume that the reverberation time stays below 500 ms. Therefore, only classic ASR techniques with adaptation using data recorded in the test environment will be considered in this study.

Background Noise. When the noise source perturbing the signal of inter-est is known, various noise removal techniques can be employed [19]. It is then possible to dedicate a microphone to record the noise source and to estimate the impulse response of the room acoustic in order to cancel the noise [20]. This impulse response can be estimated through Least Mean Square or Recur-sive Least Square methods. In a previous experiment, these methods showed promising results when the noise is composed of speech or classic music [21]. However, in case of unknown noise sources, such as washing machine or blender noise, Blind Source Separation (BSS) techniques seem more suited. The audio signals captured by the microphones are composed of a mixture of speech and noise sources. Independent Component Analysis is a subcategory of BSS which attempts to separate the different sources through their statistical properties (i.e., purely data driven). This method is particularly efficient for non-Gaussian signals (such as speech) and does not need to take into account the position of the emitter or of the microphones, but it assumes signal and noise to be linearly mixed, this hypothesis seems to be not suited in realistic recordings. Therefore, despite the important effort of the community, noise separation in realistic smart home condition remains an open challenge.

3.3 Word Spotting

Spoken word detection has been extensively studied in the last decades especially in the context of spoken term detection in large speech databases and in continuous speech streams. Performances reported in the literature are good in clean conditions, especially with broadcast news data however, when experiences are undertaken in users' home conditions such as with noisy or spontaneous speech, performances decrease dramatically [22]. In [23], an Interactive Voice Response system was set up to support elderly people to deal with their medication. Over the 300 persons recruited, a third stopped the experiment because they complained about the system and only 38 persons completed the experiment.

In this study, some aspects of both spotting and Large Vocabulary Continuous Speech Recognition are considered. A Large Vocabulary Continuous Speech Recognition system was used in the approach to increase the recognition robustness. Language and acoustic models adaptation and multisource based recognition were investigated. Finally, we designed an original approach which integrates word matching directly inside the ASR system to improve the detection rate of domotic order, this will be described in Sect. 6.5.

4 Recorded Corpus and Experimental Framework

One experiment was conducted to acquire a multimodal corpus by recording individuals performing activities of daily living in a smart home. The speech part of the corpus, called the SWEET-HOME *speech corpus*, is composed of utterances of domotic orders, distress calls and anodin sentences in French recorded using several microphones set in the ceiling of the smart home. This corpus was used to tune and to test a classic ASR system in different configurations. This section briefly introduces the smart home, the SWEET-HOME *speech corpus*. The monosource ASR system is described in Sect. 5.

4.1 Data Acquisition in the Smart Home

The DOMUS smart home. The SWEET-HOME speech corpus was acquired in realistic conditions, i.e., in a smart-home and in distant speech condition inside the DOMUS smart home. This smart home was designed and set up by the Multicom team of the Laboratory of Informatics of Grenoble to observe users' activities interacting with the ambient intelligence of the environment. Figure 2 shows the

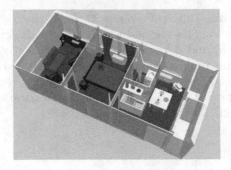

Fig. 2. The DOMUS Smart Home used during the SWEET-HOME project

details of the flat. It is a thirty five square meters suite flat including a bathroom, a kitchen, a bedroom and a study, all equipped with sensors and effectors.

More than 150 sensors, actuators and information providers are managed in the flat. The flat is fully usable and can accommodate a dweller for several days so that it is possible to act on the sensory ambiance, depending on the context and the user's habits. The technical architecture of DOMUS is based on the KNX bus system (KoNneX), a worldwide ISO standard (ISO/IEC 14543) for home and building control. The flat has also been equipped with 7 radio microphones for the need of the SWEET-HOME project; the microphones are set into the ceiling (2 per room except for the bathroom). Audio data can be recorded in real-time thanks to a dedicated PC embedding an 8-channel input audio card [13]. The sample rate is 16kHz and the bandwith 8kHz. It must be noticed that the distance between the speaker and the closest microphone is about 2 m when he is standing and about 3 m when he is sitting. Figure 3 shows the position of the microphones and of some sensors in the flat.

Corpus Recording. 21 persons (including 7 women) participated to a 2-phase experiment to record, among other data, speech corpus in the DOMUS smart home. To make sure that the audio data acquired would be as close as possible

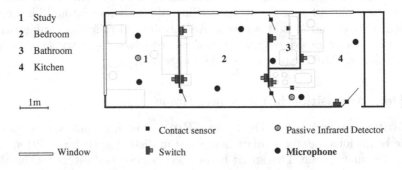

Fig. 3. The DOMUS Smart Home and the position of the sensors

to real daily living sounds, the participants performed several daily living activities. Each experimental session lasted about 2 h. The average age of the participants was 38.5 ± 13 years (22–63, min-max). No instruction was given to any participant about how they should speak and in which direction. Consequently, no participant emitted sentences directing their voice to a particular microphone.

A visit, before the first phase of the experiment, was organized to make the participants accustomed to the home in order to smoothly perform the experiment. During this first phase, participants uttered forty predefined French casual sentences on the phone such as "Allo" (*Hello*), "J'ai eu du mal à dormir" (*I slept badly*) but were also free to utter any sentence they wanted (some did speak to themselves aloud). Then, the first phase consisted in following a scenario of activities without condition on the time spent and the manner of achieving them (having a breakfast, listening to music, get some sleep, clean up the flat using the vacuum, etc.). Note that the microphone of the telephone was not recorded, only the 7 microphones set on the ceiling were used.

The second phase consisted in reading aloud a list of 44 sentences:

- 9 distress sentences such as "A l'aide" (*Help*), "Appelez un docteur" (*call a doctor*);
- 3 orders such as "Allumez la lumière" (*turn on the light*);
- 32 colloquial sentences such as "Le café est très chaud" (*The coffee is hot*).

This list was read in 3 rooms (study, bedroom, and kitchen) under three conditions: no background noise, vacuum on or radio on. 396 sentences were recorded but only those in the clean condition were used in this paper, the noisy condition records having been designed for other experiments.

4.2 The SWEET-HOME French Speech Corpus

Only the sentences uttered in the study during the phone conversation of the phase 1 were considered. For the phase 2 record, only the sentences uttered in the kitchen without additional noise (vacuum or radio) were considered. Each speaker did not follow strictly the instructions given at the beginning of the experiment, therefore this corpus was indexed manually. Some hesitations and word repetitions occurred along the records. Moreover, when two sentences were uttered without a sufficient silence between them, they were considered as one sentence. A complete description of the corpus according to each speaker is given in Table 1. The SWEET-HOME speech corpus is made of 862 sentences uttered by 21 persons in the first phase, 917 sentences in the second phase; it lasts for each channel 38 min 46 s in the case of the first phase, and 40 min 27 s in the case of the second phase. The SNR (Signal-to-Noise Ratio) is an important parameter which was used for the combination of several sources. For Phase 1 (when the speaker was in the study) mean SNR was 21.8 dB/20.0 dB (channels 6 and 7), for Phase 2 (when the speaker was in the bedroom) mean SNR was 22.1 dB/22.1 dB (channels 4 and 5).

Table 1. SWEET-HOME speech corpus description

Spkr. ID	Phase 1			Phase 2		
	Duration (s)	SNR mean (dB)	SNR mean (dB)	Duration (s)	SNR mean (dB)	SNR mean (dB)
	Channel 6 or 7	Channel 6	Channel 7	Channel 4 or 5	Channel 4	Channel 5
1	145.78	23.5	22.1	96.66	24.7	26.2
2	119.36	22.6	21.0	110.42	21.2	22.0
3	112.08	14.8	12.2	119.76	15.9	16.7
4	141.32	16.5	16.5	119.04	22.1	24.0
5	159.32	29.7	26.8	122.21	26.8	28.6
6	122.10	17.7	16.1	108.61	19.7	18.7
7	110.90	19.0	17.5	116.00	20.7	21.2
8	114.54	20.3	19.0	114.64	18.9	20.6
9	121.58	26.8	24.7	135.36	24.5	25.3
10	77.50	20.3	18.0	104.54	23.4	18.8
11	106.52	20.2	21.0	105.76	20.6	23.9
12	90.48	24.5	21.1	108.44	25.1	24.3
13	96.46	26.2	19.9	116.52	17.3	13.2
14	97.74	17.7	17.7	113.40	18.5	15.3
15	96.48	22.6	21.4	101.98	25.0	26.9
16	96.86	21.4	17.6	106.72	18.2	10.7
17	111.08	21.7	20.0	144.46	28.3	24.6
18	169.14	20.0	19.0	124.52	23.0	24.2
19	146.98	25.1	23.4	125.58	24.4	22.4
20	89.80	27.5	24.8	120.60	29.0	27.4
21	99.48	19.5	19.2	109.56	17.4	14.4
Average	115.50	21.8	20.0	115.47	22.1	20.4

The databases recorded in the course of the SWEET-HOME project are devoted to voice controlled home automation, they will be distributed for an academic and research use only [24].

5   Monosource ASR Techniques

The architecture of an ASR is described by Fig. 4. A first stage is the audio interface in charge of acoustical feature extraction in consecutive frames. The next 3 stages working together are:

- the phoneme recognizer stage;
- the word recognition stage constructing the graph of phonemes; and
- the sentence recognition stage constructing the graph of words.

The data associated with these stages are respectively the acoustic models, the phonetic dictionary and the language models. The output of the recognizer is made of the best hypothesis lattices.

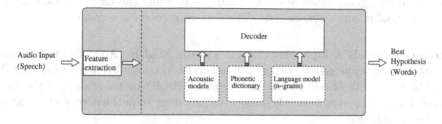

Fig. 4. General organisation of an ASR

5.1 The Speeral ASR System

The ASR system used in the study is Speeral [25]. The LIA (Laboratoire d'Informatique d'Avignon) speech recognition engine relies on an A^* decoder with HMM-based context-dependent acoustic models and trigram language models. HMMs are classic three-state left-right models while state tying is achieved by using decision trees. The acoustic features, for each 30 ms-length frame with 20 ms overlay (10 ms-time shift), were composed of 12 Perceptual Linear Predictive coefficients, the energy, and the first and second order derivatives of these 13 parameters, this represent in total 39 parameters. The acoustic models were trained on about 80 h of annotated French speech. If the participants were elderly people, the use of adapted data would be required [26], but this was not the case for this study. Given the targeted application of SWEET-HOME the computation time should not be a breach of real-time use. Thus, the $1 \times$ RT Speeral configuration was used. This this configuration, by using a strict pruning scheme, the time spent by the system to decode one hour of speech signal is real-time.

Language Models. Two language models were built: the generic and the specialized models. The *specialized* language model was estimated from the sentences that the 21 participants had to read during the experiment (domotic orders, casual phrases, etc.). The *generic* language model was estimated on about 1000 M of words from the French newspapers *Le Monde* and *Gigaword*.

5.2 Baseline System

In order to propose a **baseline system**, the adaptation of both acoustic and language models were tested. Then, to improve the robustness of the recognition, multi-streams ASR was tested. Finally, a new variant of a driven decoding algorithm was used in order to take into account *a-priori* information and several audio channels for each speaker.

The phase 1 of the corpus was used for development and acoustic model adaptation to the speaker while the phase 2 was used for performances estimation. Results obtained on the phase 2 of the corpus were analysed using two measures: the Word Error Rate (WER) and the Classification Error Rate (CER). The WER is a good measure of the robustness, while the CER corresponds to the main goal of our research (i.e., detection of *predefined* sentences).

Acoustic Models Adaptation: MAP Versus MLLR. Acoustic models were adapted for each speaker by using two methods: Maximum A Posteriori (MAP) and Maximum Likelihood Linear Regression (MLLR) by using data of the first phase. These data were perfectly annotated, allowing to perform correct targeted speaker adaptation.

The Maximum Likelihood Linear Regression (MLLR) is used when a limited amount of data per class is available. MLLR is an adaptation technique that uses small amounts of data to train a linear transform which warps the Gaussian means so as to maximize the likelihood of the data: acoustically close classes are grouped and transformed together. In the case of the Maximum a posteriori approach (MAP), initial models are used as informative priors for the adaptation.

Table 2 shows different results with and without acoustic models adaptation. Results are presented for the two best streams (high SNR). Experiments were carried out with the generic language model (GLM) lightly interpolated with *predefined* sentences (PS) presented in the next section. Without acoustic adaptation, the best average WER is about 36 %. The results show that MAP is not very performing in this case. With MAP, the WER about 27 %. The best average WER is about 18 % with MLLR adaptation, which is the best choice for sparse and noisy data whatever the channel.

Two aspects explain the MAP performance:

– The noisy environment is not adapted to MAP adaptation [27].
– The lack of parameter tying in the standard MAP algorithm implies that the adaptation is not robust.

Linguistic Variability. Large vocabulary model languages such as the *generic* language model, are known to perform poorly on specific tasks because of the large number of equi-probable hypotheses. Better recognition can be obtained by reducing the overall linguistic space by estimating a language model on the expected sentences such as with the *specialized* language model. However, such a language model would be probably too specific when the speaker deviates from the original transcript. To benefit from the two language models, we propose a linear interpolation scheme where specific weights are tested on specialized and generic language models. The reduction of the linguistic variability thanks to the contribution of known *predefined* sentences is explored. Therefore, we interpolated the specialized model with the generic large vocabulary language model.

Two schemes of linear interpolation were considered: in the first one, the *generic* model had a strong weight while in the second one, the impact of the *generic* model was low. The ASRs were assessed after MLLR adaptation using the data of phase 1 of the corpus. Table 2 presents the WER with the generic language model (Baseline). As expected, the baseline language model obtained poor results: about 74 %. Without reliable information, the ASR system, in noisy, speaker independent and large vocabulary condition is unable to perform good recognition.

Table 2. Average WER according to different configurations by using monosource techniques

Method	WER stream 1 channel 4 (%)	WER stream 2 channel 5 (%)
Generic LM	75.3	73.4
Interpolated LM	38.8	35.0
Interpolated LM with MAP adaptation	28.5	25.9
Interpolated LM with MLLR adaptation	18.6	18.0
Specialized LM with MLLR adaptation	19.2	19.0

With the specialised language model the system is able to detect more *predefined* sentences. However, when the speaker deviates from the scenario, the language model is unable to find the correct uttered sentence. The specialised language model was thus too specific.

Finally, a light (10 %) interpolated language model led to the best results. This model combined the generic language model (with a 10 % weight) and the specialised model (with 90 % weight). These results show that a decoding based on a language model mainly learnt from the *predefined* sentences improves significantly the WER. The best WER is obtained when a generic language model is also considered: when the speaker deviates, the generic language model makes it possible to correctly recognise the pronounced sentences.

5.3   Conclusion About Monosource ASR

Speeral ASR system was evaluated taking into account realistic distant-speech conditions and in the context of a home automation application (voice command). The system had to perform ASR with several constraints and challenges. Indeed, the noisy, distant-speech conditions, speaker independent recognition, continuous analysis and real-time aspects, the analysis system must operate in more difficult conditions than with the classic head-set one. Therefore, it is clear that obtained results are insufficient and must be improved, multichannel analysis is an avenue worth exploring.

The application conditions also make it possible for the ASR system to benefit from multiple audio channels, from a reduced vocabulary and from the hypothesis that only one speaker should utter voice commands. Lightly interpolated language model and a MLLR acoustic adaptation did improve significantly the ASR system performance. In the next section, we propose several techniques based on this baseline in order to perform multisource ASR.

6   Techniques for Multisource Speech Recognition and Sentence Detection

Multisource ASR can improve the recognition performances thanks to information extracted in more than one channel. The ROVER method presented in Sect. 6.1 analyses the outputs of ASR performed on all channels separately. In the DDA method presented in Sect. 6.2, the information of one channel is used to guide the analysis on another channel. We also present an improved DDA method in Sect. 6.3 were *a priori* information about the task is taken into account.

6.1   ROVER

At the ASR combination level, a ROVER [28] was applied. ROVER is expected to improve the recognition results by providing the best agreement between the most reliable sources. It combines systems output into a single word transition network. Then, each branching point is evaluated with a vote scheme. The words with the best score are selected (number of votes weighted by confidence measures). However, this approach necessitates high computational resources when several sources need to be combined and real time is needed (in our case, 7 ASR systems must operate concurrently).

A baseline ROVER was tested using all available channels without *a priori* knowledge. In a second step, an *a priori* confidence measure based on the SNR was used: for each decoded segment s_i from the ith ASR system, the associated confidence score $\phi(s_i)$ was computed according to Eq. 1 where $R()$ is the function computing the SNR of a segment and s_i is the segment generated by the ith ASR system:

$$\phi(s_i) = 2^{R(s_i)} / \sum_{j=1}^{7} 2^{R(s_j)} \tag{1}$$

For each annotated sentence a silence period I_{sil} at the beginning and the end is taken around the speech signal period I_{speech}. The SNR is thus evaluated through the function $R()$ according to Eq. 2.

$$R(S) = 10 * log(\frac{\sum_{n \in I_{speech}} S[n]^2}{|I_{speech}|} / \frac{\sum_{n \in I_{sil}} S[n]^2}{|I_{sil}|}) \tag{2}$$

Finally, a ROVER using only the two best channels overall was tested in order to check whether other channels contain redundant information and whether good results can be reached with low computational cost.

The ROVER combination led to great improvements. The results show that the ROVER made ASR more robust with an average WER of 13.0 %. This aspect shows the complementarity of the streams. However, the ROVER stage increased the computation time proportionally to the number of ASR systems used. Given that the objective of the project is to build a real-time and affordable solution, computational resources are limited. Moreover, ROVER combination for two streams reduces the problem to picking the word with the highest confidence when two systems disagree. Thus, when the recogniser confidence scores are not reliable, the ROVER between two streams does not perform well and the final performance is likely to be similar to a single system. Thus, we propose in the next section a method allowing low-cost computations with only two streams, based on the Driven Decoding Algorithm. In the following, ROVER results are used as baseline.

6.2   Driven Decoding Algorithm

The Driven Decoding Algorithm (DDA) [29,30] is able to simultaneously align and correct the imperfect ASR outputs [31]. DDA has been implemented within Speeral: The ASR generates assumptions as it walks the phoneme lattice. For each new step, the current assumption is aligned with the approximated hypothesis. Then, a matching score α is computed and integrated within the language model:

$$\tilde{P}(w_i|w_{i-1}, w_{i-2}) = P^{1-\alpha}(w_i|w_{i-1}, w_{i-2}) \tag{3}$$

where $\tilde{P}(w_i|w_{i-1}, w_{i-2})$ is the updated trigram probability of the word w_i given the history w_{i-2}, w_{i-3}, and $P(w_i|w_{i-1}, w_{i-2})$ is the initial probability of the trigram. When the trigram is aligned, α is at a maximum and decreases according to the misalignments of the history (values of α must be determined empirically using a development corpus).

In the DOMUS smart home, uttered sentences were recorded using two microphones per room. Thus, two microphones can be used as input to DDA in order to increase the robustness of the ASR systems as presented in Fig. 5. We propose

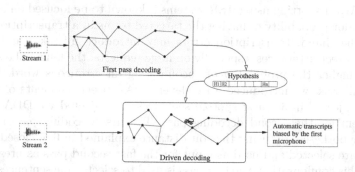

Fig. 5. Driven Decoding Algorithm used with two streams: The first stream drives the second stream

Table 3. ASR system recognition WER by using multisource techniques

Method	WER (%)$^{\pm SD}$
Baseline	$18.3^{\pm 12.1}$
Oracle Baseline	$17.7^{\pm 10.3}$
ROVER Full	$20.6^{\pm 8.5}$
ROVER 2 channels + SNR	$13.0^{\pm 6.6}$
ROVER +SNR	$\mathbf{12.2^{\pm 6.1}}$
DDA +SNR	$11.4^{\pm 5.6}$
DDA 2 levels + SNR	$\mathbf{8.8^{\pm 3.7}}$

to use a variant of the DDA where the output of the first microphone is used to drive the output of the second one. This approach presents two main benefits:

- The second ASR system speed is boosted by the approximated transcript (only $0.1 \times RT$)
- While a ROVER does not allows to combine efficiently two systems without confidence scores, DDA combines easily the information

The Fig. 5 explains the Driven Decoding solution: the first Speeral pass on the stream 1 is used to drive a second pass on the stream 2, allowing to combine the information of the two streams.

Results using the 2-stream DDA are presented in Table 3. In most cases, DDA generated hypotheses that led either to the average WER of the two initial streams or to better WER. The average WER is 11.4 %. We propose to extend this approach in the next section by driving the ASR system by *a priori* sentences selected on the first stream.

6.3   Two Level DDA

In the previous approach, the first stream of decoding was used to drive the second one: DDA aims to refine the decoding achieved during the first stream decoding. Word spotting using ASR systems is known to be focused on accuracy, since the prior probability of having the targeted terms in a transcription is low. On the other hand, transcription errors may introduce mistakes and lead to misses of correct utterances, especially on large requests: the longer the searched term, the higher the probability of encountering an erroneous word. In order to limit this risk, we introduced a two-level DDA: speech segments of the first pass are projected in $3 - best$ spotted sentences and injected via DDA into the ASR system for the second decoding pass. The first decoding pass allows to generate hypotheses. By using the edit distance explained in 6.5, closed spotted sentences are selected and used as input for the fast second pass as presented in Fig. 6. In this configuration, the first pass is used to select some sentences used to drive the second pass. In the Fig. 6, the first system outputs "Allumer la lumière"

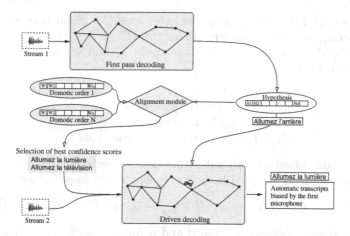

Fig. 6. Driven Decoding Algorithm used with two streams and *a priori* sentences: The first stream drives the second stream according to a refine selection of spotted sentences

(*Turn on the light*). The edit distance allows to find two close sentences: "Allumez la lumière" and "Allumez la télévision" (*Turn on the TV*). These sentences drive the second pass and allows one to find the correct output "Allumez la lumière".

Results using this approach are showed in Table 3. According to the WER, this approach improved significantly the ASR system quality, by taking advantage of the *a priori* information assessed by the *predefined* spotted sentences. WER is improved significantly for all speakers: the mean WER is 8.8 %. By using the two streams available the ASR system is able to combine them efficiently. The best results are obtained with the two level approach were the ASR system is driven by both the first stream and the potential spotted sentences. The next section investigates the impact of each previous proposed method on the detection of pronounced sentences.

6.4   Multisource Speech Recognition: Results

For each approach, the presented results are the average over the 21 speakers (plus standard deviation for the WER). For the sake of comparison, results of a baseline and an oracle baseline systems are provided. The baseline system outputs the best decoding amongst 7 ASR systems according to the highest SNR. The oracle baseline is computed by selecting the best WER for each speaker. The best results are achieved with DDA because the search for the best hypothesis in the lattice uses data from several channels and has more information than when decoding for each channel.

6.5   Detection of Predefined Sentences

In order to spot sentences into automatic transcripts T of size m, each sentence of size n from *predefined* sentences H was aligned with T by using a Dynamic

Time Warping (DTW) algorithm at the letter level [32]. Sequences were aligned by constructing an n-by-m matrix where the (i^{th}, j^{th}) element of the matrix contained the distance between the two words T_i and H_j using the distance function defined below.

$$
\begin{aligned}
d(T_i, H_j) &= 0 \text{ if } T_i = H_j \\
d(T_i, H_j) &= 3 \text{ in the insertion cases} \\
d(T_i, H_j) &= 3 \text{ in the deletion cases} \\
d(T_i, H_j) &= 6 \text{ in the substitution cases}
\end{aligned}
\tag{4}
$$

The deletion, insertion and substitution costs were computed empirically. The cumulative distance $\gamma(i, j)$ between H_j and T_i is computed as:

$$
\gamma(i, j) = d(T_i, H_j) + min\{\gamma(i - 1, j - 1), \gamma(i - 1, j), \gamma(i, j - 1)\}
\tag{5}
$$

Each *predefined* sentence is aligned and associated with an alignment score: the percentage of well aligned symbols (here letters). The sentence with the best score is then selected as best hypothesis.

This approach takes into account some recognition errors such as word declination or light variations (téléviseur, télévision etc.). Moreover, miss-decoded word are often orthographically close from the good one (due to the close pronunciation).

To test the detection of *a-priori* pronounced sentences, such as domotic orders (e.g., "allume la lumière"), the detection methods were applied in the following ASR configurations:

- Baseline: Speeral system with acoustic and language model adaptation.
- ROVER: Consensus vote between all streams.
- DDA1: DDA drived with the first stream.
- DDA2: DDA drived by the first stream and the spotted sentences.

The three systems based on ROVER and DDA gave the best performances, with respectively 88.2 %, 87,4 % and 92.5 % of correct classifications while the baseline system obtains 85 % of correct classification. It can be observed that the 2-level DDA based ASR system was able to detect more spotted sentences with less computational time and with more accuracy than the ROVER based one.

Sentence Detection: Results. In all best-configurations, *predefined* sentence recognition showed a good accuracy: the baseline recognition gave 85 %. It can be observed that in other configurations the spotting task correlated well with the WER. Thereby, ROVER and the two DDA configurations led to a significant improvement over the baseline. The best configuration based on the two-level DDA gave 92.5 % of correct classifications.

6.6 Discussion and Future Works

The goal of this study is to provide a path for vocal command recognition improvement with a focus on two aspects: distance speech recognition and sentence spotting. A distant speech French corpus was recorded with 21 speakers playing scenarios of activities of daily living in a real flat, this corpus is made of colloquial sentences, vocal commands and distress sentences. This realistic corpus was acquired in a 4-room flat equipped with microphones set in the ceiling thanks to 21 speakers. Several ASR techniques were evaluated, such as our novel approach called Driven Decoding Algorithm (DDA). They gave better results than the baseline and other approaches. Indeed, they analyse the signal on the two best SNR channels and the use of a priori knowledge (specified vocal commands and distress sentences) increases the recognition rate in the case of true positive sentences and doesnt introduce false positive.

Evaluation in Real Conditions. The technology developed in this study was then tested thanks to two other experiments in an Ambient Assisted Living context at the end of the SWEET-HOME project. These experiments involved 16 non-aged participants for the first one and 11 aged or visually impaired people for the second one [33]. Each participant followed a scenario including various situations and activities of the daily life. The objective of these experiments was to evaluate the use of voice command for home automation in distant speech conditions, in real-time and in context aware conditions [34]. Unfortunately, we were not able to integrate the DDA method in time in the real-time analysis software PATSH before the beginning of these experiments. Therefore, the performance of the system was still low, the Home Automation Command Error Rate was about 38 % [33], but the results showed there is room for improvement. But, although the participants had to repeat, sometimes up to three times, the voice command, they were overall very excited about commanding their own home by voice. These results highlight the interest of the methods discussed above and especially DDA2 that chooses among available channels those that have the best SNR in order to refine the data analysis. One of the biggest problems were the response time which was unsatisfactory (for 6 participants out of 16) and the mis-understanding of the system which implied to repeat the order (8/16). These technical limitations were reduced when we improved the ASR memory management and reduced the search space. After this improvement, only one participant with special needs complained about the response time.

Interest of the Recorded Corpus. During these experiments, all data were recorded. This acquired corpus was used to evaluate the performance of the audio analysis methods presented in this chapter. It constitutes a precious resource for future work. Indeed, one of the main problems that impede researches in this domain is the need for a large amount of annotated data (for analysis, machine learning and benchmark). It is quite obvious that the acquisition of such datasets is highly expensive both in terms of material and of human resources. For instance, in the experiment presented in Sect. 4, the acquisition and the annotation of the 33-hours corpus costed approximatively 70 k€.

Therefore, the SWEET-HOME multimodal corpus is a dataset recorded in realistic conditions in DOMUS, the fully equipped Smart Home with microphones and home automation sensors presented in Sect. 4.1 will be available for the research community [24]. This corpus was recorded thanks to participants which performed Activities of Daily living (ADL). This corpus is made of a multimodal subset, a French home automation speech subset recorded in Distant Speech conditions, and two interaction subsets, the first one being recorded by 16 persons without disabilities and the second one by 6 seniors and 5 visually impaired people. This corpus was used in studies related to ADL recognition, context aware interaction and distant speech recognition applied to home automation controlled through voice.

Future Projects. Our future project aims to develop a system capable of operating under the conditions encountered in an apartment. For this we must firstly integrate BSS techniques to reduce the noise present in the everyday life context and secondly improve the DDA2 method to detect and recognize the voice commands as well as distress calls.

7   Application of Speech Processing for Assistive Technologies

The applications of speech processing may present a greet benefit for smart homes and Ambient Assisted Living (see Sect. 7.1) but Augmentative and Alternative Communication (AAC) retains involvement from a broad community of researchers (see Sect. 7.2).

7.1   Smart Home and AAL

Anticipating and responding to the needs of persons with loss of autonomy with ICT is known as Ambient Assisted Living (AAL). ICT can contribute to the prevention and/or compensation of impairments and disabilities, to improve the quality of life, safety, communication and social inclusion of end users. They must relieve the isolation and caregiver burden. They also participate in the modernization of health and social services by facilitating home or institutional organization of professional care, their implementation, their tolerance and performance [35]. In this domain, the development of smart homes is seen as a promising way of achieving in-home daily assistance [1]. Health Smart Home has been designed to provide daily living support to compensate some disabilities (e.g., memory help), to provide training (e.g., guided muscular exercise) or to detect potentially harmful situations (e.g., fall, gas not turned off). Basically, a health smart home contains sensors used to monitor the activity of the inhabitant. Sensor data are analyzed to detect the current situation and to execute the appropriate feedback or assistance.

A rising number of studies about audio technology in smart home were conducted. This includes speech recognition [36–39], sound recognition [3, 40, 41], speech synthesis [42] or dialogue [7, 8, 11, 43]. These systems are either embedded into the home automation system or in a smart companion (mobile or not) or both as in Companions [44] or CompanionAble [41] projects.

However, given the diverse profiles of the users (e.g., low/high technical skill, disabilities, etc.), complex interfaces should be avoided. Nowadays, one of the best interfaces, is the VoiceUser Interface (VUI), whose technology has reached a stage of maturity and that provides interaction using natural language so that the user does not have to learn complex computing procedures [10]. Moreover, it is well adapted to people with reduced mobility and to some emergency situations (hand free and distant interaction). Indeed, a home automation system based on voice command will be able to improve support and well-being of people in loss of autonomy. But, despite the interest presented by sound analysis techniques, the use of ASR for voice command for home automation in a real environment is still an open challenge.

Voice-User Interface in domestic environment has recently gained interest in the speech processing community as exemplified by the rising number of smart home projects that considers Automatic Speech Recognition (ASR) in their design [5,6,8,37–39,45–49]. However, though VUIs are frequently employed in close domains (e.g., smart phone) there are still important challenges to overcome [3]. Indeed, the task imposes several constraints to the speech technology:

- distant speech conditions [16],
- hand free interaction,
- adaptation to potential users (elderly),
- affordable by people who can have low resources,
- noise conditions in the home,
- real-time,
- respect of privacy.

In recent years, the research community shows an increased interest with regards to the analysis of the speech signal in noisy conditions like the organizing of Challenges *CHiME* shows. The first CHiME Challenge held in 2011 was the first concerted evaluation of ASR systems in a real-world domestic environment involving both reverberation and highly dynamic background noise made up of multiple sound source [50]. The second CHiME Challenge in 2013 was supported by the IEEE AASP, MLSP and SL Technical Committees [51]. The configuration considered by this Challenge was that of speech from a single target speaker being binaurally recorded in a domestic environment involving multisource background noise. These challenges reported here are still no close enough to real conditions and future editions of the challenge will attempt to move closer to realistic conditions.

Ageing has effects on the voice and movement of the person and thereby, aged voice is characterized by some specific features such as imprecise production of consonants, tremors, hesitations and slower articulation [52]. Some studies have shown age-related degeneration with atrophy of vocal cords, calcification of laryngeal cartilages, and changes in muscles of larynx [53,54]. For there reason, some authors highlight that ASR performance decreases with elderly voice. This phenomenon has been observed in the case of English, European Portuguese, Japanese and French [26,55–57]. Vipperla et al. [58] made a very useful and interesting longitudinal study by using records of defence speech delivered in the

Supreme Court of the United States over a decade by the same judges. This study showed that an adaptation to each speaker can get closer to the scores of non-aged speakers but this implies that the ASR must be adapted to each speaker. Nevertheless, some authors established that many other effects can also be responsible for ASR performance degradation such as decline in cognitive and perceptual abilities [59,60].

Moreover, since smart home systems for AAL often concern distress situations, it is unclear whether distress voice will challenge the applicability of these system. Speech signal contains linguistic information but it may be influenced by the health, the social status and the emotional state [61,62]. Recent studies suggests that ASR performance decreases in case of emotional speech [63,64], however it is still an under-researched area. In their study, Vlasenko et al. [63] demonstrated that acoustic models trained on read speech samples and adapted to acted emotional speech could provide better performance of spontaneous emotional speech recognition.

Moreover, such technology must be validated in real smart homes and with potential users. At this time, validation studies in such realistic conditions are rare [33]. In the same way, there are few user studies reported in the literature and related to speech technology application [10], they are generally related to ICT [65].

7.2 Assistive Technologies

The field of Augmentative and Alternative Communication (AAC) is multidisciplinary and vast, its focus is to develop methods and technologies to aid communication for people with complex communications needs [66]. Potential users are elderly and all people who may acquire a disability or have a degenerative disability which affects communication, this disability can result from both motor and cognitive impairments (i.e., paralysis, hearing or visual impairment, brain injury, Alzheimer...).

Speech and language processing play a major role to improve function for people with communication facilities [67]. This is highlighted by the publication of special issues of journals and by the regular organisation of workshops and conferences on this topic. In 2009, the third issue of the ACM Transactions on Accessible Computing was devoted to AAC (Volume 1, Issue 3). In 2011, the relationship between assistive technology and computational linguistics was formalized with the formation of an ACL Special Interest Group on Speech and Language Processing for Assitive Technology (SIG-SLPAT[3]) which gained SIG status from the International Speech Communication Association (ISCA). The last workshops SIG-SLPAT bringing together Computational Linguistics, Speech Processing and Assistive Technologies took place in Montreal, Quebec (2012), in Grenoble, France (2013) and in Baltimore, U.S. (2014). In the same way, a special session of Interspeech[4] "Speech technologies for Ambient Assisted Living"

---

[3] http://www.slpat.org/.
[4] http://www.interspeech2014.org/.

is organized in 2014. This special session aims at bringing together researchers in speech and audio technologies with people from the ambient assisted living and assistive technologies communities to meet and foster awareness between members of either community, discuss problems, techniques and datasets, and perhaps initiate common projects.

Regarding speech recognition, the most important challenges are related to the recognition of speech uttered by elderly, dysarthric or cognitively impaired speakers.

8   Future Outlook

Future challenges have been outlined in the previous Sect. 7. These challenges are essentially related to scientific and technological problems to solve, but the human aspect must not be neglected.

8.1   Scientific and Technical Challenges

In real home environment the audio signal is often perturbed by various and undetermined noises (e.g., devices, TV, music, roadwork...). But this also shows us the challenges to obtain a usable system that will not be set-up in lab conditions but in various and noisy ones. Of course, in the future, smart homes could be designed specifically to limit these effects but the current smart home development cannot be successful if we are not able to handle these issues when equipping old-fashioned or poorly insulated home. Finally, one of the most difficult problems is the blind source separation. Some techniques developed in other areas of signal processing may be considered to analyze speech captured with far-field sensors and to develop a Distant Speech Recogniser (DSR) such as blind source separation, independent component analysis (ICA), beam-forming and channel selection.

Two main categories of audio analysis are generally targeted: daily living sounds and speech. These categories represent completely different semantic information and the techniques involved for the processing of these two kinds of signal are quite distinct. However, the distinction can be seen as artificial and there is a high confusion between speech and sounds with overlapped spectrum. For instance, one problem is to know whether scream or sigh must be classified as speech or sound.

Moreover, the system must react as quickly as possible to a vocal order. For example, if the user says "Nestor allume la lumière" (Nestor turn on the light), the sentence duration is about 1s, and the processing time last generally between 1.5 and 2 s. This duration seems low but this is not true in real conditions when the user in the obscurity is waiting for the light. Thus, optimisation are needed to obtain fast recognizers.

8.2   Human Aspect

One of the main challenges to overcome for successful integration of VUI in AAL, is the adaptation of the system to the elderly users. Indeed, the ageing process is characterised by a decay of the main bio-physiological functions, affecting the social role and the integration of the ageing person in the society. Overall elderly people will be less inclined to adapt to a technology and its limitation (e.g., the constraint to pronounce words in a certain way) than younger adults and will present a very diverse set of profiles that make this population very difficult to design for.

For the elderly, there is a balance between the benefit of a monitoring through sensors and the correspondent intrusion into privacy. The system has to be protected against intrusion and has to make sure that the information reaches only the right people or can not go out of the smart home.

This is the most important aspect because if the system is not accepted by its potential users, it will never be used in practice.

Acknowledgments. This work is part of the SWEET-HOME project supported by the French National Research Agency (Agence Nationale de la Recherche / ANR-09-VERS-011).

References

1. Chan, M., Estève, D., Escriba, C., Campo, E.: A review of smart homes- present state and future challenges. Comput. Methods Programs Biomed. **91**(1), 55–81 (2008)
2. Vacher, M., Portet, F., Rossato, S., Aman, F., Golanski, C., Dugheanu, R.: Speech-based interaction in an AAL context. Gerontechnology **11**(2), 310 (2012)
3. Vacher, M., Portet, F., Fleury, A., Noury, N.: Development of audio sensing technology for ambient assisted living: applications and challenges. Int. J. E-Health Med. Commun. **2**(1), 35–54 (2011)
4. Katz, S., Akpom, C.: A measure of primary sociobiological functions. J. Health Serv. **6**(3), 493508 (1976)
5. Badii, A., Boudy, J.: CompanionAble - integrated cognitive assistive & domotic companion robotic systems for ability and security. In: 1st Congrés of the Société Française des Technologies pour l'Autonomie et de Gérontechnologie (SFTAG 2009), pp. 18–20, Troyes (2009)
6. Filho, G., Moir, T.: From science fiction to science fact: a smart-house interface using speech technology and a photorealistic avatar. Int. J. Comput. Appl. Technol. **39**(8), 32–39 (2010)
7. Gödde, F., Möller, S., Engelbrecht, K.P., Kühnel, C., Schleicher, R., Naumann, A., Wolters, M.: Study of a speech-based smart home system with older users. In: International Workshop on Intelligent User Interfaces for Ambient Assisted Living pp. 17–22 (2008)
8. Hamill, M., Young, V., Boger, J., Mihailidis, A.: Development of an automated speech recognition interface for personal emergency response systems. J. Neuro-Engineering Rehabil. **6**(1), 26 (2009)

9. Vacher, M., Chahuara, P., Lecouteux, B., Istrate, D., Portet, F., Joubert, T., Sehili, M.E.A., Meillon, B., Bonnefond, N., Fabre, S., Roux, C., Caffiau, S.: The SWEET-HOME project: audio technology in smart homes to improve well-being and reliance. In: 35th Annual International Conference of the IEEE Engineering in Medicine and Biology Society (EMBC 2013), Osaka, Japan, pp. 7298–7301, July 2013

10. Portet, F., Vacher, M., Golanski, C., Roux, C., Meillon, B.: Design and evaluation of a smart home voice interface for the elderly: acceptability and objection aspects. Pers. Ubiquit. Comput. **17**(1), 127–144 (2013)

11. López-Cózar, R., Callejas, Z.: Multimodal dialogue for ambient intelligence and smart environments. In: Nakashima, H., Aghajan, H., Augusto, J.C. (eds.) Handbook of Ambient Intelligence and Smart Environments, pp. 559–579. Springer, Berlin (2010)

12. Koskela, T., Väänänen-Vainio-Mattila, K.: Evolution towards smart home environments: empirical evaluation of three user interfaces. Pers. Ubiquit. Comput. **8**, 234–240 (2004)

13. Vacher, M., Portet, F., Fleury, A., Noury, N.: Challenges in the processing of audio channels for ambient assisted living. In: IEEE HealthCom 2010, Lyon, France, pp. 330–337, 1–3 July 2010

14. Mäyrä, F., Soronen, A., Vanhala, J., Mikkonen, J., Zakrzewski, M., Koskinen, I., Kuusela, K.: Probing a proactive home: challenges in researching and designing everyday smart environments. Hum. Technol. **2**, 158–186 (2006)

15. Edwards, W., Grinter, R.: At home with ubiquitous computing: seven challenges. In: Abowd, G., Brumitt, B., Shafer, S. (eds.) Ubicomp 2001. LNCS, vol. 2201, pp. 256–272. Springer, Heidelberg (2001)

16. Wölfel, M., McDonough, J.W.: Distant Speech Recognition. Wiley, New York (2009)

17. Deng, L., Acero, A., Plumpe, M., Huang, X.: Large-vocabulary speech recognition under adverse acoustic environments. In: ICSLP-2000, vol. 3, pp. 806–809. ISCA, Beijing, China (2000)

18. Baba, A., Lee, A., Saruwatari, H., Shikano, K.: Speech recognition by reverberation adapted acoustic model. In: ASJ General Meeting, pp. 27–28 (2002)

19. Michaut, F., Bellanger, M.: Filtrage adaptatif: théorie et algorithmes. Hermes Science Publication, Lavoisier (2005)

20. Valin, J.M.: On adjusting the learning rate in frequency domain echo cancellation with double talk. IEEE Trans. Acoust. Speech Signal Process. **15**(3), 1030–1034 (2007)

21. Vacher, M., Fleury, A., Guirand, N., Serignat, J.F., Noury, N.: Speech recognition in a smart home: some experiments for telemonitoring. In: Corneliu Burileanu, H.N.T. (ed.) From Speech Processing to Spoken Language Technology, pp. 171–179. Publishing House of the Romanian Academy, Constanta (2009)

22. Vacher, M., Fleury, A., Serignat, J.F., Noury, N., Glasson, H.: Preliminary evaluation of speech/sound recognition for telemedicine application in a real environment. In: Proceedings of the InterSpeech, pp. 496–499 (2008)

23. Reidel, K., Tamblyn, R., Patel, V., Huang, A.: Pilot study of an interactive voice response system to improve medication refill compliance. BMC Med. Inform. Decis. Mak. **8**, 46 (2008)

24. Vacher, M., Lecouteux, B., Chahuara, P., Portet, F., Meillon, B., Bonnefond, N.: The Sweet-Home speech and multimodal corpus for home automation interaction. In: The 9th edition of the Language Resources and Evaluation Conference (LREC), Reykjavik, Iceland, pp. 4499–4506 (2014)

25. Nocera, P., Linares, G., Massonié, D., Lefort, L.: Phoneme lattice based A* search algorithm for speech recognition. In: Sojka, P., Kopeček, I., Pala, K. (eds.) TSD 2002. LNCS (LNAI), vol. 2448, pp. 301–308. Springer, Heidelberg (2002)
26. Aman, F., Vacher, M., Rossato, S., Portet, F.: Speech recognition of aged voices in the AAL context: detection of distress sentences. In: The 7th International Conference on Speech Technology and Human-Computer Dialogue, SpeD 2013, Cluj-Napoca, Romania, pp. 177–184 (2013)
27. Wang, Y., Zhu, X.: A new approach for incremental speaker adaptation. In: Proceedings of the International Symposium on Chinese Spoken Language Processing (ISCSLP 2000), pp. 163–166 (2000)
28. Fiscus, J.G.: A post-processing system to yield reduced word error rates: recognizer output voting error reduction (ROVER). In: Proceedings of the IEEE Workshop ASRU, pp. 347–354 (1997)
29. Lecouteux, B., Linarès, G., Estève, Y., Mauclair, J.: System combination by driven decoding. In: Proceedings of the IEEE International Conference on Acoustics, Speech and Signal Processing ICASSP 2007, vol. 4, pp. IV-341–IV-344 (2007)
30. Lecouteux, B., Linarès, G., Estève, Y., Gravier, G.: Generalized driven decoding for speech recognition system combination. In: Proceedings of the IEEE International Conference on Acoustics, Speech and Signal Processing ICASSP 2008, pp. 1549–1552 (2008)
31. Lecouteux, B., Linarès, G., Nocéra, P., Bonastre, J.: Reconnaissance de la parole guidée par des transcriptions approchées. In: Journées d'Etudes sur la Parole (JEP 2006), Dinard, France, pp. 53–56 (2006)
32. Berndt, D., Clifford, J.: Using dynamic time warping to find patterns in time series. In: Workshop on Knowledge Discovery in Databases (KDD 1994) pp. 359–370 (1994)
33. Vacher, M., Lecouteux, B., Istrate, D., Joubert, T., Portet, F., Sehili, M., Chahuara, P.: Experimental evaluation of speech recognition technologies for voice-based home automation control in a smart home. In: 4th Workshop on Speech and Language Processing for Assistive Technologies, Grenoble, France, pp. 99–105 (2013)
34. Chahuara, P., Portet, F., Vacher, M.: Making context aware decision from uncertain information in a smart home: a Markov logic network approach. In: Augusto, J.C., Wichert, R., Collier, R., Keyson, D., Salah, A.A., Tan, A.-H. (eds.) AmI 2013. LNCS, vol. 8309, pp. 78–93. Springer, Heidelberg (2013)
35. Franco, A.: Conférence invitée: Nouveaux paradigmes et technologies pour la santé et l'autonomie (invited conference: new paradigms and technologies for health and autonomy) [in french]. In: JEP-TALN-RECITAL 2012, Workshop ILADI 2012: Interactions Langagières pour personnes Agées Dans les habitats Intelligents (ILADI 2012: Language Interaction for Elderly in Smart Homes), pp. 1–2. ATALA/AFCP, Grenoble, France, June 2012
36. Vacher, M., Lecouteux, B., Portet, F.: Recognition of voice commands by multi-source ASR and noise cancellation in a smart home environment. In: EUSIPCO (European Signal Processing Conference), Bucarest, Romania, pp. 1663–1667, 27–31 August 2012
37. Gemmeke, J.F., Ons, B., Tessema, N., hamme, H.V., van de Loo, J., Pauw, G.D., Daelemans, W., Huyghe, J., Derboven, J., Vuegen, L., Broeck, B.V.D., Karsmakers, P., Vanrumste, B.: Self-taught assistive vocal interfaces: an overview of the ALADIN project. In: Interspeech 2013, pp. 2039–2043 (2013)

38. Christensen, H., Casanueva, I., Cunningham, S., Green, P., Hain, T.: homeService: Voice-enabled assistive technology in the home using cloud-based automatic speech recognition. In: 4th Workshop on Speech and Language Processing for Assistive Technologies (2013)
39. Cristoforetti, L., Ravanelli, M., Omologo, M., Sosi, A., Abad, A., Hagmueller, M., Maragos, P.: The DIRHA simulated corpus. In: The 9th edition of the Language Resources and Evaluation Conference (LREC), Reykjavik, Iceland, pp. 2629–2634 (2014)
40. Rougui, J., Istrate, D., Souidene, W.: Audio sound event identification for distress situations and context awareness. In: Annual International Conference of the IEEE Engineering in Medicine and Biology Society, EMBC 2009, Minneapolis, USA, pp. 3501–3504 (2009)
41. Milhorat, P., Istrate, D., Boudy, J., Chollet, G.: Hands-free speech-sound interactions at home. In: Proceedings of the 20th European Signal Processing Conference (EUSIPCO), pp. 1678–1682, August 2012
42. Lines, L., Hone, K.S.: Multiple voices, multiple choices: older adults' evaluation of speech output to support independent living. Gerontechnology J. 5(2), 78–91 (2006)
43. Wolters, M.K., Georgila, K., Moore, J.D., MacPherson, S.E.: Being old doesn't mean acting old: how older users interact with spoken dialog systems. TACCESS 2(1), 1–31 (2009)
44. Cavazza, M., de la Camara, R.S., Turunen, M.: How was your day?: a companion ECA. In: AAMAS, pp. 1629–1630 (2010)
45. Istrate, D., Vacher, M., Serignat, J.F.: Embedded implementation of distress situation identification through sound analysis. J. Inf. Technol. Healthc. 6, 204–211 (2008)
46. Charalampos, D., Maglogiannis, I.: Enabling human status awareness in assistive environments based on advanced sound and motion data classification. In: Proceedings of the 1st international conference on PErvasive Technologies Related to Assistive Environments, pp. 1:1–1:8 (2008)
47. Popescu, M., Li, Y., Skubic, M., Rantz, M.: An acoustic fall detector system that uses sound height information to reduce the false alarm rate. In: Proceedings 30th Annual International Conference of the IEEE-EMBS 2008, pp. 4628–4631, 20–25 August 2008
48. Lecouteux, B., Vacher, M., Portet, F.: Distant speech recognition in a smart home: comparison of several multisource ASRs in realistic conditions. In: Association, I.S.C. (ed.) Interspeech 2011 Florence, pp. 2273–2276. Florence, Italy (2011)
49. Bouakaz, S., Vacher, M., Bobillier-Chaumon, M.E., Aman, F., Bekkadja, S., Portet, F., Guillou, E., Rossato, S., Desserée, E., Traineau, P., Vimon, J.P., Chevalier, T.: CIRDO: smart companion for helping elderly to live at home for longer. IRBM 35(2), 101–108 (2014)
50. Barker, J., Vincent, E., Ma, N., Christensen, H., Green, P.: The PASCAL CHiME speech separation and recognition challenge. Comput. Speech Lang. 27(3), 621–633 (2013)
51. Vincent, E., Barker, J., Watanabe, S., Le Roux, J., Nesta, F., Matassoni, M.: The second 'CHiME' speech separation and recognition challenge: an overview of challenge systems and outcomes. In: 2013 IEEE Automatic Speech Recognition and Understanding Workshop, Olomouc, Czech Republic, December 2013
52. Ryan, W., Burk, K.: Perceptual and acoustic correlates in the speech of males. J. Commun. Disord. 7, 181–192 (1974)

53. Takeda, N., Thomas, G., Ludlow, C.: Aging effects on motor units in the human thyroarytenoid muscle. Laryngoscope **110**, 1018–1025 (2000)
54. Mueller, P., Sweeney, R., Baribeau, L.: Acoustic and morphologic study of the senescent voice. Ear Nose Throat J. **63**, 71–75 (1984)
55. Vipperla, R.C., Wolters, M., Georgila, K., Renals, S.: Speech input from older users in smart environments: challenges and perspectives. In: Stephanidis, C. (ed.) Universal Access in HCI, Part II, HCII 2009. LNCS, vol. 5615, pp. 117–126. Springer, Heidelberg (2009)
56. Pellegrini, T., Trancoso, I., Hämäläinen, A., Calado, A., Dias, M.S., Braga, D.: Impact of age in ASR for the elderly: preliminary experiments in European Portuguese. In: Torre Toledano, D., Ortega Giménez, A., Teixeira, A., González Rodríguez, J., Hernández Gómez, L., San Segundo Hernández, R., Ramos Castro, D. (eds.) IberSPEECH 2012. CCIS, vol. 328, pp. 139–147. Springer, Heidelberg (2012)
57. Baba, A., Yoshizawa, S., Yamada, M., Lee, A., Shikano, K.: Acoustic models of the elderly for large-vocabulary continuous speech recognition. Electron. Commun. **87**(2), 49–57 (2004)
58. Vipperla, R., Renals, S., Frankel, J.: Longitudinal study of ASR performance on ageing voices. In: Proceedings of Interspeech 2008, Brisbane, pp. 2550–2553 (2008)
59. Baeckman, L., Small, B., Wahlin, A.: Aging and memory: cognitive and biological perspectives. In: Birren, J.E., Schaie, K.W. (eds.) Handbook of the Psychology of Aging, 5th edn, pp. 349–377. Academic Press, San Diego (2001)
60. Fozard, J., Gordont-Salant, S.: Changes in vision and hearing with aging. In: Birren, J.E., Schaie, K.W. (eds.) Handbook of the Psychology of Aging, 5th edn, pp. 241–266. Academic Press, San Diego (2001)
61. Audibert, N., Aubergé, V., Rilliard, A.: The prosodic dimensions of emotion in speech: the relative weights of parameters. In: Proceedings of Interspeech 2005, Lisbon, Portugal, pp. 525–528 (2005)
62. Vlasenko, B., Prylipko, D., Philippou-Hübner, D., Wendemuth, A.: Vowels formants analysis allows straightforward detection of high arousal acted and spontaneous emotions. Proc. Interspeech **2011**, 1577–1580 (2011)
63. Vlasenko, B., Prylipko, D., Wendemuth, A.: Towards robust spontaneous speech recognition with emotional speech adapted acoustic models. In: 35th German Conference on Artificial Intelligence (KI-2012), Saarbrücken, Germany, pp. 103–107, September 2012
64. Aman, F., Auberge, V., Vacher, M.: How affects can perturbe the automatic speech recognition of domotic interactions. In: Workshop on Affective Social Speech Signals, Grenoble, France, pp. 1–5 (2013)
65. Ziefle, M., Wilkowska, W.: Technology acceptability for medical assistance. In: PervasiveHealth, pp. 1–9, March 2010
66. McCoy, K., Waller, A.: Introduction to the special issue on AAC. ACM Trans. Access. Comput. **1**(3), 1–34 (2009)
67. McCoy, K., Arnott, J., Ferres, L., Fried-Oken, M., Roark, B.: Speech and language processing as assistive technologies. Comput. Speech Lang. **27**, 1143–1146 (2013)

A User-Centered Design Approach to Physical Motion Coaching Systems for Pervasive Health

Norimichi Ukita[1]($\boxtimes$), Daniel Kaulen[2], and Carsten Röcker[2]

[1] Nara Institute of Science and Technology, Takayama, Ikoma, Nara 8916-5, Japan
`ukita@is.naist.jp`
[2] RWTH Aachen University, Campus-Boulevard 57, 52074 Aachen, Germany
`roecker@comm.rwth-aachen.de`

Abstract. Our goal is to develop a system for coaching human motions (e.g., for rehabilitation and daily health maintenance). This paper focuses on how to coach a user so that his/her motion gets closer to the good template of a target motion. It is important to efficiently advise the user to emulate the crucial features that define the good template. The proposed system (1) automatically mines the crucial features of any kind of motion from a set of motion features and (2) gives the user feedback about how to modify the motion through an intuitive interface. The crucial features are mined by feature sparsification through binary classification between the samples of good and other motions. An interface for motion coaching is designed to give feedback via different channels (e.g., visually, aurally), depending on the type of error. To use the total system, all the user must do is just move and then get feedback on the motion. Following experimental results, open problems for future work are discussed.

Keywords: Motion coaching · Error feedback · Physical rehabilitation

1 Introduction

1.1 Background

The number of people suffering from chronic diseases is constantly rising [1–3]. Today, more than three quarters of the elderly population are suffering from chronic diseases, independent of the economic, social, and cultural background [4]. However, not only the prevalence of chronic illnesses increases with age but also the likeliness of suffering from physical as well as mental disabilities. Statistical data from Great Britain [5] shows that around half of all disabled persons are 65 years or older.

A serious problem closely connected with declining physical abilities is an increased risk of falls. Statistics of the World Health Organization [6] show that approximately one third of the people over 65 years and half of the people over 80 years of age fall each year. Similar data is reported by Nehmer et al. [7]. Around 20 % to 30 % of the falls lead to serious injuries with long-term consequences for the patients [8]. Statistical data from the UK [9] shows that falls are the major cause for disability in the age group of people over 75 and a leading cause of mortality due to injury. The most common serious injuries related

© Springer International Publishing Switzerland 2015
A. Holzinger et al. (Eds.): Smart Health, LNCS 8700, pp. 189–208, 2015.
DOI: 10.1007/978-3-319-16226-3_8

to falls in older people are hip fractures, which result in annual costs of over 2 billion Euros for England alone [10].

The demographic change, which can be observed in most industrialized countries around the globe, does not only lead to an increased number of elderly people but also contributes to a continuous decline of the working population. For example, it is expected that the working force in Europe will decrease by 48 million people until 2050 while the dependency ratio is expected to double, reaching 51 % in the same time [11]. Consequently, the ratio between the working population and older citizens above 65 will shrink from currently 4:1 to only 2:1 in the coming 40 years. This development will inevitably result in a reduction of the number of people who can provide care to older and disabled people [8]. Together with the financial constraints that most are currently facing, it will become increasingly difficult to find enough caregivers for the growing number of elderly people [12].

In this context, pervasive homecare environments are often cited as a promising solution for providing automated and personalized healthcare solutions for a growing number of elderly people [7,10,12]. Pervasive healthcare environments are usually equipped with different types of sensors for automated data capturing as well as different types of output devices including large screens [13–15], mobile devices [16,17], and ambient displays [18,19]. Over the last decade, several prototype systems have been developed (e.g., [2–5,8,11]), which demonstrate the potential of such environments for individually supporting different user groups [6,20].

Within this paper, we describe the development of an automatic motion coaching system which makes use of typical input and output technologies available in pervasive homecare environments in order to provide new user-centered training and rehabilitation concepts [9]. For easy-to-use coaching systems [1], it is important to efficiently advise a user to emulate the crucial features that define the good template. This is because many other features of the target motion might be varied among individuals, but those variations give less impacts on evaluating the target motion. The proposed method automatically mines the crucial features of any kind of motion. The crucial features are mined based on feature sparsification through binary classification between the samples of good and other motions. The following section provides a more detailed overview of the proposed system.

1.2   Our Approaches and Related Work

Motion Measurement. We aimed at developing a user-centered system for coaching human movement. For motion measurement in the laboratory stage, multi-camera systems, [21–23], allow us to acquire highly accurate results, but they are too expensive for realizing pervasive health systems. We have seen a tremendous improvement of commercial real-time motion tracking devices. Systems like Microsoft Kinect, Nintendo Wiimote, or PlayStation Move provide low-cost solutions for end-users in home environments. The proposed system utilizes an inexpensive depth-measurement sensor (i.e., Microsoft Kinect) in order to get high-measurement accuracy without devices attached to the body for easy-to-use operation.

Motion Coaching Systems. During the last years, several motion coaching systems have been developed. Most systems focus on a special type of motion or exercise. This is due to the fact that there are tremendous differences between motions that have to be considered when analyzing motion data programmatically.

A review of several virtual environments for training in ball sports was introduced in [24]. They stressed that coaching and skill acquisition usually involve three distinct processes: conveying information (i.e., observational learning), structuring practice (i.e., contextual inference), and the nature and administration of feedback (i.e., feedback frequency, timing, and precision). Additionally, general possibilities when to provide feedback were identified. Concurrent feedback (during), terminal feedback (immediately following), or delayed feedback (some period after) can be used to assist the subject in correcting the motion.

One recent concurrent feedback approach was taken by Velloso et al. [25]. Another example for concurrent feedback was presented by Matsumoto et al. [26] who combined visual and haptic feedback. Even though their device greatly improved the performance, it was very awkward to perform the exercises with it due to its weight.

How to assist weightlifting training by tracking the exercises with a Kinect and using delayed feedback is proposed by Chatzitofis et al. [27]. However, there is still need for a human trainer to interpret those values in order to give feedback to the subject. The tennis instruction system developed by Takano et al. [28] also uses a delayed feedback approach but the focus is put on the process of observational learning. Due to the absence of any explicit feedback in [28], it is hard to determine how to actually correct the motion.

An example for terminal feedback can be found in [29] where the focus is put on the correct classification of motion errors while feedback is given immediately after the completion of the motion. However, this only allows the correction of previously known and trained error types.

To systematically analyze possible designs of motion coaching systems, the related work can be classified in a three-dimensional design space of multimodality [30]. The modality (visual, auditory, haptic) is chosen depending on the type of input that the computer or human needs to perceive or convey information.

A single system generally consists of multiple points in this design space (represented as a connected series of points). For example, the system developed by Chatzitofis et al. [27] can be controlled with mouse and keyboard (haptic input of control), visualizes performance metrics (visual output of data), and captures motion data by using the Kinect system (visual input of data).

In some cases, the differentiation between output of control and data is not unambiguous. Nevertheless, this can still be visualized. For example, in [25] the output of an arrow indicating the direction in which to move the left or right arm can be regarded as both, output of data and control. In the following, this type of visualization will be referred to as output of control.

2   Glossary

Depth sensor is an optical sensor that measures 3D distance from the sensor to 3D points in a scene. The measured results are obtained as a gray-scale image in which each pixel value represents the 3D distance. The examples of the depth image are shown in Fig. 1 (i.e., "Depth images" in the figure). There are several kinds of depth sensors, which are classified by a mechanism for measuring 3D distance.

Expensive but accurate sensors are based on Time-Of-Flight (TOF) measurement. A TOF sensor measures 3D distance by measuring the lapse of time after the sensor emits light and before the light returns to the sensor.

Some other depth sensors are based on triangulation. Unlike human eyes that observe a 3D point from different view points for triangulation (which is often called stereo vision), many triangulation-based depth sensors emit light and observe it from a different viewpoint for triangulation. This approach allows us to easily measure 3D distance because point correspondence is easy; in stereo vision, on the other hand, we must make a pixel correspondence between different views (i.e., different images) based on noisy image features so that pixels observing the same 3D point are paired.

Structured-light based sensors are also popular. These sensors emit a known spatial light pattern and observes it. Based on its deformation projected on a 3D surface in a scene, depth measurement can be achieved.

Kinect is a world-wide popular depth sensor developed by Microsoft. It can capture color and depth images simultaneously. Its depth measurement is based on the structured-light mechanism.

Motion capture system is used for obtaining the 3D human pose of a real person. A number of commercial products have been already developed, but all of them are still expensive. Several kinds of motion capture systems have been developed, namely optical systems with passive/active markers, inertial systems, mechanical systems, and magnetic systems.

Support Vector Machine (SVM) is a pattern classifier [31]. Any pattern is computationally expressed by a vector. In pattern classification, each pattern is attributed to a class (e.g., "good" or "bad").

3D Human Pose (aka a 3D skeleton) is computationally represented by a set of 3D joint positions and links that connect physically-connected joints. Its examples are illustrated in Fig. 1 (i.e., "Pose sequence" in the figure).

3   State-of-the-Art

3.1   System Overview

Figure 1 illustrates the overview of the proposed system consisting of two steps.

An offline model-learning step is performed before users are coached by the system. In this step, two kinds of computational models are trained. For learning

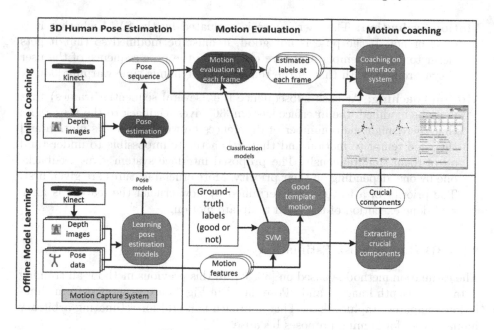

Fig. 1. Overview of the system.

the pose estimation model (i.e., "Pose models" in Fig. 1) that represents the relationship between human poses and features extracted from depth images, the samples of a target motion are captured by a synchronized Kinect and motion capture system (i.e., "Kinect" and "Motion capture system" of "Offline model learning" in Fig. 1). The pose classification model ("Classification models" in Fig. 1) is acquired by the Support Vector Machine [32] ("SVM" in Fig. 1) to evaluate whether the human pose at each frame is good or not.[1] In addition, the crucial features of the target motion (i.e., "Crucial components" in Fig. 1) are mined by a sparse coding regularization in the SVM.

In an online coaching step, with the model learned beforehand, the system observes the motion of a user with a Kinect camera (i.e., "Kinect" of "Online coaching" in Fig. 1), estimates the human pose at every frame (i.e., "Pose estimation" in Fig. 1), evaluates whether or not each pose is required to be modified (i.e., "Motion evaluation at each frame" in Fig. 1), and coaches the user. In the online coaching step, the three modules interact with a user as follows:

3D human pose estimation: A 3D human pose at each frame is estimated from a depth image captured by a Kinect. The estimation method is based on [33,34]. The accuracy of the pose estimation is improved by using real pose data captured by the motion capture system instead of synthesized CG data employed in [33,34].

---

[1] We assume that a target motion can be classified into good and other motions. For example, any motion in rehabilitation should be as correct (i.e., good) as possible.

Motion evaluation: The user's pose is evaluated by the SVM whether it is good or not. If the pose is not good, it must be modified so that it gets closer to a good template. Before evaluation, the pose sequence of the user is synchronized with that of the template by dynamic time warping [35].

Motion coaching: At each subsequence (i.e., several sequential frames) that must be modified, the interface system [36] gives feedback to the user. Note that there might be a number of differences between the user's motion and the good template motion and that it is actually impossible to understand all of them simultaneously. The proposed interface system gives feedbacks one by one, depending on their priority. More crucial features are given first. The priority of a feature is determined by how crucial the feature is for a well done execution of the good template motion.

3.2 3D Human Pose Estimation

The estimation method is based on [33,34]. In this previous method, all training data (i.e., "Depth images" and "Pose data" in Fig. 1) are generated from simulation computer graphics data. This approach is useful for estimating arbitrary human poses for gaming proposes because

- it is difficult to collect the synchronized human pose and depth data of a large variety of arbitrary human poses, and
- even if the pose estimation error is relatively large due to modeling errors of a variety of human poses, it might still be acceptable for gaming purposes.

In contrast to pose estimation for gaming purposes, for motion coaching it should be more accurate. In particular, accurate pose estimation is required for rehabilitation purposes.

In the proposed system, accuracy in pose estimation is improved by using real observation data of human motions. The real depth images and human data are captured by Kinect and a motion capture system. The left and right images in Fig. 2 show a 3D point cloud computed from a captured depth image and a skeletal human pose, respectively.

From a technical point of view, spatial alignment and temporal synchronization between the point cloud and the pose are required.

Temporal Synchronization. Since a moving human body is captured by two independent sensors, their captured data must be synchronized; a depth image and pose data in the same frame of an image sequence and a pose sequence must be captured at the same moment.

Unfortunately, Kinect does not have a hardware synchronization mechanism. Instead, in the proposed system a software synchronization between those two data sets is established.

For this synchronization, a predefined motion is performed by a subject. This predefined motion is required to have a key frame that can be easily identified in both depth image and pose sequences. The depth image and pose sequences are

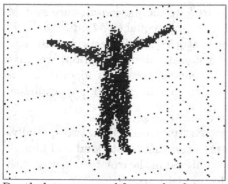

Depth data extracted from a depth image captured by Kinect

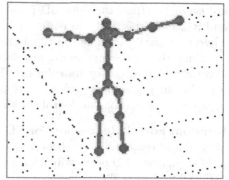

Human pose data (skeleton) obtained by a motion capture system, IGS-190

Fig. 2. Real depth and pose data, necessary to create a 3D pose model.

synchronized so that each of their key frames is a first frame in each sequence. After the first frame, f_I-th frame of the image sequence is temporally aligned with $f_P = \frac{F_P}{F_I}(f-1)+1$-th frame, where F_P and F_I denote the frames-per-second of the motion capture system and Kinect, respectively. In the experiments shown in this paper, the subjects had to raise their right arm so that the key frame where the hand was located in the highest position could be identified.

Spatial Alignment. Kinect and the motion capture system have their own coordinate systems. They must be aligned in order to completely overlap the 3D point cloud and the pose of a subject.

Assume that the temporal synchronization is established. Spatial alignment is achieved by translating and rotating the coordinate system of one of the two sensors (i.e., in our experiments the motion capture system) so that the 3D positions of several key points coincide with each other between the two coordinate systems. Since the number of unknown parameters is 6 (i.e., 3 degrees of freedom in translation and 3 degrees of freedom in rotation), at least 2 pairs of corresponding points between the point cloud and the human pose are needed for estimating those unknown parameters; each pair gives us 3 equations (i.e., x, y, and z matching).

The following Eq. (1) expresses the translation and rotation of a 3D point $\boldsymbol{M}$:

$$\boldsymbol{M}' = \boldsymbol{T} + \boldsymbol{R}\boldsymbol{M}, \tag{1}$$

$$\boldsymbol{T} = (t_x, t_y, t_z)^T, \tag{2}$$

$$\boldsymbol{R} = \begin{pmatrix} 1 & 0 & 0 \\ 0 & \cos(\alpha) & -\sin(\alpha) \\ 0 & \sin(\alpha) & \cos(\alpha) \end{pmatrix} \begin{pmatrix} \cos(\beta) & 0 & \sin(\beta) \\ 0 & 1 & 0 \\ -\sin(\beta) & 0 & \cos(\beta) \end{pmatrix} \begin{pmatrix} \cos(\gamma) & -\sin(\gamma) & 0 \\ \sin(\gamma) & \cos(\gamma) & 0 \\ 0 & 0 & 1 \end{pmatrix} \tag{3}$$

Here, t_x, t_y, t_z, α, β, and γ are 6 unknown parameters. Given a 3D position $\boldsymbol{M}_P$ of the human pose, these 6 parameters are optimized so that $\boldsymbol{M}'_P$ is equal to the corresponding 3D position $\boldsymbol{M}_I$ of the point cloud. Note that $\boldsymbol{M}_P$ and $\boldsymbol{M}_I$

are extracted from the same 3D point captured by the motion capture system and Kinect, respectively. In reality, M'_P might not be equal to M_I due to noise. Therefore, the 6 parameters are optimized so that $\|M'_P - M_I\|$ gets close to zero.

Since the above-mentioned problem is a non-linear optimization, we have a variety of options for its solution. The LevenbergMarquardt algorithm was used in our experiments. If three or more corresponding points are available, parameter estimation can be robust to noise.

Random Forest Regression for 3D Pose Estimation. Given two spatially-aligned and temporally-synchronized sequences (i.e., 3D point cloud and human pose sequences), 3D pose estimation can be achieved in the exact same way with [34]. All frames in the sequences are used for model learning.

With the model learned, we can obtain the 3D human pose at each frame only from a depth image captured by the Kinect. The sequence of the estimated human poses is employed for motion evaluation described in the following section.

3.3   Mining Crucial Features for Motion Evaluation

Mining Crucial Features via Sparse Coding. For evaluating the motion of a user (i.e., classifying the motion to good or other motions), the SVM is used in the proposed system. This classification is performed with a number of features that represent the 3D pose and the motion of a human body. Since (1) the system should be applicable to any kind of motion and (2) we do not know which features of a target motion are crucial for defining the target motion, it is better to exhaustively use all features that possibly represent a body motion. In experiments, the concatenation of the following components was used as a 621D feature vector which consists of:

- 3D positions of all joints (3D × 18 joints = 54D)
- 3D velocities of all joints (3D × 18 joints = 54D)
- 3D accelerations of all joints (3D × 18 joints = 54D)
- 3D displacement between any pairs of joints (3D × 153 = 459D).

From these 621 features, the proposed method automatically mines which body parts and/or motions are crucial for improving the movement of a user. This mining is achieved by the sparse coding regularization in the SVM, as proposed in [37]. In classification, the inner product of the feature vectors of a test pose (denoted by v) and the weight vector w is computed. If the inner product is above/below 0, the test pose is regarded as a positive/negative class (e.g., good/others). Therefore, components with a larger absolute value in w correspond to crucial features that have a large impact on the inner product. In learning the SVM, the l_1-regularized logistic regression [37] is employed so that the gap between larger and smaller absolute values of w gets much greater.

This sparsification can be regarded as dimensionality reduction because the dimensions with smaller values can be neglected. For dimensionality reduction, many other techniques have been proposed (e.g., PCA, LLE [38], Isomap [39], GPLVM [40]). Those techniques, however, cannot provide a user intuitive feedbacks for understanding how to modify the motion. This is because these techniques project a vector from a high-dimensional space to a low-dimensional space defined by an arbitrary subspace in the high-dimensional space. That is, each axis in the low-dimensional space might correspond to multiple axes in the original high-dimensional space. As a result, even if a motion feature corresponding to only one axis in a subspace obtained by PCA or similar techniques is selected, a user might be required to move the body as follows: "you should move the right hand, the right elbow, the left toe, and the hip so that ...". On the other hand, in the proposed method, only one motion feature (e.g., "the right hand" or "the right elbow") is selected from the low-dimensional space generated by the sparse coding regularization.

Experiments of Feature Mining. Experiments were conducted with baseball pitching motions[2] captured from 34 people; 13 good (i.e., expert) players and 21 beginners. From these 34 people, 445 sequences were captured in total. Both pose estimation and classification models were trained by the data of 33 people, and the data of the remaining one person was used for testing. Note that all 621 features were normalized.

The following two ways were tested for selecting crucial motion features:

(a) **Naive selection:** The distance between features of a user's pose and a good template is computed at each feature component (e.g., 3D position of the right hand); the distance at i-th feature is denoted by d_f. Features having the larger distance are regarded as crucial features.

(b) **Selection with the sparsification:** d_f is multiplied with the weight of f-th feature (i.e., f-th component of w). Features having the larger product are regarded as crucial features.

Motions selected by the above two criteria, (a) and (b), were checked by expert players. In examples shown in Fig. 3, naive selection recommended the left toe velocity as the most crucial motion (i.e., (a) in Fig. 3), while the right hand was selected by the proposed method (i.e., (b) in Fig. 3). It is natural that the motion of the hand holding a ball is more important for pitching. The experts also validated the selection of the proposed method.

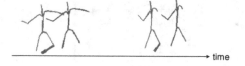

(a) Crucial feature of naive selection (i.e., left toe velocity)

(b) Crucial feature selected by the proposed method (i.e., right hand velocity)

Fig. 3. Visual feedbacks illustrating the difference between the user's motion (shown with red) and the good template (shown with blue) in pitching motions (Colour figure online).

---

[2] To validate the system, a sport motion is a good example because its exercise is important for skill proficiency of beginners as well as rehabilitation of experts.

Experiments of Using Features for Motion Evaluation. We also demonstrate the effectiveness of the sparsification in motion evaluation. The mean classification rate of all 445 sequences, each of which was evaluated by leave-one-out cross-validation, is computed. The means over all frames were 67 % and 76 % in (a) and (b), respectively. These results demonstrate the effectiveness of the sparsification also in motion classification. This effect is gained because a low-dimensional feature space allows us to improve the generalizing capability of classifiers such as the SVM, as described in [41].

3.4   Motion Coaching Interface

Just a simple visualization of a motion difference (e.g., Fig. 3) might not be intuitive for motion coaching, depending on the type of motion error. This section discusses what kind of feedback is appropriate for each type of motion error.

Interface Design. To combine the ideas of motion errors and different types of motion feedback, a prototype system was implemented that enables first experiments with some of the proposed feedback types.

JavaFX was used as an underlying framework since it allows fast creation of user interfaces with JavaFX Scene Builder and provides built-in support for animations and charts. For the user to be able to concentrate on the visualization, the system takes two synchronized motion sequence files that contain information about joint positions at each point in time as input. Synchronized in this context means that frame number i in the template motion corresponds with frame number i in the comparison motion. Figure 4 shows a screenshot of the system. In this interface, joints that are not relevant for a special motion can be de-selected manually.

Motion Errors and Feedback Types. The first step when thinking about how to provide motion error feedback is to become aware of different types of

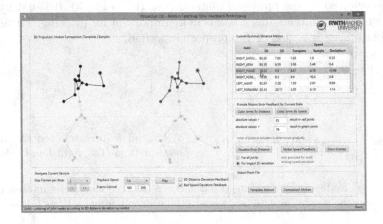

Fig. 4. Screenshot of the motion coaching system.

motion errors (i.e., deviation between a template and comparison motion) that need to be addressed. To that extent, it is obvious to differentiate between the spatial and temporal dimension.

When just considering the spatial dimension, there are three main types of motion errors that can occur. First, the absolute position of a joint can be wrong. When only the spatial collocation of several joints is important, the relative position of them should be taken into account instead. For example, a clapping motion can be defined only by the spatial relationship between the palms (i.e., the palms touch each other or not). The last main error type is a wrong angle between neighboring joints. Naturally, the angle is influenced by the actual positions of the joints, but it is expected that a different type of visualization is required depending on whether the focus is put on the angle or the absolute joint position.

In a next step, several general ways to provide feedback by using different modalities were elaborated.

The most natural but technically the most complex way when using the visual channel is to either extract only the human body or to use the complete real scene and overlay it with visual feedback (e.g., colored overlay of body parts depending on the distance error). The natural scene reduces the cognitive load for the subject as the mapping between the real world and the visualization is trivial. Displaying the human body as a skeleton makes this mapping a bit harder but allows to put the focus on the motion itself. To compare a template with a comparison motion, the abstracted skeletons can be visualized side by side or in an overlaid manner, as shown in Fig. 5. It is expected that the overlaid view is mainly applicable when trying to correct very small motion errors. At a higher abstraction level, performance metrics such as speed or distance deviation per joint or body part can be displayed textually or graphically (i.e., with the aid of charts). There is, however, no information on how to correct the motion and the subjects need to interpret those values to improve their motion. To overcome this weakness, it is desirable to be able to visualize instructions (i.e., visual output of control) that guide users in correcting their motion. Two possible

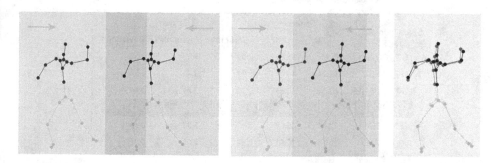

Fig. 5. Visualization of two skeletons, one captured online and one of a template motion. Left: side-by-side comparison. Right: overlay.

approaches are simple textual instructions [42] or graphical instructions such as arrows indicating the direction in which the motion should be corrected [25].

Audio feedback can be used in several ways to give motion error feedback. Spoken instructions (i.e., auditory output of control) are one possible way to which most people are already used to from real training situations. Note that the bandwidth of the auditory channel is much lower than the one of the visual channel and therefore not much information can be provided at the same time. Nevertheless, the audio feedback has the big advantage that it easily catches human attention and users do not have to look in a special direction (e.g., for observing a screen). In terms of auditory output of data, different parameters of sound (i.e., frequency, tone, volume) can be modified to represent special motion errors. A first step in this direction was taken by Takahata et al. [43] in a karate training scenario.

Another important point of research is the question of how to motivate people to use a motion coaching system. As it is commonly accepted that the use of multiple modalities increases learning performance (see [44], for example), a motion coaching system should aim at addressing multiple senses. Therefore, several of the ideas above are combined in the proposed interface.

The use of haptic output devices is not treated as applicable for a motion coaching system used to teach a wide range of different exercises due to two main reasons: First, there is no reliable and generic way to translate instructions into haptic patterns (see [45], for example). Second, specially adapted hardware is required to provide appropriate haptic feedback, which is then often considered disturbing [26].

Multimodal Feedback Types Visual Output of Data 1 – Metrics (Textual). The performance metrics illustrated in Fig. 6 provide basic information such as 3D and 2D distance deviations per joint and a comparison of the template and sample speed per joint. Due to the perspective projection of the real-world 3D coordinates to the joint positions in the visualized 2D skeleton on

Current Euclidian Distance Metrics

Joint	Distance		Speed		
	3D	2D	Template	Sample	Deviation▼
LEFT_FOOT	82.03	15.73	2.61	3.19	0.58
LEFT_HAND	82.29	4.9	2.94	3.45	0.51
LEFT_FOOT_HEEL	80.38	10.63	2.75	3.21	0.46
LEFT_LEG	85.63	9.86	2.64	3.08	0.44
LEFT_FOREARM	82.67	16.68	2.52	2.87	0.35
RIGHT_HAND	80.75	10.81	2.67	2.89	0.22

Fig. 6. Distance and speed metrics for a single pair of frames for currently loaded motion sequences.

the screen, it may occur that there are large 3D deviations that are not recognizable in the skeleton representation. The data helps to get an understanding of this relation and allows for a very detailed motion analysis. Nevertheless, this high precision is not necessarily needed for a motion coaching scenario and a subject may only use this type for terminal or delayed feedback.

Visual Output of Data 2 – Metrics (Graphical). Charts are used to visualize distance and speed metrics over time. Multiple joints can be selected to be included in a single chart to compare the respective deviations. From a motion coaching perspective, this type of feedback is mainly suited for terminal or delayed feedback. Figures 7 and 8 visualize the deviations of the distance and the speed (between the template and comparison motion) of two different joints for a small frame interval, respectively. As real-world data is often subject to large fluctuations, values are smoothed for visualization purposes by calculating a weighted average for the k-step neighborhood (k between 5 and 10), see an

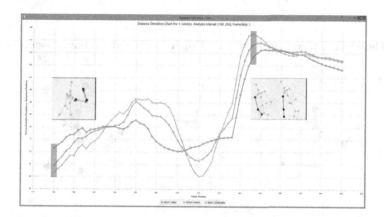

Fig. 7. Distance deviation chart for right forearm (selected series)and right hand.

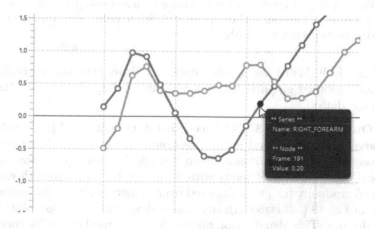

Fig. 8. Speed deviation chart for right forearm (selected series) and right hand.

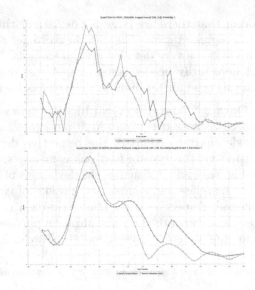

Fig. 9. The effect of temporal smoothing. Upper: original data. Lower: smoothed data.

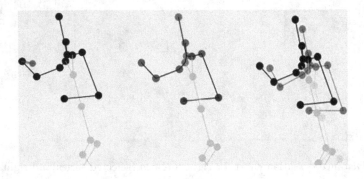

Fig. 10. Exemplary skeleton-based distance error visualizations (left: colored joint overlay, center: overlay of template and comparison skeleton, right: static result of animated joint moving to its correct position).

example in Fig. 9. While the original data was noisy (the upper graph in the figure), its smoothed graph is better for understanding the motion (the lower graph in the data).

Visual Output of Data 3 – Colored Joint Overlay. All joints with deviations larger than upper and lower thresholds, which are given manually, are respectively colored in red and green (applicable for speed and distance deviations). The coloring of joints with values in between those thresholds is determined gradually (i.e., vary from red over orange to green). An example can be found in Fig. 10 (left skeleton): the largest deviations occur for joints located in the right arm. This visualization approach can be used either for concurrent, terminal, or delayed feedback and allows to easily determine joints with high deviations.

Visual Output of Data 4 – Skeleton Overlay. Visualizing the template and comparison skeleton in an overlaid manner (instead of side by side which is the default behavior of the proposed system) turned out to be only suitable to correct very small motion errors. Otherwise the mapping between the intended and actual joint position is not directly visible. Oftentimes, it is hard to differentiate between the two skeletons. To overcome this weakness, the opacity value of the template is lower than the one of the comparison skeleton (see Fig. 10, center).

Visual Output of Control – Distance Error Animation. So far, no direct information on how to correct the motion was given. The initial idea of Velloso et al. [25] that uses directed arrows to indicate how to correct the motion was adapted and replaced by an animated joint that moves to its correct position and thus gradually changes its color from red (wrong position) to green (correct target position is reached). Even though this is still a quite technical representation, this approach is considered to be more natural than using arrows (see Fig. 10, right). However, it is only applicable for terminal or delayed feedback.

Auditory Output of Control – Speed Feedback. For the most striking speed deviation, a verbal feedback phrase is provided by using a text-to-speech library. However, even if humans are used to this type of auditory feedback, such a specific per-joint feedback is not applicable in practice. Therefore, several joints are clustered to body parts and feedback is provided accordingly (e.g., "Move your right arm faster" instead of "Move your right hand and elbow faster"). Auditory feedback in general is best suited for concurrent feedback.

Combination of Visual and Auditory Output of Data. As stressed in the previous section, per-joint speed feedback is regarded as too technical. In this approach that combines visual and auditory output, joints are clustered to body parts (by using the charts for analyzing deviation dependencies) and considered as a whole during motion error feedback. The animated illustration is embedded in a video playback of the motion sequences and supported by corresponding speech output, as illustrated in Fig. 11. Note that the coloring allows to easily determine the affected body part and the blinking speed of the highlighted joints depicts the type of speed deviation (too fast: fast blinking, too slow: slow blinking).

4   Open Problems

Our goal is to develop a user-centered physical motion coaching system which can be used for supporting private rehabilitation and training. For this coaching system, this chapter described (1) accurate 3D human pose estimation, (2) mining crucial motion features for efficient coach, and (3) intuitive motion-error feedback interface.

For 3D human pose estimation, its accuracy is improved by using real observation data (i.e., 3D point cloud captured by Kinect and 3D human pose data

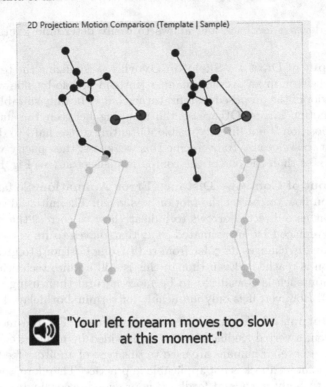

Fig. 11. Example of embedded multimodal speed feedback in motion sequence playback (Note: text in the figure is provided by speech output and is not visualized).

obtained by a motion capture system) as training data. Since the two data are captured independently by different devices, spatial alignment and temporal synchronization are inevitable. While the system proposed in this chapter achieves these alignment and synchronization, the following questions remain open:

- Frame rate: Are the frame rates of the Kinect and the motion capture system completely identical?
- Drift: Does the 3D pose obtained by the motion capture system temporally drift at all?
- Frame(s) for temporal synchronization: Are the frames of the coordinate systems of the Kinect and the motion capture system appropriate for spatial alignment? Are there measurement errors in that frame? Would another frame be better suited for the alignment? Would it be better to use multiple frames for the alignment to cope with drift?

The crucial motions are mined by the sparse coding regularization during training of the SVM that classifies target motions into good or not. The weight vector of the SVM shows which features are crucial for classifying whether a user's motion is good or not. In particular, the sparse coding regularization allows us to enhance the difference between crucial and non-crucial features.

In reality, however, it is not so easy to extract only crucial features correctly from a huge number of possible features. While the ultimate goal of the system is to apply to any kind of motion fully automatically, it might be possible to reduce the possible features manually, based on knowledge of the motion so that only meaningful features (i.e., features that might be crucial) remain. Otherwise, for realizing a fully-automatic system, we might be able to reduce the possible features independently of the motion, based on the structure and general kinematics of a human body.

From a technical point of view, important issues for developing an intuitive motion-error feedback interface are not clear yet. In particular, how to automatically select a feedback type depending on the motion is an open problem. We need extensive user tests in order to address this.

5 Future Outlook

Future work for improving feature mining includes using knowledge of a human body (e.g., kinematics and joint structures) as heuristics, extensive user tests, and verification with many other kinds of motions. In terms of using the knowledge of a human body, it is expected that the knowledge is helpful for mining more discriminative features. Since this knowledge does not depend on the type of motion, usability of the system is not damaged.

For an intuitive interface system, different ways to provide motion error feedback were analyzed. The results from this first prototype can be used for an initial evaluation that may allow to exclude several feedback possibilities or reveal the need for analyzing others in more detail.

However, technology acceptance is a quite complex phenomenon and the success of a motion coaching system does not only depend on the interface alone. Final statements are only possible when a complete system has been developed and tested in detail. The development of such a system requires an interdisciplinary approach with scientific contributions from the fields of machine learning, computer vision, human-computer interaction, and psychology.

References

1. Campana, F., Moreno, A., Riano, D., Laszlo, Z.: K4care: Knowledge-based homecare eservices for an ageing europe
2. Laleci, G.B., Dogac, A., Olduz, M., Tasyurt, I., Yuksel, M., Okcan, A.: Spahire: A multi-agent system for remote healthcare monitoring through computerized clinical guidelines. In: Agent Technology and E-Health (2007)
3. Villar, A., Federici, A., Annicchiarico, R.: K4care: Knowledge-based homecare eservices for an ageing europe. In: Agent Technology and E-Health (2007)
4. Vergados, D.J., Alevizos, A., Mariolis, A., Caragiozidis, M.: Intelligent services for assisting independent living of elderly people at home. In: PETRA (2008)
5. Population Censuses and Surveys Office: General Household Survey 1994 (1995)
6. World Health Organization: Active Aging: A Policy Framework (2012)

7. Nehmer, J., Becker, M., Karshmer, A.I., Lamm, R.: Living assistance systems: an ambient intelligence approach. In: ICSE, pp. 43–50 (2006)

8. de Ruyter, B.E.R., Pelgrim, E.: Ambient assisted-living research in carelab. Interactions 14(4), 30–33 (2007)

9. Health Education Authority: Older People - Older People and Accidents, Fact Sheet 2 (1999)

10. Torgerson, D., Dolan, D.J.: The cost of treating osteoporotic fractures in the united kingdom female population

11. EU: The Demographic Future of Europe - From Challenge to Opportunity. Commission Communication (2006)

12. Adam, S., Mukasa, K.S., Breiner, K., Trapp, M.: An apartment-based metaphor for intuitive interaction with ambient assisted living applications. In: BCS HCI (1) (2008)

13. Röcker, C.: User-centered design of intelligent environments: Requirements for designing successful ambient assisted living systems. In: The Central European Conference of Information and Intelligent Systems (2013)

14. Röcker, C.: Smart medical services: a discussion of state-of-the-art approaches. International Journal of Machine Learning and Computing

15. Röcker, C., Ziefle, M.: Current approaches to ambient assisted living. In: The International Conference on Future Information Technology and Management Science and Engineering (2012)

16. Röcker, C., Maeder, A.: User-centered design of smart healthcare applications. Electron. J. Health Inf. 6(2), 1–3 (2011)

17. Röcker, C.: Designing ambient assisted living applications: an overview of state-of-the-art implementation concepts. In: The International Conference on Information and Digital Engineering (2011)

18. Ziefle, M., Röcker, C., Holzinger, A.: Medical technology in smart homes: Exploring the user's perspective on privacy, intimacy and trust. In: COMPSAC Workshops, pp. 410–415 (2011)

19. Röcker, C., Ziefle, M., Holzinger, A.: Social inclusion in aal environments: Home automation and convenience services for elderly users. In: The International Conference on Artificial Intelligence (2011)

20. Röcker, C.: Intelligent environments as a promising solution for addressing current demographic changes. Int. J. Innov. Manage. Technol. 4(1), 76–79 (2013)

21. Ukita, N., Hirai, M., Kidode, M.: Complex volume and pose tracking with probabilistic dynamical models and visual hull constraints. In: ICCV (2009)

22. Ukita, N., Kanade, T.: Gaussian process motion graph models for smooth transitions among multiple actions. Comput. Vis. Image Underst. 116(4), 500–509 (2012)

23. Ukita, N.: Simultaneous particle tracking in multi-action motion models with synthesized paths. Image Vis. Comput. 31(6–7), 448–459 (2013)

24. Miles, H.C., Pop, S., Watt, S.J., Lawrence, G.P., John, N.W.: A review of virtual environments for training in ball sports. Comput. Graph. 36(6), 714–726 (2012)

25. Velloso, E., Bulling, A., Gellersen, H.: Motionma: motion modelling and analysis by demonstration. In: CHI (2013)

26. Matsumoto, M., Yano, H., Iwata, H.: Development of a motion teaching system using an immersive projection display and a haptic interface. In: WHC. (2007)

27. Chatzitofis, A., Vretos, N., Zarpalas, D., Daras, P.: Three-dimensional monitoring of weightlifting for computer assisted training. In: VRIC (2013)

28. Takano, K., Li, K.F., Johnson, M.G.: The design of a web-based multimedia sport instructional system. In: AINA Workshops (2011)

29. Chen, Y.J., Hung, Y.C.: Using real-time acceleration data for exercise movement training with a decision tree approach. Expert Syst. Appl. **37**(12), 7552–7556 (2010)
30. O'Sullivan, D., Igoe, T.: Physical computing (2004)
31. Cortes, C., Vapnik, V.: Support-vector networks. Mach. Learn. **20**(3), 273–297 (1995)
32. Chang, C.C., Lin, C.J.: Libsvm: a library for support vector machines. ACM TIST **2**(3), 27 (2011)
33. Shotton, J., Fitzgibbon, A.W., Cook, M., Sharp, T., Finocchio, M., Moore, R., Kipman, A., Blake, A.: Real-time human pose recognition in parts from single depth images. In: Cipolla, R., Battiato, S., Farinella, G.M. (eds.) Machine Learning for Computer Vision. Studies in Computational Intelligence, vol. 411, pp. 119–135. Springer, Heidelberg (2011)
34. Girshick, R.B., Shotton, J., Kohli, P., Criminisi, A., Fitzgibbon, A.W.: Efficient regression of general-activity human poses from depth images. In: ICCV (2011)
35. Myers, C.S., Rabiner, L.R.: Comparative study of several dynamic time-warping algorithms for connected-word recognition. Bell Syst. Tech. J. **60**(7), 1389–1409 (1981)
36. Ukita, N., Kaulen, D., Röcker, C.: Towards an automatic motion coaching system: feedback techniques for different types of motion errors. In: International Conference on Physiological Computing Systems (2014)
37. Li, L.J., Su, H., Xing, E.P., Li, F.F.: Object bank: a high-level image representation for scene classification and semantic feature sparsification. In: NIPS (2010)
38. Roweis, S.T., Saul, L.K.: Nonlinear dimensionality reduction by locally linear embeddin. Science **290**(5500), 2323–2326 (2000)
39. Tenenbaum, J.B., de Silva, V., Langford, J.C.: A global geometric framework for nonlinear dimensionality reduction. Science **290**(5500), 2319–2323 (2000)
40. Lawrence, N.D.: Probabilistic non-linear principal component analysis with gaussian process latent variable models. J. Mach. Learn. Res. **6**, 1783–1816 (2005)
41. Cristianini, N., Shawe-Taylor, J.: An Introduction to Support Vector Machines and Other Kernel-based Learning Methods. Cambridge University Press, Cambridge (2010)
42. Kelly, D., McDonald, J., Markham, C.: A system for teaching sign language using live gesture feedback. In: FG (2008)
43. Takahata, M., Shiraki, K., Sakane, Y., Takebayashi, Y.: Sound feedback for powerful karate training. In: NIME (2004)
44. Evans, C., Palacios, L.: Using audio to enhance learner feedback. In: International Conference on Education and Management Technology (2010)
45. Spelmezan, D., Borchers, J.: Real-time snowboard training system. In: CHI Extended Abstracts (2008)

Reading

46. Ukita, N., Kaulen, D., Röcker, C.: Towards an automatic motion coaching system: feedback techniques for different types of motion errors. In: International Conference on Physiological Computing (2014)
47. Ukita, N., Kaulen, D., Röcker, C.: Mining crucial features for automatic rehabilitation coaching systems. In: International Workshop on User-Centered Design of Pervasive Healthcare Applications (2014)

48. Holzinger, A., Ziefle, M., Röcker, C.: Pervasive Health - State-of-the-Art and Beyond. Springer, London (2014)
49. Varshney, U.: Pervasive Healthcare Computing: EMR/EHR. Wireless and Health Monitoring. Springer, United States (2009)
50. Röcker, C., Ziefle, M.: Smart Healthcare Applications and Services: Developments and Practices. IGI Publishing, Niagara Falls (2011)
51. Bardram, J., Mihailidis, A., Wan, D.: Pervasive Computing in Healthcare. CRC Press Inc., Boca Raton (2006)
52. Röcker, C., Ziefle, M.: E-Health, Assistive Technologies and Applications for Assisted Living: Challenges and Solutions. IGI Publishing, Niagara Falls (2011)
53. Jähn, K., Nagel, E.: E-Health. Springer, Berlin (2003)
54. Ziefle, M., Röcker, C.: Human-Centered Design of E-Health Technologies: Concepts. Methods and Applications. IGI Publishing, Niagara Falls (2011)
55. Coronato, A., De Pietro, G.: Pervasive and Smart Technologies for Healthcare: Ubiquitous Methodologies and Tools. IGI Publishing, Niagara Falls (2011)

Linking Biomedical Data to the Cloud

Stefan Zwicklbauer$^{(\boxtimes)}$, Christin Seifert, and Michael Granitzer

University of Passau, Innstraße 33, 94032 Passau, Germany
{Stefan.Zwicklbauer,Christin.Seifert,Michael.Granitzer}@uni-passau.de

Abstract. The application of Knowledge Discovery and Data Mining approaches forms the basis of realizing the vision of Smart Hospitals. For instance, the automated creation of high-quality knowledge bases from clinical reports is important to facilitate decision making processes for clinical doctors. A subtask of creating such structured knowledge is entity disambiguation that establishes links by identifying the correct semantic meaning from a set of candidate meanings to a text fragment. This paper provides a short, concise overview of entity disambiguation in the biomedical domain, with a focus on annotated corpora (e.g. CalbC), term disambiguation algorithms (e.g. abbreviation disambiguation) as well as gene and protein disambiguation algorithms (e.g. inter-species gene name disambiguation). Finally, we provide some open problems and future challenges that we expect future research will take into account.

Keywords: Linked data cloud · Entity disambiguation · Text annotation · Natural language processing · Knowledge bases

1 Introduction

The amount of digital data, also called the digital universe, grows rapidly, amounting to 4.4 Zetabytes in 2013[1]. Thus, medical doctors and biomedical researchers of today are confronted with increasingly large volumes of high-dimensional, heterogeneous and complex data from various sources, which pose substantial challenges to the computational sciences [1]. Overall, the majority of such information (e.g. medical reports) is transmitted through unstructured documents [2], more suitably defined as non-standardized data [3]. The task of Knowledge Discovery is to extract implicit, previously unknown, and potentially useful information from such unstructured data [4].

The application of Knowledge Discovery and Data Mining approaches forms the basis of realizing the vision of *Smart Hospitals* [1,5]. A prominent example is the (automated) creation of high-quality knowledge bases (KB) from clinical reports. The Comparative Toxicogenomics Database (CTD) [6], for instance, is a high-quality data base for researching the influence of chemicals on human health, but is manually curated and therefore restricted in its coverage of the

---

[1] The digital universe of opportunities http://www.emc.com/collateral/analyst-reports/idc-digital-universe-2014.pdf.

© Springer International Publishing Switzerland 2015
A. Holzinger et al. (Eds.): Smart Health, LNCS 8700, pp. 209–235, 2015.
DOI: 10.1007/978-3-319-16226-3_9

documents annotated by experts. Providing high-quality, automatic methods for populating the KB from clinical reports would facilitate decision making processes for clinical doctors [1]. The demand for automatic methods is also reflected in the natural language processing challenges posed by various initiatives, like the BioCreative initiative[2] and the BioNLP shared tasks [7]. For instance, in the domain of biomedical research, the understanding of two-component regulatory systems (TCSs), a mechanism widely used by bacteria to sense and respond to the environment, can be facilitated [8]. TCSs are of particular interest for infectious disease researchers including virulence, response to antibiotics, quorum sensing and bacterial cell attachment [9].

For these purposes, the recognition and assignment of symptoms, chemicals, genes, proteins etc. to a unique identifier in a KB is an important subtask. This chapter gives an overview of the state-of-the art of linking unstructured biomedical data to the Linked Data Cloud, with a special emphasis on biomedical entity disambiguation.

The remainder of the chapter is structured as follows: Sect. 2 defines the technical terms required for understanding the chapter. Section 3 gives a clear definition of the problem that should be solved and illustrates why linking biomedical entities to the cloud is a challenging task by examples. Section 4 then provides the foundations for understanding the reviewed algorithms by exemplifying the data structures used by disambiguation methods. The state-of-the-art review in Sect. 5 is divided into four subsections:

- The state of the biomedical Linked Data Cloud is described in Sect. 5.1,
- Section 5.2 presents annotated corpora for training linking algorithms,
- Algorithms for biomedical term disambiguation are reviewed in Sect. 5.3,
- Algorithms for gene and protein disambiguation are presented in Sect. 5.4.

The chapter concludes with an overview of open problems in Sect. 6 and an outlook on future work is given in Sect. 7.

2   Glossary and Key Terms

Automatic Term Recognition (ATR) Recognition and linking of terms to domain specific data bases [10], synonym to ↑ NED.

Disambiguation The process of linking a ↑ surface form to a ↑ URI.

Entity A modeled abstract or concrete object of the real world, for example a specific gene. In the context of ↑ disambiguation also called label [11].

Knowledge Base (KB) describes a knowledge repository that stores facts about the world. Knowledge bases can be coarsely classified into structured and unstructured knowledge bases depending on the form of the data representation. An orthogonal classification is specific for general-purpose knowledge bases, depending on the type of knowledge stored.

---

[2] http://www.biocreative.org.

Linked (Open) Data describes the concept of providing semantic information for data sets. The goal is to support automatic sharing and linking pieces of the data on a semantic level. The basic technologies for Linked Data are ↑ URIs and ↑ RDF. Linked Open Data (LOD) encompasses the idea that these data sets should be openly accessible.

Linked (Open) Data Cloud subsumes the (openly accessible) data sets represented as ↑ Linked Data.

Named Entity A modeled, concrete object of the real world, referenced by proper names or acronyms in the text. Originally introduced in the Message Understanding Conference (MUC) Challenges, the commonly agreed types were person, location and organization, later date and time, measures and email addresses were added [12]. Depending on the application domain, other domain-specific named entities exist. These are for instance names of drugs or proteins in the biomedical domain.

Named Entity Recognition (NER) The process of identifying a ↑ named entity, i.e. identifying that a surface form represents a named entity (but not yet knowing, which entity exactly).

Named Entity Disambiguation (NED) The process of linking a ↑ surface form representing a ↑ named entity to a unique meaning [13].

Resource Description Framework (RDF) is a general concept for the semantic description of resources. The building blocks of RDF are triplets consisting of subject (the thing that is described), the object (to which it is related) and a relation (specifying the relationship between subject and object). Relations are unidirectional. All parts of a triplet are uniquely identifiable by the means of ↑ URIs.

Surface Form refers to the piece of textual information (words or phrases) that should be linked to a semantic entity [14,15]. Also called mention, entity mention, mention occurrence, spot [11], or lemma [16].

Uniform Resource Identifier (URI) is a string of characters identifying a resource. The most prominent example is the Uniform Resource Locator (URL) used in the World Wide Web.

Word Sense Disambiguation (WSD) The process of linking a ↑ surface form to a unique entry in a dictionary. In general, the linked ↑ surface forms are not ↑ entities. Consider for instance the different meanings of the word "mind" (depending on the context it could be used as verb or noun and may have different meanings in each grammatical form.).

3   Problem Statement

Entity annotators undertake a crucial processing step in producing structured knowledge. They "ground" the underlying texts with respect to an adequate semantic representation. The entity annotation task can be subdivided into the following two sub steps:

- **Entity Recognition:** The identification of short-and-meaningful sequences of terms, also called surface forms, which can be linked to entities in a catalog.
- **Entity Disambiguation:** The annotation of surface forms with unambiguous identifiers (entities) drawn from a catalog.

Entity Recognition. Entity recognition forms the first step of creating entity annotations. It identifies proper nouns that can be linked to a semantic meaning. Proper nouns often exhibit *structural ambiguity* that complicates the correct identification. For example, the components of "Victoria and Albert Museum and IBM and Bell Laboratories" look identical. The term "and" is part of the name of the museum in the first example, but a conjunction joining two computer company names in the second [17]. The task of named entity recognition (NER) focuses on identifying surface forms in a text which are the names of things, such as person, organization, gene or protein names. Overall, (named) entity recognition is a well studied research topic. State-of-the-art algorithms for generic knowledge entities score ≈90 % of F-measure [18], while accuracy of biomedical NER strongly depends on the entities' types (e.g. proteins, genes, diseases) [19].

Entity Disambiguation. The task of entity disambiguation establishes links between identified surface forms and entities within a catalog (KB) and faces the problem of *semantic ambiguity* [17]. Formally, entity disambiguation inherently involves resolving many-to-many relationships. Multiple distinct surface forms may refer to the same entity. Simultaneously, multiple identical surface forms may refer to distinct entities [20]. Figure 1 shows a specific example of this relationship. We assume a sentence containing the surface forms "Ford" and "CART" (depicted in the yellow rectangle). Both surface forms may refer to different entities, e.g. Ford by itself could be an actor (Harrison Ford), the

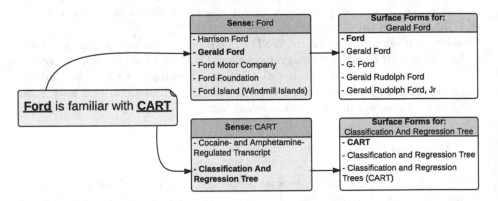

Fig. 1. Surface forms (bold) within a sentence (yellow rectangle) may refer to different entities (rectangles in the middle) depending on the context. Additionally, an entity may be addressed by various surface forms (rectangles on the right) (Colour figure online).

38th President of the United States (Gerald Ford), an organization (Ford Motor Company) or a place (Ford Island). In our context, we assume "Gerald Ford" to be the correct entity, which may be expressed in several ways, e.g. "Gerald Rudolph Ford, Jr.". However, similar to NER, the task of named entity disambiguation (NED) focuses on surface forms constituting the names of special entity classes. The ever-increasing publication rate of biomedical documents now means that entity disambiguation in the biomedical domain is becoming more and more important. Biomedical NED is constrained to biomedical entities only, but is extremely challenging [21] since a surface form

1. could refer to another type of biomedical entity, such as a protein or phenotype, e.g. the mouse gene "hair loss".
2. could be other types of concepts in closely related domains, such as the clinical field, e.g. the mouse gene "diabetes".
3. could be the same as common English words, e.g. fly genes "can" and "lie".
4. could refer to several, different genetic entities, either from the same or from other species, e.g. cow or chicken.

In biomedical entity disambiguation, genes and gene products (i.e. proteins) form an important class of entities. To map surface forms of these entity classes to an entity within a KB, it is important to identify what organisms (species) the genes and proteins belong to, and on what species the experiments are carried out to understand particular biological phenomena. There are dozens of species commonly used in biological studies, such as Escherichia coli, Caenorhabditis elegans, Drosophila melanogaster, Homo sapiens and hundreds more are frequently mentioned in biological research papers. For example, without context, "tumor protein p53" may associate to over 100 proteins across 23 species[3]. To identify the proteins (i.e. the underlined terms) in the following sentence, knowing the "focus" species of the article is not sufficient, as they belong to three different species: human, mouse and rat.

The amounts of human and mouse CD200R-CD4d3+4 and rCD4d3+4 protein on the microarray spots were similar ...

The authors of [21] investigated the extent of the ambiguity problem in the biomedical domain. They obtained genes from 21 species and quantified naming ambiguities within and across species, with English words and with medical terms. The results revealed that official gene symbols display negligible ambiguity within a specific species (0.02 % regarding uppercase letters) and a high ambiguity across-species (14.20 %). Additionally, the results showed a moderate ambiguity rate with general English words (0.57 %) and medical terms (1.01 %). The analysis of correct gene disambiguation results within abstracts of biomedical research paper also showed a very high number of ambiguous genes across species [21] (85.1 %).

Overall biomedical NED is a challenging task and thus has attained much attention in research in the last decade.

---

[3] Querying RefSeq database (http://www.ncbi.nlm.nih.gov/refseq/). The number of species was manually counted.

4   Entity Representation

A crucial factor for creating a disambiguation system is the way entities are represented within a KB. Generally an entity can be defined intensionally, i.e. through a set of describing properties, or extensionally, i.e. through instances and usage in documents [22]. In the following we differentiate more precisely between these representations and give examples of how entities might be represented within disambiguation KBs in practice.

4.1   Intensional Description

An intensional definition of an entity can be understood as a thesaurus or logical representation, as it is provided by Linked Open Data repositories. In the context of entity disambiguation, KBs comprising intensionally defined entities are referred to as *entity-centric KBs* [23]. Formally, an entity-centric KB can be described as

$$Kb_{\mathrm{ent}} = \{e_0, ..., e_n | e_i \in E, n \in \mathbb{N}\} \tag{1}$$

The set of all entities available in the entity-centric KB Kb_{ent} is denoted as E, with e_i being a single entity [23]. All entities $e_i \in Kb_{\mathrm{ent}}$ usually provide a unique primary key ID which combines the name of the knowledge source as well as its identifier in the knowledge source. Additionally, a variable number of fields k contain domain-independent attributes, e.g. descriptions, and domain-dependent information, e.g. the sequence length of genes. Formally, such an entity can be denoted as

$$e_{\mathrm{i}} = (ID, Field_1, ..., Field_k) \tag{2}$$

Table 1 shows a specific example of how the entity "Phenylalanyl-tRNA–protein transferase" might be represented in an entity-centric KB. The entity contains standard attributes, i.e., name, synonyms, description, link to web resource, type, as well as occurrence information. More specifically, all referenced surface forms for this entity and the respective amount of occurrences with this surface form are stored in *Occurrences*. The field *Cooccurrences* contains surface forms of entities that appeared near the described entity in any text and the amount of appearances of the respective surface form in the context range (i.e. 300 words).

4.2   Extensional Description

An extensional entity definition resembles information on the usage context of an entity. For instance, natural language text documents annotated with entities can be used as such usage context. KBs containing extensional entity definition are referred to as *document-centric KBs* [23]. Formally, a document-centric KB is defined as

$$Kb_{\mathrm{doc}} = \{d_0, ..., d_n | d_i \in D, n \in \mathbb{N}\} \tag{3}$$

An entry d_i in a document-centric KB Kb_{doc} consists of the document content representing a text string and a list of annotations of surface forms $t^l_{e_i}$, with

Table 1. Example of an entity-centric KB entry

Field	Content
ID	UNQ9A741
Name	Phenylalanyl-tRNA–protein transferase
Synonyms	Leucyltransferase
Description	Functions in the N-end rule pathway of protein degradation where it conjugates Leu, Phe and, less efficiently, Met from aminoacyl-tRNAs to the N-termini of proteins
Mainlink	http://www.uniprot.org/uniprot/Q9A741
Type	Caulobacter
Occurrences	aat:::3
Co-Occurrences	substrate:::3, Leu::::6, Phe:::6

l denoting the lth annotation in the document. Annotated surface forms are described by their position in the document and a list of their entity references. An entry in a document-centric KB is denoted as

$$d_i = (Document, \{(Start, End, \{ID\}), ...\}) \qquad (4)$$

Table 2 shows an example of a biomedical document containing the surface form "'Myeloma'" in a document-centric KB. The document's content is subdivided in *title* and *titleandtext*, which is a concatenation of the document's title and main content. Furthermore, all available annotations (and its respective properties) are stored in the field *Annotations*. The field ID depicts a unique document identifier.

Table 2. Example of a document-centric KB entry

Field	Content
ID	174996
Title	Antibody therapy for treatment of multiple myeloma
Abstract	Monoclonal antibody therapy antibody therapy has emerged as a viable treatment option for patients with lymphoma and some leukemias. It is now beginning to be...
TitleAndAbs	Antibody therapy for treatment of multiple myeloma. Monoclonal antibody therapy antibody therapy has emerged as a viable treatment option for patients with...
Keywords	Myeloma::43::50::diso:umls:C0026764:T191:diso

5   State-of-the-Art

In this section the state-of-the-art is reviewed along three dimensions. First, we review the state of the biomedical linked data cloud in Sect. 5.1. Second, we describe available annotated corpora for training algorithms in Sect. 5.2. Third, we review the algorithms for for biomedical term disambiguation in Sect. 5.3 and for gene and protein disambiguation in Sect. 5.4. We note that we do not describe and review text (pre-)processing steps (e.g. tokenization, normalization, stemming) which are necessary for entity recognition and disambiguation. An overview of relevant steps for text processing in the biomedical domain can be found in [1].

5.1   The Biomedical Linked Data Cloud

According to the "State of the LOD Cloud 2014"[4] the Linked Open Data cloud comprises 1014 data sets, 83 (8.19 %) belong to the life sciences domain as of April 2014. Data sets use different vocabularies, proprietary or non-proprietary. Proprietary vocabularies are only used by one data set and thus are not useful for interlinking differently linked data repositories. Non-proprietary vocabularies are used by at least two data sets and comprise only 41.76 % of all encountered 649 vocabularies. In terms of data sets, 23.17 % (241) data sets use proprietary vocabularies, but also nearly all of the data sets (99.87 %) use non-proprietary vocabularies. In the life sciences this amount is slightly higher. 35 different proprietary vocabularies are used in 26 data sets (these amount to 29.21 % of all life sciences data sets). Only 28.57 % of these data sets are fully linkable to other data sets, i.e. can be fully interpreted by automatic mechanisms. 65.71 % of these data sets are not linkable at all.

5.2   Annotated Corpora

This section presents an overview of annotated corpora for biomedical entity disambiguation. We omitted corpora that were not, or are no longer publicly available.

GENIA Corpus

The GENIA corpus [24], released in 2003, contains ≈2000 MEDLINE abstracts from the domain of molecular biology. The corpus is freely available for download[5]. The MEDLINE abstracts were collected by querying PubMed for the three MeSH terms "human", "blood cells", and "transcription factors". They were syntactically and semantically annotated, resulting in six different sub-corpora corresponding to the specific annotations:

---

[4] http://linkeddatacatalog.dws.informatik.uni-mannheim.de/state/.
[5] http://www.nactem.ac.uk/genia/genia-corpus.

Table 3. Statistics of the GENIA corpus (term annotations)

	GENIA
Documents	2,000
Document Type	MEDLINE abstract
Surface Forms	89,862
Release Date	2003 (version 3.0)

- Part-of-Speech annotation subcorpus,
- Constituency (phrase structure) syntactic annotation subcorpus,
- Term annotation subcorpus,
- Event annotation subcorpus,
- Relation annotation subcorpus,
- Coreference annotation subcorpus.

Linguistic structures are annotated with biological terms from the GENIA ontology in the term annotation subcorpus, which represents the corpus for entity disambiguation. Table 3 provides an overview of the GENIE term annotation subcorpus.

BioCreative Corpora

The BioCreative (Critical Assessment of Information Extraction in Biology) community has released various annotated corpora since 2004. The data sets are freely available for non-commercial purposes[6].

GM Corpus (BioCreative I and II): The BioCreative I data set [25] for the Gene Mention (GM) task was released in 2005 and consists of sentences from MEDLINE abstracts annotated with gene mentions. The provided sentences have already been tokenized. The BioCreative II data set [26] is an extended and refined version of the BioCreative I data set and was released in 2008. The changes include an addition of 5000 sentences, a review of the annotations with $\approx$13 % changes and linkage of the gene mentions to either the GENE or ALTGENE KB. Further, in the BioCreative II data set the sentences were not tokenized a-priori. An overview of the basic statistics for the BioCreative I+II data sets can be found in Table 4.

Table 4. Statistics of the GM I and II corpus (aggregated training, test and development set)

	GM I	GM II
Documents	1,500	2,000
Document Type	MEDLINE abstract	MEDLINE abstract
Surface Forms	1,800	44,500
Release Date	2005	2008

---

[6] http://www.biocreative.org/resources/.

Table 5. Statistics of the ChemDNER corpus (aggregated training, test and development set)

	ChemDNER
Documents	10,000
Document Type	PubMed abstract
Surface Forms	84,355
Entities	19,805
Release Date	2013

ChemDNER Corpus (BioCreative IV): The ChemDNER (Chemical and Drug Named Entity Recognition) corpus [27], released by the BioCreative community in 2013 (part of BioCreative IV), contains PubMed abstracts manually annotated with chemical compounds and drugs. Each abstract was annotated by at least two experts with an overall inter-annotater agreement of 91 %, thus the corpus can be considered a gold standard for chemical NER. Table 5 provides a summary statistics of the corpus with all values aggregated over training, test and development set. More details on corpus construction and statistic can be found in [27].

BC4GO Corpus (BioCreative IV): The Gene Ontology (GO) corpus [28] was released by the BioCreative community in 2013 as part of the BioCreative IV challenge. The corpus consists of 200 annotated full-text articles from PMC. The task associated with this corpus involves extracting gene function terms and the associated evidence sentences. Table 6 provides an overview of the corpus.

CalbC Corpus

The CalbC (Collaborative Annotation of a Large Biomedical Corpus) corpus is a very large, community-wide shared text corpus annotated with biomedical entity references [29]. CalbC represents a silver standard corpus which results from the

Table 6. Statistics of the BC4GO corpus (aggregated training, test and development set)

	BC4GO
Documents	200
Document Type	PMC full-texts
Gene mentions	5,162
Entities (Genes)	665
GO term mentions	5,275
Entities (GO terms)	1,311
Release Date	2013

harmonization of automatically generated annotations and is freely accessible[7]. The data set is released in 3 different sizes: small (CalbCSmall), big (CalbCBig) and pilot, with the former two being the most widely used. Table 7 provides an overview of the basic properties of CalbCSmall and CalbCBig. A comparison regarding the overlap of entities within both corpora shows that a very high percentage of entities occurs in both data sets. Hence, there are few entities which occur in CalbCBig but are not present in the small corpus. In contrast to other disambiguation corpora like Dbpedia, a surface form may be linked to more than one entity resource per annotation. Due to a comprehensive taxonomy and classification system a surface form provides 9 entity annotations on average. Figure 2 presents an overview of the distribution of surface forms and their corresponding entities. The histogram axis showing the number of entities is truncated at 40 entities due to very few existing surface forms which contain a lot of different meanings (maximum 9895). Nearly half of all surface forms may attain between 2 and 7 different entities. The other half of surface forms attains up to 9895 different entity meanings. Figure 3 shows an overview of the distribution of surface forms over entities. More than 10,000 different surface forms address general entities like "kinase" or "protein".

Table 7. Statistics of the CalbCSmall and CalbCBig corpora

	CalbCSmall	CalbCBig
Documents	174,999	714,282
Document Type	MEDLINE abstract	MEDLINE abstract
Surface Forms	2,548,900	10,304,172
Unique Surface Forms	50,725	101,439
Entities	37,309,221	96,526,575
Unique Entities	453,352	308,644
Used Unique Entities	265,532	228,744
Namespaces	14	16
Release Date	2011	2011

CRAFT Corpus

The CRAFT (Colorado richly annotated full text) corpus [30] is an annotated corpus consisting of 67 full-text journal articles from the biomedical domain. The corpus contains ≈100,000 annotations from the biomedical domain, linking it to 7 different repositories (Chemical Entities of Biological Interest, Cell Ontology, Entrez Gene, Gene Ontology, NCBI Taxonomy, Protein Ontology and Sequence Ontology). Table 8 provides an overview of the data set. The corpus is licenced under the Creative Commons Attribution 3.0 license (CC BY) and is available online[8].

---

[7] http://www.calbc.eu/.
[8] http://bionlp-corpora.sourceforge.net/CRAFT/.

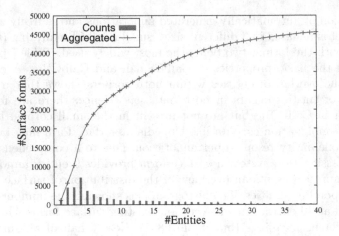

Fig. 2. Distribution of surface forms and their corresponding entities

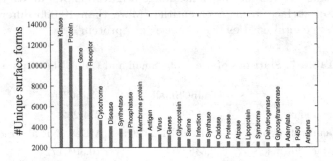

Fig. 3. Number of entity annotations (Only entities annotated for more than 2000 different entities are shown.)

BioNLP Shared Tasks Corpera

The BioNLP Shared Tasks corpora originates from the GENIA corpus (see above). In 2004, 2009 and 2011, the initiative covering different natural language tasks for the biomedical domain released several corpora. The data sets are available online[9]. Here, we describe subcorpora from the release in 2011 [8], which is also publicly available[10].

EPI Corpus: The EPI corpus (Epigenetics and Post-translational Modifications) was crafted to research automatic extraction of events related to epigenetic changes. The corpus consists of 1,200 MEDLINE abstracts, annotated with entities representing proteins or genes. Additional annotations are made for events (e.g. hydroxylation, DNA methylation), and event modifications (e.g.

---

[9] http://www.nactem.ac.uk/genia/shared-tasks.
[10] http://2011.bionlp-st.org/.

Table 8. Statistics of the CRAFT corpus

	CRAFT
Documents	67
Document Type	PubMed full-texts
Surface Forms	≈100,000
Namespaces	7
Unique Entities	4,319
Release Date	2012

catalysis, positive regulation, negation or speculation). An overview of the EPI corpus is presented in Table 9.

Table 9. Statistics of the EPI corpus from the BioNLP Shared Task (aggregated training, test and development set)

	EPI
Documents	1,200
Document Type	PubMed abstract
Surface Forms (Protein, Gene)	15,190
Surface Forms (Event)	3,714
Surface Form (Modification)	369
Release Date	2011

ID Corpus: The ID (infectious diseases) corpus was designed to study the molecular mechanism of infectious diseases. It consists of 30 full-text documents from the PMC data base. The documents are annotated with five types of entities (protein, two-component system, regulon-operon, chemical and organism), event types (e.g. for example gene expression, binding, regulation) and modifications. The latter indicates whether a statement is a speculation or a negation. Table 10 provides an overview of the ID corpus.

CDT Corpus

The Comparative Toxicogenomic Database (CTD) [6] is a publicly available database[11] containing the following types of manually curated annotations:

– Chemical-gene interactions,
– Chemical-disease associations,

---

[11] http://ctdbase.org/.

Table 10. Statistics of the ID corpus from the BioNLP shared Task (aggregated training, test and development set)

	ID
Documents	30
Document Type	PMC full-texts
Surface Forms (Entity)	12,740
Surface Forms (Event)	3,714
Surface Form (Modification)	369
Release Date	2011

– Gene-disease associations,
– Chemical-phenotype associations.

The manual data collection started in 2004 and is constantly updated. An overview of the data sets as of July 2014 can be found in Table 11.

Table 11. Statistics of the CDT corpus (figures correspond to the version from July 2014)

	CDT
Documents	109,701
Document Type	PubMed full-texts
Chemicals	13,446
Diseases	6,347
Genes	36,393
Release Date	Silent releases, constantly updated

5.3   Biomedical Term Disambiguation

Biomedical term disambiguation focuses on disambiguating all classes of biomedical entities (e.g. medical terms, abbreviations, genes, chemicals). Official biomedical symbols display only a moderate degree of ambiguities with general English words, medical terms and concepts [21]. Thus, the number of works resolving these ambiguities is limited.

String Matching Algorithms. String Matching algorithms are able to map case-sensitive surface forms to the respective KB entries. The work by Tsuruoka et al. [31] focused on learning a string similarity measure from a dictionary with logistic regression. The experiments were conducted on several large-scale gene and protein name dictionaries. Results showed that a logistic regression-based similarity measure outperforms existing similarity measures like Hidden Markov

Model [32], SoftTFIDF [33], Jaro-Winkler [34] and Levenshtein in dictionary look-up tasks.

Another work from Rudniy et al. [35] describes the problem of mapping entities in biomedical data to the UMLS Metathesaurus. The work introduces the Longest Approximately Common Prefix (LACP) method as an algorithm for approximate string matching that runs in linear time. The authors compare the LACP method to nine other well-known string matching algorithms (e.g. TF-IDF [36], Jaro-Winkler [34], Needleman-Wunsch [37]) in terms of precision and performance. As a result, LACP outperforms all nine string similarity methods in both disciplines, performance and accuracy. It attains the best F1 values (up to 92 %) when evaluated on three out of the four data sets.

A major disadvantage of these approaches is the non-availability of disambiguation techniques. In other words, if surface forms are ambiguous these algorithms are hardly able to determine the potential entity candidate.

Abbreviation Disambiguation. There are a number of systems that have been developed to map biomedical abbreviations to appropriate entities. Methods for mapping abbreviations to full forms fall into two broad categories [38]: abbreviations are linked to entities with the help of pattern or rules when the entities' full forms appear nearby in the text [39,40], or statistical disambiguation methods choose entities for an abbreviation based on the context the abbreviation occurs in [38,41].

The intention of the AbbRe system [39] (Abbreviation Recognition and Extraction) was to map abbreviations to entities when the entities' full forms are explicitly defined in biomedical full-text articles. AbbRE operates through a set of manually annotated rules assigning matches between letters in the abbreviations and words in the full form. AbbRE was evaluated in full-text biomedical articles and found to have 70 % recall and 95 % precision.

Yu et al. [38] proposed the first model that resolves the problem of abbreviation ambiguity in full-text journal articles. The approach is built upon the earlier work AbbRe and presents a semi-supervised method that applies MEDLINE as a knowledge source for disambiguating abbreviations and acronyms in full-text biomedical journal articles. The authors trained supervised learning algorithms (i.e. Naive Bayes and Support Vector Machines) on 11 million MEDLINE abstracts which were annotated with AbbRe first.

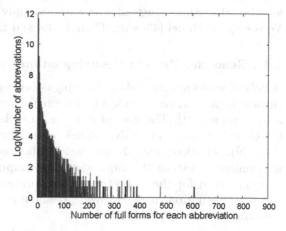

Fig. 4. Distribution (from eleven million MEDLINE records) of the numbers of abbreviations paired with different numbers of full forms [38].

Figure 4 shows the distribution of the numbers of abbreviations paired with different numbers of full forms occurring in the annotated MEDLINE abstracts. The abbreviations "or" and "ca" correspond to the largest numbers of different full forms. Overall, the authors report up to 92 % precision when disambiguating biomedical abbreviations.

General Biomedical Term Disambiguation. Few works focused on general biomedical term disambiguation, which comprises all kinds of biomedical surface forms that can be linked to an entity (i.e. medical terms, gene names, abbreviations).

The work of Chen et al. [42] presents a simple method for biomedical term disambiguation, which can be viewed as a context-based classification approach. Instead of directly using all of a words' surrounding words, the authors only select certain words with high "discriminating" capabilities as features. By using this method, unimportant surrounding words are discarded to improve disambiguation quality. The top-n influential context terms are used as feature vector. These feature vectors serve as input to a classification method for creating classifiers (i.e. Support Vector Machine, Naive Bayes, Ripper and C4.5), which map each surface form to an entity in the KB. A major contribution of this method is its unique way of selecting the features of the ambiguous terms and building feature vectors.

Zwicklbauer et al. [23] investigated biomedical entity disambiguation with entity- and document-centric KBs. The authors state that document-centric KBs outperform laboriously constructed entity-centric KBs if an adequate amount of annotations is available. In this context, they investigated to which degree disambiguation results depend on the quality of entity repositories [23]. They showed that the quality of disambiguation results with an entity-centric KB is distinguished from the use of different repositories and biomedical subdomains (e.g. UMLS, Uniprot, Entrez Gene). A major limitation is the non-use of machine learning algorithms. Instead, the authors apply standard approaches like the Vector Space Model [43] with TF-IDF [36] and BM-25 [44].

5.4   Gene and Protein Disambiguation

A bulk of works specialized on disambiguating genes and proteins, which constitutes a challenging task due to a high degree of ambiguous gene/protein mentions across species [21]. The goal of gene and protein disambiguation, a subtask of the Gene Normalization (GN) process (also comprises gene and protein recognition [45]), is to determine the unique identifiers of genes and proteins mentioned in scientific literature. A unique identifier comprises a unique species id as well as a unique id for the respective gene or protein. Basically, the gene and protein disambiguation (in the following denoted as gene disambiguation) faces the following ambiguity problems:

1. Gene-Protein name ambiguity: a surface form may refer either to a gene or a protein, but is unambiguous within the set of all genes or proteins across all species.

2. Intra-species gene name ambiguity: a surface form could be the identifier of several genes or proteins belonging to a specific species when the species identifier is provided.
3. Inter-species gene name ambiguity: a surface form could be the identifier of several genes or proteins across species.

In the following we describe the most important works addressing the respective ambiguities.

5.4.1 Gene-Protein Name Ambiguity

The simplest form of ambiguity occurs if a surface form either refers to a gene or a protein while being unambiguous within the set of all genes or proteins across all species. This assumption can be modeled as a binary classification problem which classifies the surface form into the gene or protein class.

While recent work do not *explicitly* distinguish between both classes, the authors of [46] conducted experiments on how standard classification approaches like Naive Bayes and C4.5 [47] perform on this disambiguation task. When Naive Bayes was combined with a well-chosen smoothing function, it attained $\approx 80\%$ accuracy in the classification task on different data sets. Ginter et al. [48] introduced a new classifier based on ordering and weighting the feature vectors obtained from word counts and work co-occurrence in the text. An additional improvement was attained after weighting by positions of the words in the context of annotated article abstracts downloaded from the PubMed [49] database. Pahikkala et al. [50] further improved accuracy by incorporating a weighting scheme based on distances of context words into a conventional Support Vector Machine.

Overall gene-protein classification is quite simple and thus attains accuracy values between 85% and 90% with standard approaches.

5.4.2 Intra-species Gene Name Ambiguity

It is more likely that a surface form could be the identifier of several genes or proteins belonging to a specific species when the species identifier is provided. Algorithms that resolve an intra-species gene name ambiguity do not *explicitly* distinguish between the gene and protein class. The BioCreative I and II challenges [45] were conducted to map genes from the EntrezGene KB when specific sets of species are provided. Focusing on gene recognition in text and gene disambiguation (and also on protein-protein interactions), the BioCreative II dataset is commonly used for evaluation purpose of intra-species gene-protein name ambiguity. However, by also including the gene recognition task, the result values of the evaluated systems are not applicable to the disambiguation task in general.

Semantic Approaches Xu et al. [51] proposed a gene profile-based approach which examines gene name disambiguation under several idealistic assumptions:
1. Perfect gene mentions are assumed with most being restricted to short string

gene symbols, and 2. among the possible gene candidates in their disambiguation task one candidate is always the correct answer, which ignores the fact that
an apparent gene mention in a text may not denote a gene at all [52]. However, in their approach, they extract a profile with different types of information
(e.g. context terms, context ontological semantic concepts) from each gene from
already annotated knowledge sources. Their disambiguation approach describes
an information retrieval approach which ranks the similarity scores between the
context of the surface form and the candidate gene profiles. A look at their
results, however, reveals that a plain bag-of-words approach performs almost
equally well.

A complex semantic disambiguation approach was introduced by Hakenberg
et al. [53,54]. They identify genes by using background knowledge from Entrez-
Gene, UniProt and GeneOnthology (GO). For each candidate ID that is assigned
to a gene surface form and thus to a text, the approach tries to find all information in the text and picks the ID with the highest likelihood. To calculate the
similarity based on GO terms, GO terms in the surface form context are compared with gene candidate GO terms. For each potential tuple taken from the
two sets, the system calculates a distance of the terms in the ontology tree. These
distances yield a similarity measure for two terms, even if they do not belong
to the same sub-branch or are immediate parents/children of each other. The
distance takes the shortest path via the lowest common ancestors into account,
as well as the depth of this lowest common ancestor in the overall hierarchy. The
distances for the closest terms from each set then define a similarity between the
gene and the text [54]. The approach currently achieves an F-measure of 86.4 %
on the BioCreative II gene normalization data and, thus, belongs to the best
intra-species gene name disambiguation systems.

Machine Learning Approaches. There are also a few machine-learning approaches
for intra-species gene ambiguity. One system is Azure, which is able to automatically assign gene names to their LocusLink[12] ID in previously unseen MED-
LINE abstracts [55]. Azure contains a supervised learning approach that covers
tens of thousands of genes and proteins. Apparently, it is possible to achieve
high quality gene disambiguation using scalable automated techniques. Wermter
et al. [52] developed GeNo, a highly competitive system for gene name normalization. The authors apply a Maximum Entropy string similarity measure for
candidate retrieval and calculate a semantic similarity score for checking semantic matches. Additionally, the authors show that (i) machine learning methods
perform superiorly when integrated with publicly available training data in a
well-designed manner and (ii) a simple bag-of-words semantic approach to biological background knowledge performs as well as more complex semantic disambiguation [52].

Major disadvantages for machine learning and profile-based approaches are:
As new biological entities are discovered very quickly, there may be no mention
in the previous existing literature for that sense or for that symbol. A partial

---

[12] http://www.ncbi.nlm.nih.gov/Web/Newsltr/Summer99/locus.html.

solution is to perform updates to the profiles and machine learning models regularly.

5.4.3 Inter-species Gene Name Ambiguity

In inter-species gene name ambiguity tasks the species information for genes is not provided. Hence, a surface form could be the identifier of several genes or proteins across species. The disambiguation task requires the disambiguation of species first, and the resolution of the intra species gene name ambiguity in the second step (cf. Sect. 5.4.2). Species disambiguation faces the problem that multiple species assignments may be correct and that therefore multiple correct entities may exist. Hence, determining the parameter of how many results should be retrieved for each disambiguation task is a challenge. If not explicitly mentioned the proposed algorithms return a single species with the most likelihood.

Rule-Based Approaches. A simple approach to link surface forms to a species is by looking for species words in the context. More specifically, several works use one of the following rules as a baseline system [56]:

1. Previous species word: if the word preceding an entity is a species word, assign the species ID indicated by that word to the entity.
2. Species word in the same sentence: if a species word and an entity appear in the same sentence, assign its species ID to the entity. When more than one species word co-occurs in the sentence, priority is given to the species word to the entity's left with the smallest distance. If all species words occur to the right of the entity, take the nearest one.
3. Majority vote: assign the most frequently occurring species ID in the document to all entity mentions.

A well-known system to detect the species of genes in scientific publications is GNAT and was proposed by Hakenberg et al. [54]. Their approach relies on a multi-stage procedure with descending reliability to assign species to genes. For instance, a gene and a species could occur in the same phrase, including enumerations: "rat and murine Eif4g1". If no rule can be applied, the approach checks the abstract for general mentions of kingdoms, classes, etc. The system obtained one of the best performance for the Gene Normalization task in BioCreative II.

A recent approach [57] defines a three-step species disambiguation system. First, a preprocessing step including tokenization and cue word extraction for each gene surface form is performed. Second, the algorithm estimates focus species with the proposed EF-AISF coefficient, the entity frequency-augmented invert species frequency, to calculate the relevance between the cue words of a surface form and species. The species with the highest correlation coefficient is chosen as the probable focus species. Third, an appropriate species is assigned to each gene surface form with the help of the introduced *Relational Guide Factor* which enhances the capability of species assignment. An evaluation shows that the usage of EF-AISF may significantly outperform other (machine-learning) approaches like SVMs in the task of entity species disambiguation.

Wang et al. [58] introduced and compared a number of rule-based and machine-learning based approaches to resolve species ambiguity in mentions of biomedical named entities, and demonstrated that a hybrid method achieves the best overall accuracy at 71.7%, as tested on the gold-standard ITI-TXM corpora [59]. The authors performed multiple species assignments and investigated the average rank of the first correct species annotation.

They also introduced a hybrid species information tagging system (a combination between rule-based and machine learning approach), which improved the rule-based term identification system by up to 10% [58].

Machine Learning Approaches. The authors of [60] describe a generic approach to disambiguate specific entity classes (e.g. species). Instead of classifying each individual occurrence of an entity, it classifies pair-wise relations between the surface form in question and the cue words in its adjacent context, where each cue word is assumed to bear a semantic class (e.g. a specific species). If a cue word features a "positive" relation with the surface form, the corresponding semantic tag of the cue word is assigned to the surface form. While an individual surface form may belong to a large number of semantic classes, a relation can only take one of two values: positive or negative, hence transforming a complex multi-classification problem into a less complicated binary classification task. The binary classification problem was solved with Support Vector Machines. One drawback of the relation classification systems is that they cannot cover all surface forms but only the ones with informative keywords co- occurring in the same sentence. The authors overcame that drawback by using spreading rules [60].

The approach by Harmston et al. [61] transforms a MEDLINE record into a mixture of adjacency matrices. By performing a random walk over the resulting graph, the authors are able to perform multi-class supervised classification, allowing the assignment of taxonomy identifiers to individual gene mentions. This method does not require training data for all potential classes in order to achieve high performance and does not only perform classification but also provides a probability, which serves to quantify the certainty attached to a classification. This species disambiguation approach shows significant improvements over the relation method proposed by Wang et al. [60]. Once the reliable corpora are in place, the approach can be applied in an automatic fashion without any user intervention, which will aid its employment in the context of novel organisms [61].

Wang et al. [56] compared a parser-based (e.g. Stanford parser), a supervised multi-classification [58] and a relation-based [60] species disambiguation approach. Promising results are obtained by training a machine learning model on syntactic parse trees, which is then used to decide whether an entity belongs to the model organism denoted by a neighboring species-indicating word (e.g. yeast). The parser-based approaches are also compared with a supervised classification method and results indicate that the former are a favorable choice when domain portability is of concern. The best overall performance was obtained by combining the strengths of a syntactic parser (i.e. ENJU-Genia), a relation classification model, and a supervised classification model. Their method does not function well if no species term co-occurs with the gene mentions in a sentence. Similarly, the method cannot handle the articles that lack species mentions.

A comparison between rule-based and machine learning approaches shows that machine learning approaches attain satisfying results. However, the availability of training data is often limited, and the available data sets tend to be imbalanced and, in some cases, heterogeneous.

6 Open Problems

This chapter lists the open problems for linking biomedical data to the cloud, categorized into problems with the data (Sect. 6.1) and algorithm-related problems (Sect. 6.2).

6.1 Dataset Related Problems

Annotated corpora for training linking algorithms contain surface forms linked to entities from different KBs and namespaces (e.g. Uniprot, UMLS, SnomedCT). This implies that algorithms trained on one specific corpus with its respective KBs are only able to link to these KBs. Depending on the application scenario, however, references to different KBs might be required. Although the Semantic Web standard accounts for connections between two repositories in the Linked Data Cloud by special types of relations, e.g. the owl:sameAs relation, the majority of the biomedical linked data repositories (65.71 %) is not linkable to other repositories (see Sect. 5.1). Thus, an open problem is the missing links between the various available repositories, also termed ontology alignment. High-quality automatic ontology alignment is still an open problem, while semi-automatic approaches seem to yield promising results [62], but require considerable human effort.

Further problems root in the missing provenance and licensing information of the Linked Data Cloud repositories. As described in Sect. 5.1 for the life sciences domain, only 3.37 % of the data sets provide licensing information in RDF and pose a challenge for fully automatic exploitation of these KBs. Applications using Linked Data repositories rely on the actuality and correctness of the represented knowledge, but only the minority of the life sciences data sets in the Linked Data Cloud (23.60 %) contain provenance information.

6.2 Algorithm Related Problems

Analyzing available disambiguation algorithms shows three major, important and open problems which have been addressed insufficiently so far.

Inter-domain Entity Disambiguation. Scientific literature is being published in various domains (e.g. biomedical, computer science domain). Consequently, these documents comprise entities from different domains. Generally, existing disambiguation systems are able to disambiguate entities belonging to a specific domain, either generic entities as available in Wikipedia or special knowledge entities (e.g. biomedical entities). Zwicklbauer et al. [23] showed that large-scale and heterogeneous entity KBs may mitigate disambiguation results significantly. An open problem is how different entity repositories from different domains can be combined while providing reliable disambiguation results.

Supervised or Unsupervised Classification. Disambiguation tasks (i.e. intra-species and inter-species gene name ambiguity) may be interpreted as classification tasks. Thus, many approaches rely on supervised classification, which needs a non-negligible amount of training data. The availability of training data is often limited, and the available data sets tend to be imbalanced and, in some cases, heterogeneous [60]. Another problem of making extensive use of training data is that new biological entities are discovered very quickly. There may be no surface form in the previous existing literature for that sense or for that symbol [51]. Unsupervised or rule-based algorithms are either not available or do not provide similar results as supervised algorithms [58]. The question remains how algorithms provide reliable results despite requiring less or no training data.

Multiple Species Assignments. As shown in Sect. 3, a surface form of genes or proteins may belong to several different species (e.g. the proteins in sentence "human and mouse CD200R-CD4d3+4 and rCD4d3+4 protein" belong to the species human, mouse and rat). Hence, these surface forms refer to multiple entities. Existing algorithms usually extract the corresponding species providing the highest score. Furthermore, a static threshold often denotes the top-n relevant species to be extracted. However, existing approaches lack algorithms to investigate how many and which species belong to surface forms of genes or proteins.

7   Conclusion and Outlook on Future Work

Biomedical entity disambiguation has benefited from substantial interest from researchers and from practical needs of several domains (e.g. smart hospitals, infectious disease researchers), especially in the last ten years. In this work we provide an overview of biomedical entity disambiguation, with a special focus on annotated corpora, term disambiguation algorithms as well as gene and protein disambiguation algorithms.

As stated in the section above, there is a need for disambiguation systems for entities across several domains (e.g. entities from computer science and biomedical domain). A first important step would be to investigate how to combine two KBs, comprising entities from different domains, without mitigating disambiguation results due to an increase of heterogeneity and quantity.

Another important direction to add more flexibility to disambiguation systems is in reducing the necessity of training data by intelligent algorithm design and data exploitation. Most works are built upon supervised algorithms and need a huge amount of annotated data sets. Promising approaches avoid using expensive manually annotated data for each new domain and thus achieve better portability, e.g. [60].

With the entity linking approaches becoming more and more sophisticated, the application tasks shift to more complex recognition tasks. This shift can for instance, be observed in the community challenges issued by the BioNLP consortium. Starting with 2011, the event detection task additionally involved co-reference resolution and relation identification, and assumed a correct entity disambiguation system as prerequisite [8].

Acknowledgments. The presented work was developed within the EEXCESS project funded by the European Union Seventh Framework Programme FP7/2007–2013 under grant agreement number 600601.

References

1. Holzinger, A., Schantl, J., Schroettner, M., Seifert, C., Verspoor, K.: Biomedical text mining: state-of-the-art, open problems and future challenges. In: Holzinger, A., Jurisica, I. (eds.) Interactive Knowledge Discovery and Data Mining in Biomedical Informatics. LNCS, vol. 8401, pp. 271–300. Springer, Heidelberg (2014)
2. Gantz, J., Reinsel, D.: Extracting value from chaos. Technical report. IDC iview (2011)
3. Holzinger, A.: On Knowledge Discovery and Interactive Intelligent Visualization of Biomedical Data - Challenges in Human-Computer Interaction and Biomedical Informatics. INSTICC, Rome (2012)
4. Piateski, G., Frawley, W.: Knowledge Discovery in Databases. MIT press, Cambridge (1991)
5. Holzinger, A., Jurisica, I.: Knowledge discovery and data mining in biomedical informatics: the future is in integrative, interactive machine learning solutions. In: Holzinger, A., Jurisica, I. (eds.) Interactive Knowledge Discovery and Data Mining in Biomedical Informatics. LNCS, vol. 8401, pp. 1–18. Springer, Heidelberg (2014)
6. Davis, A.P., Grondin, C.J., Lennon-Hopkins, K., Saraceni-Richards, C., Sciaky, D., King, B.L., Wiegers, T.C., Mattingly, C.J.: The comparative toxicogenomics database's 10th year anniversary: update 2015. Nucleic acids research (2014)
7. Kim, J.D., Pyysalo, S.: Bionlp shared task. In: Dubitzky, W., Wolkenhauer, O., Cho, K.H., Yokota, H. (eds.) Encyclopedia of Systems Biology, pp. 138–141. Springer, New York (2013)
8. Pyysalo, S., Ohta, T., Rak, R., Sullivan, D., Mao, C., Wang, C., Sobral, B., Tsujii, J., Ananiadou, S.: Overview of the ID, EPI and REL tasks of BioNLP shared task 2011. BMC Bioinform. **13**(Suppl 11), S2 (2012)
9. Krell, T., Lacal, J., Busch, A., Silva-Jiménez, H., Guazzaroni, M.E., Ramos, J.L.: Bacterial sensor kinases: diversity in the recognition of environmental signals. Annu. Rev. Microbiol. **64**, 539–559 (2010)
10. Krauthammer, M., Nenadic, G.: Term identification in the biomedical literature. J. Biomed. Inform. **37**(6), 512–526 (2004). Named Entity Recognition in Biomedicine

11. Kulkarni, S., Singh, A., Ramakrishnan, G., Chakrabarti, S.: Collective annotation of wikipedia entities in web text. In: Proceedings of the 15th ACM SIGKDD international conference on Knowledge discovery and data mining, KDD 2009, pp. 457–466. ACM, New York, NY, USA (2009)

12. Grishman, R., Sundheim, B.: Message understanding conference-6: A brief history. In: Proceedings of the 16th Conference on Computational Linguistics, COLING 1996, vol. 1, pp. 466–471. Association for Computational Linguistics, Stroudsburg, PA, USA (1996)

13. Gentile, A.L., Zhang, Z., Xia, L., Iria, J.: Semantic relatedness approach for named entity disambiguation. In: Agosti, M., Esposito, F., Thanos, C. (eds.) IRCDL 2010. CCIS, vol. 91, pp. 137–148. Springer, Heidelberg (2010)

14. Cucerzan, S.: Large-scale named entity disambiguation based on Wikipedia data. In: Proceedings of the 2007 Joint Conference on Empirical Methods in Natural Language Processing and Computational Natural Language Learning (EMNLP-CoNLL), pp. 708–716. Association for Computational Linguistics, Prague, Czech Republic (2007)

15. Mihalcea, R., Csomai, A.: Wikify!: linking documents to encyclopedic knowledge. In: Proceedings of the sixteenth ACM conference on Conference on information and knowledge management, CIKM 2007, pp. 233–242. ACM, New York, NY, USA (2007)

16. Limaye, G., Sarawagi, S., Chakrabarti, S.: Annotating and searching web tables using entities, types and relationships. Proc. VLDB Endow. 3(1–2), 1338–1347 (2010)

17. Wacholder, N., Ravin, Y., Choi, M.: Disambiguation of proper names in text. In: Proceedings of the Fifth Conference on Applied Natural Language Processing, ANLC 1997, pp. 202–208. Association for Computational Linguistics, Stroudsburg, PA, USA (1997)

18. Marsh, E., Perzanowski, D.: Muc-7 evaluation of ie technology: overview of results. In: Proceedings of the Seventh Message Understanding Conference (MUC-7) (1998)

19. Campos, D.: Srgio Matos. Theory and Applications for Advanced Text Mining, J.L.O. (2012)

20. Bagga, A., Baldwin, B.: Entity-based cross-document coreferencing using the vector space model. In: Proceedings of the 36th Annual Meeting of the Association for Computational Linguistics and 17th International Conference on Computational Linguistics, COLING-ACL 1998, vol. 1, pp. 79–85. Association for Computational Linguistics, Stroudsburg, PA, USA (1998)

21. Chen, L., Liu, H., Friedman, C.: Gene name ambiguity of eukaryotic nomenclatures. Bioinformatics 21(2), 248–256 (2005)

22. Ogden, C., Richards, I.A.: The Meaning of Meaning: a Study of the Influence of Language Upon Thought and of the Science of Symbolism, 8th edn. Harcourt Brace Jovanovich, New York (1923). Reprint

23. Zwicklbauer, S., Seifert, C., Granitzer, M.: Do we need entity-centric knowledge bases for entity disambiguation? In: Proceedings of the 13th International Conference on Knowledge Management and Knowledge Technologies. i-Know 2013, pp. 4:1–4:8. ACM, New York, NY, USA (2013)

24. Kim, J.D., Ohta, T., Tateisi, Y., Tsujii, J.: Genia corpusa semantically annotated corpus for bio-textmining. Bioinformatics 19(suppl 1), i180–i182 (2003)

25. Yeh, A., Morgan, A., Colosimo, M., Hirschman, L.: Biocreative task 1a: gene mention finding evaluation. BMC Bioinform. 6(Suppl 1), S16 (2005)

26. Smith, L., Tanabe, L., Johnson nee Ando, R., Kuo, C.J., Chung, I.F., Hsu, C.N., Lin, Y.S., Klinger, R., Friedrich, C., Ganchev, K., Torii, M., Liu, H., Haddow, B., Struble, C., Povinelli, R., Vlachos, A., Baumgartner, W.A., Hunter, L., Carpenter, B., Tzong-Han Tsai, R., Dai, H.J., Liu, F., Chen, Y., Sun, C., Katrenko, S., Adriaans, P., Blaschke, C., Torres, R., Neves, M., Nakov, P., Divoli, A., Maa-Lpez, M., Mata, J., Wilbur, W.: Overview of biocreative II gene mention recognition. Genome Biol. 9(Suppl 2), S2 (2008)

27. Krallinger, M., Leitner, F., Rabal, O., Vazquez, M., Oyarzabal, J., Valencia, A.: Overview of the chemical compound and drug name recognition (chemdner) task. In: BioCreative Challenge Evaluation Workshop, vol. 2. (2013)

28. Van Auken, K., Schaeffer, M.L., McQuilton, P., Laulederkind, S.J., Li, D., Wang, S.J., Hayman, G.T., Tweedie, S., Arighi, C.N., Done, J. et al.: Corpus construction for the biocreative IV go task. In: Proceedings of the BioCreative IV workshop, Bethesda, MD, USA (2013)

29. Rebholz-Schuhmann, D., Yepes, A.J.J., Van Mulligen, E.M., Kors, J., Milward, D., Corbett, P., Buyko, E., Beisswanger, E., Hahn, U.: Calbc silver standard corpus. J. Bioinform. Comput. Biol. 8(01), 163–179 (2010)

30. Bada, M., Eckert, M., Evans, D., Garcia, K., Shipley, K., Sitnikov, D., Baumgartner, W.A., Cohen, K., Verspoor, K., Blake, J., Hunter, L.: Concept annotation in the craft corpus. BMC Bioinform. 13(1), 161 (2012)

31. Tsuruoka, Y., McNaught, J., Tsujii, J., Ananiadou, S.: Learning string similarity measures for gene/protein name dictionary look-up using logistic regression. Bioinformatics 23(20), 2768–2774 (2007)

32. Smith, L.H., Yeganova, L., Wilbur, W.J.: Hidden markov models and optimized sequence alignments. Comput. Biol. Chem. 27(1), 77–84 (2003)

33. Cohen, W., Minkov, E.: A graph-search framework for associating gene identifiers with documents. BMC Bioinform. 7(1), 440 (2006)

34. Winkler, W.E.: String comparator metrics and enhanced decision rules in the fellegi-sunter model of record linkage. In: Proceedings of the Section on Survey Research, pp. 354–359 (1990)

35. Rudniy, A., Song, M., Geller, J.: Mapping biological entities using the longest approximately common prefix method. BMC Bioinform. 15, 187 (2014)

36. Salton, G., Buckley, C.: Term-weighting approaches in automatic text retrieval. Inf. Process. Manage. 24(5), 513–523 (1988)

37. Needleman, S.B., Wunsch, C.D.: A general method applicable to the search for similarities in the amino acid sequence of two proteins. J. Mol. Biol. 48(3), 443–453 (1970)

38. Yu, H., Kim, W., Hatzivassiloglou, V., Wilbur, W.J.: Using medline as a knowledge source for disambiguating abbreviations and acronyms in full-text biomedical journal articles. J. Biomed. Inform. 40(2), 150–159 (2007)

39. Yu, H., Hripcsak, G., Friedman, C.: Mapping abbreviations to full forms in biomedical articles. JAMIA 9(3), 262–272 (2002)

40. Pustejovsky, J., Castaño, J., Saurí, R., Rumshinsky, A., Zhang, J., Luo, W.: Medstract: Creating large-scale information servers for biomedical libraries. In: Proceedings of the ACL-02 Workshop on Natural Language Processing in the Biomedical Domain, BioMed 2002, vol. 3, pp. 85–92. Association for Computational Linguistics, Stroudsburg, PA, USA (2002)

41. Pakhomov, S.: Semi-supervised maximum entropy based approach to acronym and abbreviation normalization in medical texts. In: Proceedings of the 40th Annual Meeting on Association for Computational Linguistics. ACL 2002, pp. 160–167. Association for Computational Linguistics, Stroudsburg, PA, USA (2002)

42. Chen, P., Al-Mubaid, H.: Context-based term disambiguation in biomedical literature. In: Proceedings of the 19th International FLAIRS conference FLAIRS Conference, pp. 62–67 (2006)

43. Salton, G., Wong, A., Yang, C.S.: A vector space model for automatic indexing. Commun. ACM **18**(11), 613–620 (1975)

44. Spärk Jones, K., Walker, S., Robertson, S.E.: A probabilistic model of information retrieval: development and comparative experiments. Inf. Process. Manage. **36**(6), 493–502 (2000)

45. Morgan, A.A., Lu, Z., Wang, X., Cohen, A., Fluck, J., Ruch, P., Divoli, A., Fundel, K., Leaman, R., Hakenberg, J., Sun, C., Liu, H.H., Torres, R., Krauthammer, M., Lau, W., Liu, H., Hsu, C.N., Schuemie, M., Cohen, K.B.: Overview of biocreative ii gene normalization. Genome Biol. **9**(Suppl 2), S13 (2008)

46. Hatzivassiloglou, V., Dubou, P.A., Rzhetsky, A.: Disambiguating proteins, genes, and RNA in text: a machine learning approach. In: ISMB (Supplement of Bioinformatics), pp. 97–106 (2001)

47. Manning, C.D., Raghavan, P., Schütze, H.: Introduction to Information Retrieval. Cambridge University Press, New York (2008)

48. Ginter, F., Boberg, J., Järvinen, J., Salakoski, T.: New techniques for disambiguation in natural language and their application to biological text. J. Mach. Learn. Res. **5**, 605–621 (2004)

49. McEntyre, J., Lipman, D.: PubMed: bridging the information gap. CMAJ Can. Med. Assoc. J. (journal de l'Association medicale canadienne) **164**(9), 1317–1319 (2001)

50. Pahikkala, T.: Filip Ginter, J.B.: Contextual weighting for support vector machines in literature mining: an application to gene versus protein name disambiguation. BMC Bioinform. **6**(1), 157 (2005)

51. Xu, H., Fan, J.W., Hripcsak, G., Mendonça, E.A., Markatou, M., Friedman, C.: Gene symbol disambiguation using knowledge-based profiles. Bioinformatics **23**(8), 1015–1022 (2007)

52. Wermter, J., Tomanek, K., Hahn, U.: High-performance gene name normalization with geno. Bioinformatics **25**(6), 815–821 (2009)

53. Hakenberg, J., Plake, C., Royer, L., Strobelt, H., Leser, U., Schroeder, M.: Gene mention normalization and interaction extraction with context models and sentence motifs. Genome Biol. **9**(Suppl 2), S14 (2008)

54. Hakenberg, J., Plake, C., Leaman, R., Schroeder, M., Gonzalez, G.: Inter-species normalization of gene mentions with GNAT. In: ECCB, pp. 126–132 (2008)

55. Podowski, R.M., Cleary, J.G., Goncharoff, N.T., Amoutzias, G., Hayes, W.S.: Azure, a scalable system for automated term disambiguation of gene and protein names. In: CSB, pp. 415–424. IEEE Computer Society (2004)

56. Wang, X., Tsujii, J., Ananiadou, S.: Disambiguating the species of biomedical named entities using natural language parsers. Bioinformatics **26**(5), 661–667 (2010)

57. Hsiao, J.C., Wei, C.H., Kao, H.Y.: Gene name disambiguation using multi-scope species detection. IEEE/ACM Trans. Comput. Biol. Bioinform. **11**(1), 55–62 (2014)

58. Wang, X., Matthews, M.: Distinguishing the species of biomedical named entities for term identification. BMC Bioinform. **9**(Suppl 11), S6 (2008)

59. Alex, B., Grover, C., Haddow, B., Kabadjov, M., Klein, E., Matthews, M., Roebuck, S., Tobin, R., Wang, X.: The ITI TXM corpora: tissue expressions and protein-protein interactions. In: Proceedings of LREC, vol. 8, Citeseer (2008)

60. Wang, X., Tsujii, J., Ananiadou, S.: Classifying relations for biomedical named entity disambiguation. In: Proceedings of the 2009 Conference on Empirical Methods in Natural Language Processing, EMNLP 2009, vol. 3, pp. 1513–1522. Association for Computational Linguistics, Stroudsburg, PA, USA (2009)
61. Harmston, N., Filsell, W., Stumpf, M.P.H.: Which species is it? Species-driven gene name disambiguation using random walks over a mixture of adjacency matrices. Bioinformatics **28**(2), 254–260 (2012)
62. Sabol, V., Kow, W.O., Rauch, M., Ulbrich, E., Seifert, C., Granitzer, M., Lukose, D.: Visual ontology alignment system - an evaluation. In: Proceedings of SIGRAD (2012)

Towards Personalization of Diabetes Therapy Using Computerized Decision Support and Machine Learning: Some Open Problems and Challenges

Klaus Donsa[1(✉)], Stephan Spat[1], Peter Beck[1], Thomas R. Pieber[1,2], and Andreas Holzinger[3]

[1] HEALTH - Institute for Biomedicine and Health Sciences,
JOANNEUM RESEARCH Forschungsgesellschaft mbH, Graz, Austria
klaus.donsa@joanneum.at

[2] Division of Endocrinology and Metabolism, Department of Internal Medicine,
Medical University of Graz, Graz, Austria

[3] Institute for Medical Informatics, Statistics and Documentation Research Unit HCI-KDD,
Medical University Graz, Auenbruggerplatz 2/V, 8036 Graz, Austria

Abstract. Diabetes mellitus (DM) is a growing global disease which highly affects the individual patient and represents a global health burden with financial impact on national health care systems. Type 1 DM can only be treated with insulin, whereas for patients with type 2 DM a wide range of therapeutic options are available. These options include lifestyle changes such as change of diet and an increase of physical activity, but also administration of oral or injectable anti-diabetic drugs. The diabetes therapy, especially with insulin, is complex. Therapy decisions include various medical and life-style related information. Computerized decision support systems (CDSS) aim to improve the treatment process in patient's self-management but also in institutional care. Therefore, the personalization of the patient's diabetes treatment is possible at different levels. It can provide medication support and therapy control, which aid to correctly estimate the personal medication requirements and improves the adherence to therapy goals. It also supports long-term disease management, aiming to develop a personalization of care according to the patient's risk stratification. Personalization of therapy is also facilitated by using new therapy aids like food and activity recognition systems, lifestyle support tools and pattern recognition for insulin therapy optimization. In this work we cover relevant parameters to personalize diabetes therapy, how CDSS can support the therapy process and the role of machine learning in this context. Moreover, we identify open problems and challenges for the personalization of diabetes therapy with focus on decision support systems and machine learning technology.

Keywords: Personalization · Machine learning · Decision support · Diabetes mellitus

© Springer International Publishing Switzerland 2015
A. Holzinger et al. (Eds.): Smart Health, LNCS 8700, pp. 237–260, 2015.
DOI: 10.1007/978-3-319-16226-3_10

1 Introduction

Diabetes mellitus (DM) is a growing global disease which highly affects the individual patient but it also represents a global health burden with financial impact on national health care systems. In 2013 approximately 382 million people were suffering from diabetes. It is estimated that this number will have reached 592 million in 2035. In addition, approximately 175 million diabetes patients are estimated to remain undiagnosed. In the U.S., the total estimated costs for diabetes were $174 billion for the year 2007 [1–3].

DM is a chronic illness of the metabolic system leading to high blood glucose levels. DM can be classified into two main clinical categories. Type 1 diabetes mellitus (T1DM) is caused by the loss of β-cells which are responsible for the storage and release of insulin and it mainly occurs in children, adolescents and young adults. In contrast, type 2 diabetes mellitus (T2DM) is determined by insulin resistance and develops due to a progressive insulin secretory defect, mostly in elderly people with overweight or obesity [4].

In both conditions continuous medical care is required to minimize the risk of acute (e.g. ketoacidosis) and long-term complications (e.g. diabetic foot syndrome, nephropathy, retinopathy, cardiovascular diseases or stroke) [5]. T1DM can only be treated with insulin, whereas a wide range of therapeutic options are available for patients with T2DM [4]. Adhering to therapy in chronic diseases like T2DM requires active participation and is often very burdensome for patients. Furthermore the effects of non-adherence are not immediately evident. Long-term complications like a diabetic foot syndrome or retinopathy take years to develop [6]. Diabetes therapy is complex and therapy decisions comprise various medical and life-style related information.

The availability of smart health technology [7] like continuous glucose monitoring (CGM) [8], physical activity detection [9], location and movement data, image recognition for planned meals [10], data from computerized diabetes diaries offer large data sets which can be used for therapy initialization or the further improvement of the therapy of an individual person suffering from diabetes. The large amount of generated data shows the importance of knowledge discovery in data handling/processing for therapy personalization [11]. Computerized decision support systems (CDSS) aim to improve the treatment process in the hospital [12] as well as at home [13].

In this work we cope with the potential of CDSS in the personalization of diabetes therapy to support the therapy process in different health care sectors and the role of machine learning. Moreover, open problems and challenges for the personalization of the diabetes therapy focusing on CDSS and machine learning technology are identified.

2 Glossary and Key Terms

Clinical Computerized Decision Support systems (CCDSS): 'Clinical Decision Support systems link health observations with health knowledge to influence health choices by clinicians for improved health care' - this definition has been proposed by Robert Hayward of the Centre for Health Evidence.

Computerized Physician Order Entry (CPOE) is a specialized sub-category of hospital electronic patient records for the management of physician orders. Such systems in general can offer reminders or prompts or even go further and perform calculations and offer decision support [14].

Diabetes Mellitus (DM) is a group of metabolic diseases in which high blood sugar levels over a prolonged period occur. DM is classified into two main clinical categories. Type 1 diabetes mellitus (T1DM) results from the body's failure to produce enough insulin. This form was previously referred to as "insulin-dependent diabetes mellitus" (IDDM) or "juvenile diabetes". The source is unknown. In contrast, type 2 diabetes mellitus (T2DM) develops due to a progressive insulin secretory defect in mostly elderly people with overweight or obesity [4, 6].

Diabetes Therapy: The success of a diabetes therapy depends on various factors. Regular measurement of the blood glucose level is the basal requirement for patients suffering from diabetes. The amount of necessary measurements depends on the intensification of the therapy and the progress of the diabetes disease. In contrast to type 1 DM that can only be treated with insulin, a wide range of therapeutic options are available for patients with type 2 DM. These are in the best case lifestyle change with change of diet and increased physical activity, but therapy options also include oral or injectable antidiabetic drugs and insulin administration. Furthermore insulin therapy itself opens a wide variety of different treatment options. The options range from an once-daily injection of a basal insulin dose (least intensive insulin therapy) to basal-bolus-insulin therapy, where a basal insulin dose and several bolus insulin doses are administered every day (intensified insulin therapy).

Glycated Hemoglobin (HbA1c) is a laboratory parameter which serves as a biomarker for the average blood glucose levels in patients over the previous 2 to 3 months prior to the measurement. In specific situations it can also be used as a measure of compliance with diabetes therapy. In diabetes mellitus, higher amounts of glycated hemoglobin have been associated with increased risk for microvascular complications (nephropathy, retinopathy) and to a lesser extend with macrovascular complications [6].

Glycemic Variability (GV) is the fluctuation of the blood glucose values and it is used as an indicator for the quality of diabetes management, as a high GV leads to increased risk of hypo- and hyperglycemic episodes.

Machine Learning (ML) is an algorithm-based and data-driven technique to automatically improve computer programs by learning from experience. Training of machine learning is performed by the estimation of unknown parameters of a model by using training sets. Literature separates between three main ML groups: supervised, unsupervised and reinforced learning.

3 Personalization of Diabetes Therapy

Individualized glycemic management of diabetes patients using insulin or oral antidiabetics is only possible due to recent advances in diabetes therapy, which increased the therapy safety and efficacy. The development of new insulin analogs led to a more predictable behavior of the drugs' blood glucose lowering effect [15, 16]. The first type of oral antidiabetic agents were developed in France in the 1940s [6]. Since then a multitude of new oral antidiabetic agents has been developed using different pharmacological and physiological strategies. Furthermore a paradigm shift happened in diabetes therapy over the past decades which led to patient empowerment and therapy personalization due to improved patient education.

The choice of therapy and potential personalization especially depends on the DM type. T1DM patients exclusively get insulin treatment. They either receive insulin via pump or by multiple daily injections. Here, personalization is possible by fine-tuning the parameters which drive the algorithms for the patient's individual insulin dose calculation [17]. Patients with a high risk of developing T2DM (pre-diabetes) are treated by lifestyle changes (diet change and increase of physical activity). T2DM patients have a broader array of therapeutic choices. Early onset of T2DM is treated by lifestyle changes or oral antidiabetic agents. If an intensification of the diabetes therapy is necessary different strategies involving insulin are treatment options. Here, personalization is possible by setting different treatment goals for the different stages of intensification (stepwise approach) of the insulin therapy [4, 16]. Less intensive insulin therapies comprise fixed insulin doses once a day, either adjusted by the physician at the next routine appointment or by the patient according to a schema. More intensive insulin regimens require multiple insulin doses per day and the consideration of carbohydrate intake and correction insulin for blood glucose levels outside of a target range. Here, personalization is also possible by fine-tuning the parameters which drive the algorithms for the patient's insulin dose. These algorithms are usually less complex than the ones used for T1DM and consequently they allow fewer options for personalization.

Recent guidelines recommend individualized diabetes therapy goals for people with DM [4]. In the current position statement for the management of T2DM the American Diabetes Association (ADA) and the European Association for the Study of Diabetes (EASD) placed great emphasis on patient-centered and personalized diabetes care [18]. Personalization of glycemic control targets is based on clinical parameters, including age, duration of DM, prevailing risk of hypoglycemia, presence of DM associated complications or co-morbidities and eco-system components [19]. In specific situations, the patient's glycated hemoglobin (HbA1c) serves as a measure of adherence with diabetes therapy. It is a biomarker for average blood glucose levels over the 2 to 3 months prior to the measurement. In diabetes therapy, certain blood glucose target values and HbA1c targets are defined for the patient's therapy. These targets are also determined by the choice of the patient's therapy option. Insulin for example is very effective in lowering HbA1c but insulin administration also increases the risk of hypoglycemia [16].

Individual therapy goals are set to avoid co-morbidities caused by poor glycemic control. To avoid the deterioration of a retinopathy, a better glucose control which means achievement of lower blood glucose levels and HbA1c targets is recommended [20, 21].

Two other important factors in personalizing diabetes therapy are age and diabetes duration. Consequently, lower targets should be achieved in younger patients to reduce the long-term risk of DM associated complications. In contrast, therapy should aim for safer targets and achieving them more slowly in older patients [22].

The setting in which the therapy is performed also strongly influences the therapy targets. Patients in a nursing home setting have typically less stringent targets to avoid hypoglycemia and less frequent blood glucose monitoring compared to patients in intensive care units [23]. Even though the exact therapy goals for patients in intensive care units are discussed controversially, intensive insulin therapy to maintain blood glucose at lower targets reduces morbidity and mortality in critically ill patients [24, 25].

In this article we focus on personalization of diabetes treatment rather than on all strategies of Personalized Medicine for Diabetes (PMFD), because widespread adoption of this global approach will only occur when the identification of risk factors through genotype or through biomarkers is accompanied by an effective therapy [26]. PMFD uses information about the genetic makeup of a person with diabetes to customize strategies for preventing, detecting, treating and monitoring their diabetes.

The vast amount of parameters for personalization makes diabetes management increasingly complex and diabetes complications remain a great burden to individual patients and the society [27]. Therefore it is hypothesized that the quality of these medical decisions can be enhanced by personalized decision support tools that summarize patient clinical characteristics, treatment preferences and ancillary data at the point of care [28].

4   Towards Personalization Using Decision Support Systems

Diabetes therapy takes place in different health care sectors. Every sector has different goals for the patients' diabetes therapy, as mentioned in the previous chapter. This results in specialized solutions for diabetes management available on the market, each specifically targeting a particular sector. Diabetes decision support systems are used in the following sectors:

1. *Patient self-management*

    a. *At home*
    b. *Primary care*
    c. *Outpatient care*

2. *Institutional care*

    a. *Nursing homes*
    b. *Hospital*

        i. *Inpatient care*
        ii. *Intensive care*

Decision support aiding health care professionals can primarily be found in insti-tutional care, whereas decision support targeting decisions performed by patients can mostly be found in the patient self-management sector. DM patients outside of insti-tutional care settings are on average younger, more independent and the focus of the therapy lies predominately on the diabetes disease. Patients in institutional care are primarily not admitted because of having DM, but for the complications associated with having DM (diabetic foot syndrome, nephropathy, retinopathy, cardiovascular diseases or stroke). DM is mostly regarded as concomitant disease and should therefore cause the least possible additional effort. Strategies for personalization of the diabetes therapy are therefore very different in the health care sectors. The following chapters summarize decision support systems and tools which facilitate a personalization of the diabetes therapy.

4.1 Diabetes Decision Support Applications for Self-Management

Medication support and therapy control: Self-management of the patient's insulin therapy requires the frequent measurement of blood glucose levels and the adjustment of the patient's medication. In *insulin therapy,* the calculation of the required insulin dose involves the use of more or less complicated mathematical formulas. Therefore mathematical aides, integrated into insulin pumps and glucose meters, have been devel-oped which model evidence based protocols for insulin dosage [29], so called *Automated Bolus Calculators (ABC)*. A recent review summarized the current state of the art on 'Glucose meters with built-in automated bolus calculator' [30]. The authors concluded that ABC incorporated in glucose meters can be regarded as bringing real value to insulin treated patients with diabetes. Software apps are not recommended up to now as they generally are of poor quality [31]. ABC allow very detailed personalization of the insulin dosing decision support. Aside from blood glucose levels, ABC also consider carbohy-drate intake and physical activity or health events to estimate insulin requirements. 'Automated' bolus calculation means that no manual bolus calculation is necessary. The identification of the correct parameters for personalization of the bolus calculation is a very individual and time consuming process for every user [29].

In the context of insulin-based diabetes therapy, a *controller* is an algorithm that controls the blood glucose values by titrating the amount of insulin. ABC are either rule or model based open-loop diabetes control methods. Independent of the used diabetes control method, it is categorized *open-loop system,* when a patient has the final power of decision [32].

Artificial pancreas systems are used for automated insulin injections. This type of diabetes control is characterized as *closed-loop.* Using these systems, model-predictive control algorithms are applied which use predictions of future glucose levels to estimate insulin requirement in insulin-pump therapy [33]. In these applications the input for the prediction models is continuous glucose monitoring data of T1DM patients.

Models of glucose dynamics for predictive purposes can mainly be divided into two categories; physiologically-oriented models and data-driven methods. The latter approach can furthermore be divided into time series analysis, using auto regressive models and machine learning methodologies [34]. Physiological models for blood glucose estimations are very accurate for short time predictions. They achieve a predictive capacity with a root mean square error (RMSE) of 3,6 mg/dl for a prediction horizon of 15 min [35]. Main advantages of these models compared to data-driven models are that there is no need to train these models and that their output is physiologically explainable. The main disadvantage is that if the difference is not explainable with the input variables no personalization of the algorithm is possible. *Data-driven glucose prediction* is a relatively new methodology compared to physiological glucose prediction. Similar to the development of the personal computer these technologies advanced in the late 1990s [36]. Main advantages of these models are that they are adaptive (self-learning) and patient specific without the need for developing a physiological model. Main disadvantages are that the system depends on the training data quality (garbage in and garbage out problem) and that the output of the system is not physiologically explainable.

For artificial pancreas systems relatively short prediction horizons and therefore a comprehensive monitoring using CGM are needed to enable closed-loop diabetes control [37]. But also patients without CGM which are not so intensively monitored could benefit from the prediction of future blood glucose levels. In [38–40] the authors devised an engine that predicts the expected blood glucose level at the next meal and the pending risks of hypoglycemia. They performed a study for safety and efficacy of using predicted data in dosing decision support for routine patient care. The prediction engine was used in patients who were referred to begin basal-bolus-insulin therapy. HbA1c levels fell significantly from 9.7 ± 1.7 % (baseline) to 7.9 ± 1.2 % (end of study), and hypoglycemia dropped fourfold.

Decision support tools for physicians: The patient's diabetes therapy is performed in close collaboration with primary care physicians and/or outpatient clinics. In [41] a computer application which helps primary care physicians in diabetes therapy decision making was developed and validated in a cluster-randomized clinical trial. The application was used to make decisions when starting, continuing or changing insulin and its dosage. The HbA1c in the intervention group was significantly reduced by the use of the decision support application (–0.69 %; $p = 0.001$). Electronic decision support tools for primary care physicians are summarizing information about patients' diabetes state, they provide reminders to required diabetes care and a support to patient education [42]. In [66] a CDSS was designed to help outpatient clinicians manage glycaemia in patients with T2DM. A rule-based expert system generates recommendations for changes in therapy and accompanying explanations. As mentioned earlier, T2DM is in contrast to T1DM a disease where a variety of different treatment options exist. Therefore, the system considers 9 classes of medications and 69 regimens with combinations of up to 4 therapeutic agents. The program is integrated in a web-based system for diabetes case management and supports a method for uploading data from glucose meters via telephone network. The system provides a report to the clinician regarding the overall quality of glycemic control and identifies problems, e.g., hyperglycemia, hypoglycemia, glycemic variability, and insufficient data.

Therapy aids and lifestyle support: To aid diabetes patients in the difficult task of estimating the correct personalized insulin requirement and to meaningful perform personalized control of therapy several tools are available.

Carbohydrate estimation: The success of the patient's insulin therapy is significantly dependent on the correct estimation of how nutrition influences insulin requirements [43]. This relationship is used in insulin therapy and it is called the *Carbohydrate Factor*. The factor is patient specific and may vary over the time of the day. Once accurate patient specific factors have been developed for different times of the day, correct estimation of the number of carbohydrates in a meal represents another obstacle in insulin therapy. Many patients might not estimate carbohydrates accurately and commonly either over or underestimate carbohydrates in a given meal [44, 45]. Another source of inaccuracy in estimating the patient's insulin requirement for meals based on carbohydrate counting is the composition of foods. Not only the number of carbohydrates influences the physiological glycemic response but also how the meal is absorbed. For example rich-in-fat meals need more time to be absorbed. Therefore these meals lead to prolonged hyperglycemia or the risk of hypoglycemia, if the insulin dose to cover the expected blood glucose rise for these meals is administered at once [46]. To approach the these problems, bolus calculators with nutrition data base software integrated into an insulin pump have been developed which are able to control the type of bolus [47]. In rich-in-fat meals the bolus is administered using a wave profile to administer insulin over a longer period of time compared to a single bolus.

For easier estimation of the meals' carbohydrate content, it has been proposed to implement nutrition data bases in food recognition systems. These systems use machine learning algorithms to categorize images of food [10, 48]. Therefore it is possible to identify the food by taking a picture of the meal using a smartphone. The systems are now able to detect food with an accuracy of up to 81 %. The final systems for diabetes therapy should include food segmentation such that images with multiple food types can also be addressed. Furthermore, to be eligible for diabetes therapy, the food volume should be estimated using multi-view reconstruction and the carbohydrate content should be calculated based on the computer vision results and nutrition data bases.

Activity recognition: The patient's insulin requirement and therefore the blood glucose levels are strongly influenced by the amount of physical activity and the health status. In diabetes therapy, establishing health benefits from physical activity is primarily done on the basis of self-reported data; typically surveys asking patients to recall what physical activity they performed according to their diabetes treatment plan. This is usually performed in T2DM patients. In T1DM patients using bolus calculators, physical activity often plays a major role in insulin calculation. The extent of change rate of the insulin dose depends on the intensity and duration of physical activity and varies among the patients [49]. Currently, this estimation process is very imprecise due to inaccurate reporting of physical activities. One solution to improve the accuracy of reporting could be automated activity recognition. Such systems consist of [50]:

(1) A sensing module that continuously gathers information about activities using accelerometers, microphones, light sensors, heart rate sensors, etc.
(2) A feature processing and selection module that processes the raw sensor data into features which categorize by activities.
(3) A classification module that uses the features identified in the previous data procession step to infer which activity has been performed.

Methods to predict activity-related energy expenditure have advanced from linear regression to innovative algorithms capable of determining physical activity types and the related metabolic costs. These novel techniques can measure the engagement in specific activity types [51]. Integrated into T2DM therapy, the therapy adherence to physical activity lifestyle interventions could be monitored. In T1DM, these new techniques could help to estimate the possibly required insulin reduction prior to sports using earlier recordings of similar intensive activities.

Activity recognition can also be implemented in a smart home-based health platform for behavior monitoring. In order to recognize activities being performed by smart home residents, machine learning algorithms could be used to classify sensor data streams. The smart home platform could be used to monitor the activity, diet, and exercise adherence of diabetes patients and evaluate the effects of alternative medicine and behavior regimens [52].

Lifestyle support/promotion: In T1DM patients, the loss of the insulin-producing beta cells of the islets of Langerhans in the pancreas results in the body to fail to produce insulin. T2DM is characterized by insulin resistance which, as the disease progresses, may be combined with a relatively reduced insulin secretion [6]. Therefore, the pathogenesis of T2DM, as a not rapidly progressing disease, can be prolonged by lifestyle interventions. Lifestyle intervention options are diets and/or increase of physical activity used to effectively manage patients in the pre-diabetes phase. Nevertheless, lifestyle management remains challenging for both, patients and clinicians. To track lifestyle events a variety of web- or mobile phone-based diabetes diaries are available. Petrella et al. developed a lifestyle support system which facilitates personalized, data-driven recommendations for people living with pre-diabetic and T2DM conditions [53]. The system suggests subtle lifestyle changes to improve overall blood glucose levels. To improve and support therapy adherence, a mobile phone app with lifestyle diary for coaching of the patient based on multiple psychological theories for behavior change has been recently developed. The user automatically receives generated messages with persuasive and personalized content [54]. Such systems can be used to enforce patient's therapy adherence and to help the patient to better understand their diabetes.

Pattern recognition for optimization of insulin therapy: Diabetes therapy leads to an accumulation of data. Sources are glucose data from blood glucose meters or CGM devices, records of diabetes diaries and therapy plans in more or less structured forms and data from different kinds of therapy aids like bolus calculators. The sources of data are often complex and weakly structured resulting in massive amounts of unstructured information. The data interpretation by the physicians and the patients is often performed without or with only weak decision aids. Currently few products enable data analysis using state of the art technologies which could be found for example in predictive analytics.

In a state of the art article targeting emerging applications for intelligent diabetes management, machine learning classification of blood glucose plots was highlighted [55]. The authors cope with the identification of excessive glycemic variability (EGV). The focus of diabetes therapy is to mimic physiological blood glucose profiles as close as possible. This means to avoid too high and too low blood glucose levels. But, to some extent high and low blood glucose levels are physiologically normal e.g. blood glucose rise after meals. Both upward (postprandial) and downward (interprandial) acute fluctuations of glucose around a mean value activate oxidative stress. As a consequence, it is strongly suggested that a global antidiabetic strategy should be aimed to reduce HbA1c, pre- and post-prandial glucose, as well as glucose variability to a minimum [56]. To the best of our knowledge no guideline-defined metric for classifying glycemic variability exists [57], nor a decision support system which aids in the detection of EGV [58]. Wiley et al. describe an automatic approach to detect EGV from CGM data [59]. Therefore, two physicians independently built a knowledge data base from CGM data which was used for the training of machine learning algorithms for EGV detection. The best performing prediction model achieved an accuracy of 93.8 %. The results of EGV predictions could inform clinical disease management, if a patient used CGM for the week preceding a routine appointment and therefore propose a personalization of the diabetes therapy approach.

Pattern recognition can be used to meaningfully identify blood glucose patterns, highlighting potential opportunities for improving glycemic control in patients who self-adjust their insulin [60]. Skrøvseth et al. conducted a study to identify how self-gathered data can help users to improve their blood glucose management [61]. The participants were equipped with a mobile phone application, recording blood glucose, insulin, dietary information, physical activity and disease symptoms in a minimally intrusive way. Data-driven feedback to the user in form of graphic representation of results from scale-space trends and pattern recognition methods may help patients to gain deeper insight into their disease. Blood glucose pattern analysis can also be found in ABC.

Long-term disease management: During the last decades, research in medicine has given increasing attention to the study of risk factors for diabetes complications. A practical application of risk factor studies is the development of risk assessment models (UKPDS model [62], Framingham model [63]). These models are able to provide a prediction, based on patient characteristics, of the patient's risk to develop diabetes associated complications [64].

In care management, which is facilitated from a payer perspective by health insurance companies, patients receive a personalization of care according to risk stratification. Stratification focuses on whether patients are ill enough to require ongoing support from a care manager. Having less serious chronic conditions warrant more intensive interventions to prevent them from worsening. Fairly healthy patients just need preventive care and education [65].

Risk preventive modelling enables the prognosis of future high-risk and/or high-cost patients, in patients having a chronic disease like T2DM. The models use a combination of factors, such as demographics, clinical parameters, lifestyle factors, family history of diabetes and metabolic traits [66]. Several machine learning techniques have been applied in clinical settings to predict disease progression and have shown higher accuracy for diagnosis than conventional methods [67]. Risk models have been integrated in guidelines and are increasingly advocated as tools to assist risk stratification and guide prevention and treatments decisions in diabetes care [68, 69]. It is hypothesized that with the prior knowledge of disease risk, the incidence of T2DM could be reduced considerably by implementing preventive measures in high-risk patients [4].

4.2   Diabetes Decision Support Applications for Institutional Care

Systems used in hospitals for management of diabetes care are very generic and they are designed to operate safely for the majority of patients. Currently personalization for patient characteristics plays a secondary role due to two factors: (1) A short length of stay does not allow the empiric development of patient specific factors which are crucial for the personalization of diabetes therapy. (2) Rigid hospital workflows and excessive workload of clinical personnel often prohibits the implementation of individualizations in diabetes therapies. Nonetheless, aside from these restrictions personalization is possible to some extent. Clinical computerized decisions support systems (CCDSS) often model evidence based guidelines which facilitate personalization of the estimation of medication requirements according to laboratory and demographic parameters [70–73].

Medication and workflow support: Clinical physician order entries *(CPOE)* are a specialized sub-category of hospital electronic patient records for the management of physician orders. They can be configured to support glucose management besides many other things. Such systems generally can offer reminders or prompts or go even further and perform calculations and offer decision support [14].

A recent review dealing with CCDSS' impact on healthcare practitioner performance and patient outcomes displayed significant evidence that CCDSS can positively impact healthcare providers' performance with drug ordering and preventive care reminders [74]. Furthermore, a recent diabetes guideline emphasizes the use of CCDSS and CPOE for insulin dosing [75]. This is a particularly important field of decision support because the correct handling of insulin in diabetes patients is prone to error. In a recent audit which investigated the quality of inpatient diabetes care, 36.7 % of the patients experienced at least one diabetes medication error during hospital stay [76]. A current review estimated that an adoption of CPOE systems in hospitals alone without decision support function leads to a 12.5 % reduction in medication errors [77]. A *Cochrane Review* assessed whether computerized advice on drug dosage has beneficial effects on patient outcomes compared with routine care. The review led to the conclusion that computerized advice on drug dosage (oral anticoagulants and insulin) results in a physiological parameter more often in the desired range. Furthermore, it tends to reduce the length of hospital stay compared to the length of hospital stay in routine care. Furthermore comparable or better cost-effectiveness ratios were achieved with computerized advice on drug dosage [78]. Diabetes medication CCDSS in the hospital range from administering and managing oral antidiabetic agents in non-critically ill patients to adjusting insulin infusion in critically ill patients. Insulin infusion in intensive care units is performed according to paper based nurse-directed insulin nomograms that adjust rates of insulin infusion according to the current rate of infusion and the blood glucose reading. These nomograms usually do not take patient-specific blood glucose trends into consideration and patients may oscillate between hypoglycemia and hyperglycemia [79].

By using a computerized insulin infusion algorithm in a CCDSS which also takes into account the patient's sensitivity to insulin, this system was used to safely achieve near normoglycemia in hospital inpatients. Additionally, there was lower incidence of hypoglycemia compared to initial studies [80].

The success that a CCDSS or CPOE is accepted by clinical staff greatly depends on the implementation into existing workflows [81, 82]. Automatic provision of decision support should be performed as part of the clinicians' workflow. Overall, the use of CCDSS and CPOE systems lead to a standardization of processes in clinical workflows.

Recently, a survey to map the current state of implementation of CPOE and CCDSS in Switzerland was performed. According to this survey, the introduction of CPOE in Swiss healthcare facilities is increasing. The types of CCDSS currently in service usually include only basic decision support related to drug, the co-medication or the setting, and only scarcely taking into account patient characteristics [83]. Future decision support tools must be designed to account for both clinical and patient characteristics [28].

5 Decision Support Using Machine Learning Technology

5.1 A Glimpse into Machine Learning Methods for Health Care

Advances in medical signal, image and text acquisition led to an extensive improvement of available patient-related medical data. These amounts of data make it difficult for health care professionals or patients to provide a timely treatment decision [84]. CDSS support the medical decision making process in diagnostics, therapeutics and prognostics in main medical disciplines [74]. Typical CDSS applications can be found for example in radiology, emergency medicine and intensive care, cardiovascular medicine, internal medicine or oncology [85–91].

In CDSS machine learning is an important underlying technology in many applications. For example radiology-based CDSS usually apply pattern recognition techniques based on machine learning for detection of medical conspicuities [92–94]. ECG signal processing used in cardiology is another promising machine learning approach in medical decision support applications [88, 95].

Machine learning is concerned with the question how computer programs automatically improve with experience [96]. Witten et al. [97] proposed *"Things learn when they change their behavior in a way that makes them perform better in future."* Practically, training of machine learning algorithms is performed by estimation of unknown parameters using training sets.

Duda et al. [98] separates between supervised, unsupervised and reinforced learning. In supervised learning (classification) category labels are manually assigned to each pattern by human experts. The set is divided into a training and a test set. The algorithm learns from the training set, which means that discriminating features of the patterns are identified. The test set is used for evaluation of classification quality. High accuracy means, that the features maximize the difference between patterns of different categories and underline the similarity of patterns in the same category. Typical supervised machine learning models are for example Support Vector Machines (SVM), k-Nearest Neighbors (K-NN), Decision Trees, Naïve Bayes, Random Forests and Neural

Networks. Unsupervised learning (clustering) is important if no human expert could or should label patterns. Unsupervised learning models build clusters based on the features of patterns. K-means, hierarchical clustering or expecting-maximization are typical algorithms to solve clustering problems. Reinforced learning follows a feedback mechanism. A feedback is given if a category is correct or incorrect. Based on this feedback, the algorithm should 'take new paths' and consequently improves with experience.

In the following section, typical applications of machine learning in the field of diabetes therapy are presented.

5.2 Application of Machine Learning for Diabetes Therapy

Diabetes therapy depends on medical, demographic and lifestyle-related parameters. These parameters include diabetes type, age, weight, diabetes duration, co-morbidities, blood glucose, physical activity and diet, to name a few examples. Latest innovations in sensor technology (CGM, clothes integrated movement sensors, smartphone-based image recognition) together with improved documentation effort of medical history in electronic patient records, diabetes-related patient diaries or telemonitoring systems provide large and valuable datasets for therapy-related decision making. Machine learning is regarded to be a helpful technology to support diabetes therapy. In the following, selected fields of machine learning in diabetes therapy are described.

Data-driven blood glucose prediction: No information about the physiology of diabetes is necessary in the data-driven blood glucose prediction. This is in contrast to systems which simulate the human physiology of the glucose-insulin regulatory systems. Data-driven techniques mainly rely on collected data and exploit hidden information in the data to predict future blood glucose levels [99].

With the availability and improved accuracy of tight glucose monitoring using CGM devices, research postulated the question if recent and future blood glucose values can be predicted from glucose history [100]. If this would be possible, hypoglycemic events could be detected or short and long term medication could be titrated.

The data-driven prediction of blood glucose can be considered as nonlinear regression problem between medication, food intake, exercise, stress etc. as input parameters and blood glucose value as output parameter [34]. Besides regression models [101, 102] and time series analysis [103], especially machine learning methods like artificial neural networks (ANN) [102, 104–107], support vector machines [108] and Gaussian models [105] have proven to be successful. Daskalaki et al. [109] presented a promising ANN model with a RMSE of only 4.0 mg/dl for a prediction horizon of 45 min for adults with T1DM. 94 % of the predictions were clinically accurate in the hypoglycemic range. Instead of conducting evaluation with real patients in a clinical study already measured data from patients were used for training and evaluation of the models. Thus, real patient data is needed for a final conclusion on the very good performance of the model. Pappada et al. [110] reported a RMSE of 43.9 mg/dl in his study with ten T1DM patients using a neural network model. The model predicted 88.6 % of normal glucose concentrations (>70 and <180 mg/dl), 72.6 % of hyperglycemia (>=180 mg/dl), but only 2.1 % of hypoglycemia (<=70 mg/dl) correctly within a prediction horizon of 75 min. Data-driven prediction approaches often lack on estimation of hypoglycemic and/or hyperglycemic events due to limited data on low and high blood glucose values [110]. Another problem of blood glucose prediction is the decreasing performance with increasing prediction horizon. Sufficient prediction is only possible in a 5 to 75 min. range [34, 109].

Data-driven prediction methods depend on the frequency and accuracy of available data. CGM measurements are not state-of-the-art in diabetes therapy due to the lack of accuracy and the missing reimbursement by health insurance companies [111].

Hypo-/Hyperglycemia detection: In contrast to the regression problem of blood glucose prediction, the detection of hypo- or hyperglycemic events can be treated as a typical classification problem. For a given set of input parameters, the model should detect if a hypo- or hyperglycemic event will take place. The prediction can be reduced to a binary classification problem which is easier to achieve than a continuous prediction of blood glucose values.

Sudharsan et al. [112] showed that the detection of hypo- and hyperglycemic events for patients with T2DM is achievable with high accuracy, even if only sparse blood glucose values based on self-monitored blood glucose (SMBG) readings once or twice a day are available. They trained the model with data from approximately 10 weeks. The prediction, if a hypoglycemic event will occur within the following 24 hours was achieved with a sensitivity of 92 % and a specificity of 70 %. By including medication information of the past days the specificity was improved to 90 %, although the prediction was narrowed to the hour of hypoglycemia.

Machine learning can also be used to improve the accuracy of CGM systems. Especially in the hypoglycemic range incorrect measurements can occur. Bondia et al. [113] successfully used Gaussian SVM to detect incorrect CGM blood glucose values with a specificity of approximately 93 % and sensitivity with 75 %.

Glycemic variability detection: Glycemic variability (GV), the fluctuation of blood glucose values, is an indicator for the quality of diabetes management due to increased risk of hypo- and hyperglycemic episodes [114]. In order to rate the quality of GV, numerous metrics have been defined in the last decades. Rodbard [58] rated metrics according to their importance and concluded that many metrics are overlapping. He suggested the following five metrics as the most relevant:

(1) SD_T (total variability in data set), (2a) SD_w (the average of the SDs within each day), or (2b) MAGE (average amplitude of upstrokes or downstrokes with magnitude greater than 1 SD), as a measure of within-day variability, and (3a) $SD_{b\ hh:mm}$ (average of all SDs for all times of day), or (3b) MODD (mean difference between glucose values obtained at the same time of day on two consecutive days under standardized conditions) as a measure of between-day variability.

Based on these metrics automated classification tasks can support healthcare professionals to identify patients at risk and to provide therapy suggestions [58]. Detection of GV is usually based on CGM signals which provide a comprehensive dataset of blood glucose values. Machine learning proved to be a valuable method to support the consensus building for a GV metric and to categorize CGM data according to this metric.

Marling et al. [57] applied multilayer perceptrons (MPs) and support vector machines for regressions (SVR) on 250 CGM plots of 24 h on a consensus perceived glycemic variability metric (CPGV) which have been manually classified into four CV classes (low, borderline, high, or extremely high) by twelve physicians. The manual classification was averaged and ten-fold cross validation was used for evaluation. SVR performed better than MPs. This CPGV metric obtained an accuracy of 90.1 %, with a sensitivity of 97.0 % and a specificity of 74.1 % and outperformed other metrics like MAGE or SD.

Controller for insulin-based diabetes therapy: Besides rule-based and model-based control methods, machine learning can be used to control blood glucose values. Machine learning is categorized as model-free method which means that it does not need a mathematical model of the glucose-insulin interaction [32, 115].

Zitar et al. [116] applied two different artificial neural network models; the Levenberg-Marquardt training algorithm of multilayer feed forward neural network (LM-NN) and a polynomial network (PN) as controller for insulin dose titration. Simulations were performed with a data set of 30,000 BG samples from 70 different patients. LM-NN proofed to be superior over PN. The authors stated that LM-NN has the potential to be used as model-free insulin controller.

Lifestyle support: Carbohydrate intake and physical activity are important parameters for the treatment of diabetes. While the former case increases the blood glucose values, the latter is glucose-lowering. Anthimopoulos et al. [10] presented an automated food recognition system using computer vision. They adapted the well-known bag-of-words approach from natural language processing to describe the identified features of the images. The classification was performed with three different supervised classifiers: SVM, ANN and Random Forests (RF). In total 5,000 images of typical European food-sets were available in 11 food classes. 60 % of the images were used for training and the remaining 40 % built the evaluation set. SVM performed best with an overall accuracy of 78 % for the image classification task. Future work will include automated food segmentation and food volume estimation to count carbohydrates. A smartphone-based real-time mobile food recognition system was presented by Kawano et al. [48]. They used bounding boxes to identify food items which have been classified in one of fifty food categories using SVM. Accuracy was 81.55 % taking the top five candidates into account. The automated system also showed better performance than the manual food selection from a hierarchical menu which has been tested in a small user study.

Physical activity detection is an important pre-requisite to estimate the energy expenditure. Ruch et al. [117] used a tri-accelerometer together with parameters like age, gender and weight, to train a decision tree based activity-specific prediction equation (Tree-ASPE) and an artificial neural network for energy expenditure estimation (ANNEE). Tree-ASPE outperformed ANNEE.

Ellis et al. [118] showed that RF classifier can be used to predict physical activity type and energy expenditure using accelerometers. In this study wrist accelerometers were more successful in physical activity detection, while hip accelerometers were superior in energy expenditure estimation.

6 Open Problems

In this chapter we highlight the main challenges for personalization of diabetes therapy. The focus lies on the problems regarding technical implementation rather than on the medical issues of therapy personalization.

Problem 1: Often DM is regarded with secondary importance especially in the clinical domain. This is very understandable because primarily the patients are not hospitalized because of having DM and the clinicians need to focus on the reasons for the admission. The clinicians are often not able to spend much time for the patient's diabetes therapy due to heavy workload and rigid clinical workflows. Therefore one focus in development of CDSS is the optimization of the devices' usability. In a systematic review investigating features critical to the success of CCDSS, the authors discovered that 75 % of interventions succeeded when the decision support was provided to clinicians automatically. None succeeded when clinicians were required to seek out the advice of the decision support system [82].

Problem 2: Modelling the human insulin system is a complex task. Different approaches have been developed in recent decades. The artificial pancreas is still a field of research and no end-consumer system is available on the market. The main reason for this is that precision and usability of continuous blood glucose (CGM) in daily use currently does not meet the needs for such a system.

Problem 3: Diabetes therapy is complex and varies from patient to patient. Success of diabetes therapy depends on many different factors. Nutrition intake, physical activity and current health status influences the specific therapy. Whereas T1DM can only be treated with insulin, for patients with T2DM a wide range of therapeutic options are available. The combination of factors influencing the therapy and the therapeutic options makes personalized therapy initialization and optimization a complex task. In addition, physicians and patients are often reluctant to start insulin donation and to intensify insulin treatment regimens due to the fear of hypoglycemia. Thus, the use of continuous monitoring with on-body sensors (blood glucose, nutrition intake, physical activity, health status) together with intelligent therapy prediction and optimization models can help to initiate and to optimize therapy with reduced risk of safety critical events like hypoglycemia.

Problem 4: Currently there are many freestanding software applications (apps) available for smartphones which calculate bolus doses of insulin. These apps regulate dosing of potentially dangerous insulin, which puts them in the domain of the Food and Drug Administration (FDA). But none have been approved by the FDA. Patients should not use such non-approved medical software because of the risk of being instructed to administer an unsafe dose of insulin [31]. Also in the institutional care sector, systems with decision support functionality are developed in this "grey area". CPOE systems in Europe have not yet been classified as Medical Devices [119]. A discussion is on-going whether vendors classify their products as Medical Devices Class IIa, Class I or not at all. The development process of CDSS is complicated and expensive due to requirements of Medical Device Directive (MDD) conform development.

Problem 5: Especially for the personalization of insulin therapy new sensor technologies integrated in applications like wearable devices are very promising. Using intelligent controllers which are available for example in integrated machine learning approaches [120] in combination with an arrangement of different sensors can lead to a significant improvement of insulin therapy. However, the problematic lies in the accuracy of currently available minimal intrusive sensor systems. Sensors have to be very accurate to prevent errors in insulin dose calculations. Also food and activity recognition systems have to be improved to be eligible for insulin therapy. Closed loop systems, such as artificial pancreas systems face the same problem. Currently, the biggest obstacle for safely running these systems is not the controller algorithm but the accuracy of CGM sensor systems.

Problem 6: Personalization of the patient's diabetes treatment demands patient involvement. The development of factors for personalization requires frequent documentation of relevant events (e.g. blood glucose, meals, physical activity, health status etc.) and adherence to the therapy goals. This human-in-the-loop situation demands special adaptations of CDSS [121]. For elderly, or unexperienced or less motivated patients this may quickly lead to a therapy overload. Unfortunately, the majority of T2DM patients are part of this group. The main challenge is the development of therapy aids which are as least intrusive and interactive as possible.

Problem 7: The treatment of diabetes takes place in different health care sectors (at home, outpatient care, nursing home, hospital care …). Borders between the health care sectors make it difficult to provide a decision support that can be seamless used in every sector. Consequently, the developed CDSS are focused on a special sector and usually interfaces for data-transfer are lacking. These developments make it difficult for patients and for healthcare professionals to initialize and optimize therapy. Future research should focus on cross-border treatment of patients with diabetes.

Problem 8: Machine learning is used to predict blood glucose values. As machine learning is a data-driven method quality of prediction depends on the quality of available data. Very low blood glucose (hypoglycemia) is an adverse event. Consequently, data is sparse which leads to unsatisfactory prediction results for these safety critical situations.

7   Future Outlook

Recent DM guidelines and advances in research and development of diabetes therapy highlight the importance of therapy personalization.

The ultimate goal of technical research in the field of diabetes therapy is to develop an artificial pancreas system. But as long as artificial pancreas systems are still a research field and no commercial product is available, CDSS are valuable tools to assist in the personalized decision making process. On the one hand, machine learning used within the CDSS (e.g. short-term glucose prediction, pattern recognition, physical activity detection) has proven to be a valuable method to support personalized therapy, but on the other hand it has shortcomings in terms of accuracy and usability in the daily routine (e.g. long-term blood glucose predictions, energy expenditure calculation, carbohydrate estimation).

Consequently, future CDSS using machine learning need to improve to be eligible for DM therapy. Personalization of DM therapy using CDSS is a promising future issue and various promising research routes exist.

References

1. Guariguata, L., Whiting, D.R., Hambleton, I., Beagley, J., Linnenkamp, U., Shaw, J.E.: Global estimates of diabetes prevalence for 2013 and projections for 2035. Diabetes Res. Clin. Pract. **103**, 137–149 (2014)
2. Beagley, J., Guariguata, L., Weil, C., Motala, A.A.: Global estimates of undiagnosed diabetes in adults. Diabetes Res. Clin. Pract. **103**, 150–160 (2014)
3. American Diabetes Association: Economic costs of diabetes in the U.S. in 2007. Diabetes Care **31**, 596–615 (2008)
4. American Diabetes Association: Standards of medical care in diabetes–2014. Diabetes Care **37**(Suppl. 1), S14–S80 (2014)
5. Deakin, T., McShane, C.E., Cade, J.E., Williams, R.D.R.R.: Group based training for self-management strategies in people with type 2 diabetes mellitus. Cochrane Database Syst. Rev. CD003417 (2005)
6. Berger, M.: Diabetes Mellitus. Urban & Fischer Verlag, München (2000)
7. Holzinger, A., Röcker, C., Ziefle, M.: From smart health to smart hospitals. In: Holzinger, A., Röcker, C., Ziefle, M. (eds.) Smart Health. LNCS, vol. 8700, pp. 1–19. Springer, Heidelberg (2015)
8. Battelino, T., Bode, B.W.: Continuous glucose monitoring in 2010. Int. J. Clin. Pract. Suppl. **65**, 10–15 (2011)
9. Anastasopoulou, P., Tubic, M., Schmidt, S., Neumann, R., Woll, A., Härtel, S.: Validation and comparison of two methods to assess human energy expenditure during free-living activities. PLoS One **9**, e90606 (2014)
10. Anthimopoulos, M.M., Gianola, L., Scarnato, L., Diem, P., Mougiakakou, S.G.: A food recognition system for diabetic patients based on an optimized bag-of-features model. IEEE J. Biomed. Heal. Inf. **18**, 1261–1271 (2014)
11. Holzinger, A., Dehmer, M., Jurisica, I.: Knowledge Discovery and interactive Data Mining in Bioinformatics–State-of-the-Art, future challenges and research directions. BMC Bioinf. **15**(Suppl. 6), I1 (2014)
12. Nirantharakumar, K., Chen, Y.F., Marshall, T., Webber, J., Coleman, J.J.: Clinical decision support systems in the care of inpatients with diabetes in non-critical care setting: systematic review. Diabet. Med. **29**, 698–708 (2012)
13. Cleveringa, F.G.W., Gorter, K.J., van den Donk, M., van Gijsel, J., Rutten, G.E.H.M.: Computerized decision support systems in primary care for type 2 diabetes patients only improve patients' outcomes when combined with feedback on performance and case management: a systematic review. Diabetes Technol. Ther. **15**, 180–192 (2013)
14. Ammenwerth, E., Schnell-Inderst, P., Machan, C., Siebert, U.: The effect of electronic prescribing on medication errors and adverse drug events: a systematic review. J. Am. Med. Inform. Assoc. **15**, 585–600 (2008)
15. Heise, T., Hermanski, L., Nosek, L., Feldman, A., Rasmussen, S., Haahr, H.: Insulin degludec: four times lower pharmacodynamic variability than insulin glargine under steady-state conditions in type 1 diabetes. Diabetes Obes. Metab. **14**, 859–864 (2012)
16. Paschou, S.A., Leslie, R.D.: Personalizing guidelines for diabetes management: twilight or dawn of the expert? BMC Med. **11**, 161 (2013)

17. Walsh, J., Roberts, R., Bailey, T.: Guidelines for insulin dosing in continuous subcutaneous insulin infusion using new formulas from a retrospective study of individuals with optimal glucose levels. J. Diabetes Sci. Technol. **4**, 1174–1181 (2010)

18. Inzucchi, S.E., Bergenstal, R.M., Buse, J.B., Diamant, M., Ferrannini, E., Nauck, M., Peters, A.L., Tsapas, A., Wender, R., Matthews, D.R.: Management of hyperglycemia in type 2 diabetes: a patient-centered approach: position statement of the American Diabetes Association (ADA) and the European Association for the Study of Diabetes (EASD). Diabetes Care **35**, 1364–1379 (2012)

19. Glauber, H.S., Rishe, N., Karnieli, E.: Introduction to personalized medicine in diabetes mellitus. Rambam Maimonides Med. J. **5**, e0002 (2014)

20. Ambrosius, W.T., Danis, R.P., Goff, D.C., Greven, C.M., Gerstein, H.C., Cohen, R.M., Riddle, M.C., Miller, M.E., Buse, J.B., Bonds, D.E., Peterson, K.A., Rosenberg, Y.D., Perdue, L.H., Esser, B.A., Seaquist, L.A., Felicetta, J.V., Chew, E.Y.: Lack of association between thiazolidinediones and macular edema in type 2 diabetes: the ACCORD eye substudy. Arch. Ophthalmol. **128**, 312–318 (2010)

21. Stratton, I.M., Adler, A.I., Neil, H.A., Matthews, D.R., Manley, S.E., Cull, C.A., Hadden, D., Turner, R.C., Holman, R.R.: Association of glycaemia with macrovascular and microvascular complications of type 2 diabetes (UKPDS 35): prospective observational study. BMJ **321**, 405–412 (2000)

22. Pozzilli, P., Leslie, R.D., Chan, J., De Fronzo, R., Monnier, L., Raz, I., Del Prato, S.: The A1C and ABCD of glycaemia management in type 2 diabetes: a physician's personalized approach. Diabetes Metab. Res. Rev. **26**, 239–244 (2010)

23. Valencia, W.M., Florez, H.: Pharmacological treatment of diabetes in older people. Diabetes Obes. Metab. **16**, 1192–1203 (2014)

24. Van den Berghe, G., Wouters, P.: Intensive insulin therapy in critically ill patients. New Engl. J. **345**, 1359–1367 (2001)

25. Abdelmalak, B.B., Lansang, M.C.: Revisiting tight glycemic control in perioperative and critically ill patients: when one size may not fit all. J. Clin. Anesth. **25**, 499–507 (2013)

26. Klonoff, D.C.: Personalized medicine for diabetes. J. Diabetes Sci. Technol. **2**, 335–341 (2008)

27. Raz, I., Riddle, M.C., Rosenstock, J., Buse, J.B., Inzucchi, S.E., Home, P.D., Del Prato, S., Ferrannini, E., Chan, J.C.N., Leiter, L.A., Leroith, D., Defronzo, R., Cefalu, W.T.: Personalized management of hyperglycemia in type 2 diabetes: reflections from a Diabetes Care Editors' Expert Forum. Diabetes Care. **36**, 1779–1788 (2013)

28. Wilkinson, M.J., Nathan, A.G., Huang, E.S.: Personalized decision support in type 2 diabetes mellitus: current evidence and future directions. Curr. Diab. Rep. **13**, 205–212 (2013)

29. Walsh, J., Roberts, R., Varma, C.: Using Insulin: Everything You Need for Success with Insulin. Torrey Pines Press, San Diego (2003)

30. Colin, I.M., Paris, I.: Glucose meters with built-in automated bolus calculator: gadget or real value for insulin-treated diabetic patients? Diabetes Ther. **4**, 1–11 (2013)

31. Klonoff, D.C.: The current status of bolus calculator decision-support software. J. Diabetes Sci. Technol. **6**, 990–994 (2012)

32. Lunze, K., Singh, T., Walter, M., Brendel, M.D., Leonhardt, S.: Blood glucose control algorithms for type 1 diabetic patients: a methodological review. Biomed. Signal Process. Control **8**, 107–119 (2013)

33. Turksoy, K., Cinar, A.: Adaptive control of artificial pancreas systems - a review. J. Healthc. Eng. **5**, 1–22 (2014)

34. Georga, E.I., Protopappas, V.C., Fotiadis, D.I.: Glucose prediction in type 1 and type 2 diabetic patients using data driven techniques. In: Knowledge-Oriented Applications in Data Mining (2011)
35. Hovorka, R., Chassin, L.J., Ellmerer, M., Plank, J., Wilinska, M.E.: A simulation model of glucose regulation in the critically ill. Physiol. Meas. **29**, 959–978 (2008)
36. Otto, E., Semotok, C., Andrysek, J., Basir, O.: An intelligent diabetes software prototype: predicting blood glucose levels and recommending regimen changes. Diabetes Technol. Ther. **2**, 569–576 (2000)
37. Hovorka, R., Canonico, V., Chassin, L.J., Haueter, U., Massi-Benedetti, M., Orsini Federici, M., Pieber, T.R., Schaller, H.C., Schaupp, L., Vering, T., Wilinska, M.E.: Nonlinear model predictive control of glucose concentration in subjects with type 1 diabetes. Physiol. Meas. **25**, 905–920 (2004)
38. Albisser, A.M., Baidal, D., Alejandro, R., Ricordi, C.: Home blood glucose prediction: clinical feasibility and validation in islet cell transplantation candidates. Diabetologia **48**, 1273–1279 (2005)
39. Albisser, A.M., Sakkal, S., Wright, C.: Home blood glucose prediction: validation, safety, and efficacy testing in clinical diabetes. Diabetes Technol. Ther. **7**, 487–496 (2005)
40. Albisser, A.M.: A graphical user interface for diabetes management that integrates glucose prediction and decision support. Diabetes Technol. Ther. **7**, 264–273 (2005)
41. Sáenz, A., Brito, M., Morón, I., Torralba, A., García-Sanz, E., Redondo, J.: Development and validation of a computer application to aid the physician's decision-making process at the start of and during treatment with insulin in type 2 diabetes: a randomized and controlled trial. J. Diabetes Sci. Technol. **6**, 581–588 (2012)
42. Wan, Q., Makeham, M., Zwar, N.A., Petche, S.: Qualitative evaluation of a diabetes electronic decision support tool: views of users. BMC Med. Inform. Decis. Mak. **12**, 61 (2012)
43. Smart, C.E., King, B.R., McElduff, P., Collins, C.E.: In children using intensive insulin therapy, a 20-g variation in carbohydrate amount significantly impacts on postprandial glycaemia. Diabet. Med. **29**, e21–e24 (2012)
44. Bishop, F.K., Maahs, D.M., Spiegel, G., Owen, D., Klingensmith, G.J., Bortsov, A., Thomas, J., Mayer-Davis, E.J.: The carbohydrate counting in adolescents with type 1 diabetes (CCAT) study. Diabetes Spectr. **22**, 56–62 (2009)
45. Smart, C.E., Ross, K., Edge, J.A., King, B.R., McElduff, P., Collins, C.E.: Can children with Type 1 diabetes and their caregivers estimate the carbohydrate content of meals and snacks? Diabet. Med. **27**, 348–353 (2010)
46. Smart, C.E.M., Evans, M., O'Connell, S.M., McElduff, P., Lopez, P.E., Jones, T.W., Davis, E.A., King, B.R.: Both dietary protein and fat increase postprandial glucose excursions in children with type 1 diabetes, and the effect is additive. Diabetes Care **36**, 3897–3902 (2013)
47. Pankowska, E., Blazik, M.: Bolus calculator with nutrition database software, a new concept of prandial insulin programming for pump users. J. Diabetes Sci. Technol. **4**, 571–576 (2010)
48. Kawano, Y., Yanai, K.: Real-time mobile food recognition system. In: 2013 IEEE Conference on Computer Vision and Pattern Recognition Workshops, pp. 1–7 (2013)
49. Rabasa-Lhoret, R., Bourque, J., Ducros, F., Chiasson, J.L.: Guidelines for premeal insulin dose reduction for postprandial exercise of different intensities and durations in type 1 diabetic subjects treated intensively with a basal-bolus insulin regimen (ultralente-lispro). Diabetes Care **24**, 625–630 (2001)

50. Choudhury, T., Borriello, G., Consolvo, S., Haehnel, D., Harrison, B., Hemingway, B., Hightower, J., "Pedja" Klasnja, P., Koscher, K., LaMarca, A., Landay, J.A., LeGrand, L., Lester, J., Rahimi, A., Rea, A., Wyatt, D.: The mobile sensing platform: an embedded activity recognition system. IEEE Pervasive Comput. 7, 32–41 (2008)
51. Bonomi, A.G., Westerterp, K.R.: Advances in physical activity monitoring and lifestyle interventions in obesity: a review. Int. J. Obes. (Lond) 36, 167–177 (2012)
52. Helal, A., Cook, D.J., Schmalz, M.: Smart home-based health platform for behavioral monitoring and alteration of diabetes patients. J. Diabetes Sci. Technol. 3, 141–148 (2009)
53. Petrella, R.J., Schuurman, J.C., Ling, C.X., Luo, Y.: A Smartphone-based Personalized System for Alleviating Type-2 Diabetes. American Telemedicine Association. p. P58 (2014)
54. Klein, M., Mogles, N., van Wissen, A.: Intelligent mobile support for therapy adherence and behavior change. J. Biomed. Inform. 51, 137–151 (2014)
55. Marling, C., Wiley, M., Bunescu, R., Shubrook, J., Schwartz, F.: Emerging applications for intelligent diabetes management. AI Mag. 33, 67 (2012)
56. Monnier, L., Colette, C.: Glycemic variability: should we and can we prevent it? Diabetes Care 31(Suppl. 2), S150–S154 (2008)
57. Marling, C.R., Struble, N.W., Bunescu, R.C., Shubrook, J.H., Schwartz, F.L.: A consensus perceived glycemic variability metric. J. Diabetes Sci. Technol. 7, 871–879 (2013)
58. Rodbard, D.: Interpretation of continuous glucose monitoring data: glycemic variability and quality of glycemic control. Diabetes Technol. Ther. 11(Suppl. 1), S55–S67 (2009)
59. Wiley, M., Bunescu, R.: Automatic detection of excessive glycemic variability for diabetes management. In: Machine Learning and Applications and Workshops (ICMLA), 2011 10th International Conference on Machine Learning and Applications. pp. 148–154 (2011)
60. Grady, M., Campbell, D., MacLeod, K., Srinivasan, A.: Evaluation of a blood glucose monitoring system with automatic high- and low-pattern recognition software in insulin-using patients: pattern detection and patient-reported insights. J. Diabetes Sci. Technol. 7, 970–978 (2013)
61. Skrøvseth, S.O., Arsand, E., Godtliebsen, F., Hartvigsen, G.: Mobile phone-based pattern recognition and data analysis for patients with type 1 diabetes. Diabetes Technol. Ther. 14, 1–7 (2012)
62. Stevens, R.J., Kothari, V., Adler, A.I., Stratton, I.M.: The UKPDS risk engine: a model for the risk of coronary heart disease in Type II diabetes (UKPDS 56). Clin. Sci. (Lond) 101, 671–679 (2001)
63. Wilson, P.W., D'Agostino, R.B., Levy, D., Belanger, A.M., Silbershatz, H., Kannel, W.B.: Prediction of coronary heart disease using risk factor categories. Circulation 97, 1837–1847 (1998)
64. Lagani, V., Koumakis, L., Chiarugi, F., Lakasing, E., Tsamardinos, I.: A systematic review of predictive risk models for diabetes complications based on large scale clinical studies. J. Diabetes Complications 27, 407–413 (2013)
65. Fortini, R.: Population Health Management Global Director of Healthcare Transformation, New York (2012)
66. Herder, C., Kowall, B., Tabak, A.G., Rathmann, W.: The potential of novel biomarkers to improve risk prediction of type 2 diabetes. Diabetologia 57, 16–29 (2014)
67. Choi, S.B., Kim, W.J., Yoo, T.K., Park, J.S., Chung, J.W., Lee, Y., Kang, E.S., Kim, D.W.: Screening for prediabetes using machine learning models. Comput. Math. Meth. Med. 2014, 618976 (2014)
68. MacLean, C.D., Littenberg, B., Gagnon, M.: Diabetes decision support: initial experience with the Vermont diabetes information system. Am. J. Public Health 96, 593–595 (2006)

69. Kengne, A.P., Masconi, K., Mbanya, V.N., Lekoubou, A., Echouffo-Tcheugui, J.B., Matsha, T.E.: Risk predictive modelling for diabetes and cardiovascular disease. Crit. Rev. Clin. Lab. Sci. **51**, 1–12 (2014)
70. Umpierrez, G.E., Smiley, D., Zisman, A., Prieto, L.M., Palacio, A., Ceron, M., Puig, A., Mejia, R.: Randomized study of basal-bolus insulin therapy in the inpatient management of patients with type 2 diabetes (RABBIT 2 trial). Diabetes Care **30**, 2181–2186 (2007)
71. Umpierrez, G.E., Smiley, D., Jacobs, S., Peng, L., Temponi, A., Mulligan, P., Umpierrez, D., Newton, C., Olson, D., Rizzo, M.: Randomized study of basal-bolus insulin therapy in the inpatient management of patients with type 2 diabetes undergoing general surgery (RABBIT 2 surgery). Diabetes Care **34**(Suppl.), 256–261 (2011)
72. Umpierrez, G.E., Hellman, R., Korytkowski, M.T., Kosiborod, M., Maynard, G.A., Montori, V.M., Seley, J.J., Van den Berghe, G.: Management of hyperglycemia in hospitalized patients in non-critical care setting: an endocrine society clinical practice guideline. J. Clin. Endocrinol. Metab. **97**, 16–38 (2012)
73. Umpierrez, G.E., Smiley, D., Hermayer, K., Khan, A., Olson, D.E., Newton, C., Jacobs, S., Rizzo, M., Peng, L., Reyes, D., Pinzon, I., Fereira, M.E., Hunt, V., Gore, A., Toyoshima, M.T., Fonseca, V.A.: Randomized study comparing a Basal-bolus with a basal plus correction insulin regimen for the hospital management of medical and surgical patients with type 2 diabetes: basal plus trial. Diabetes Care **36**, 2169–2174 (2013)
74. Jaspers, M.W.M., Smeulers, M., Vermeulen, H., Peute, L.W.: Effects of clinical decision-support systems on practitioner performance and patient outcomes: a synthesis of high-quality systematic review findings. J. Am. Med. Inform. Assoc. **18**, 327–334 (2011)
75. Moghissi, E.S., Korytkowski, M.T., DiNardo, M., Einhorn, D., Hellman, R., Hirsch, I.B., Inzucchi, S.E., Ismail-Beigi, F., Kirkman, M.S., Umpierrez, G.E.: American Association of Clinical Endocrinologists and American Diabetes Association consensus statement on inpatient glycemic control. Diabetes Care **32**, 1119–1131 (2009)
76. Rayman, G., National Health Service: National Diabetes Inpatient Audit 2012. United Kingdom (2013)
77. Radley, D.C., Wasserman, M.R., Olsho, L.E., Shoemaker, S.J., Spranca, M.D., Bradshaw, B.: Reduction in medication errors in hospitals due to adoption of computerized provider order entry systems. J. Am. Med. Inform. Assoc. **20**, 470–476 (2013)
78. Gillaizeau, F., Chan, E., Trinquart, L., Colombet, I., Walton, R.T., Rège-Walther, M., Burnand, B., Durieux, P.: Computerized advice on drug dosage to improve prescribing practice. Cochrane Database Syst. Rev. **11**, CD002894 (2013)
79. Yamashita, S., Ng, E., Brommecker, F., Silverberg, J., Adhikari, N.K.J.: Implementation of the glucommander method of adjusting insulin infusions in critically ill patients. Can. J. Hosp. Pharm. **64**, 333–339 (2011)
80. Davidson, P.C., Steed, R.D., Bode, B.W.: Glucommander: a computer-directed intravenous insulin system shown to be safe, simple, and effective in 120,618 h of operation. Diabetes Care **28**, 2418–2423 (2005)
81. Pearson, S.-A., Moxey, A., Robertson, J., Hains, I., Williamson, M., Reeve, J., Newby, D.: Do computerised clinical decision support systems for prescribing change practice? A systematic review of the literature (1990–2007). BMC Health Serv. Res. **9**, 154 (2009)
82. Kawamoto, K., Houlihan, C.A., Balas, E.A., Lobach, D.F.: Improving clinical practice using clinical decision support systems: a systematic review of trials to identify features critical to success. BMJ **330**, 765 (2005)
83. Carli-Ghabarou, D., Seidling, H.M., Bonnabry, P., Lovis, C.: A survey-based inventory of clinical decision support systems in computerised provider order entry in Swiss hospitals. Swiss Med. Wkly. **143**, w13894 (2013)

84. Belle, A., Kon, M.A., Najarian, K.: Biomedical informatics for computer-aided decision support systems: a survey. Sci. World J. **2013**, 769639 (2013)
85. Chen, W., Cockrell, C.H., Ward, K., Najarian, K.: Predictability of intracranial pressure level in traumatic brain injury: features extraction, statistical analysis and machine learning-based evaluation. Int. J. Data Min. Bioinform. **8**, 480–494 (2013)
86. Van Ginneken, B., ter Haar Romeny, B.M., Viergever, M.A.: Computer-aided diagnosis in chest radiography: a survey. IEEE Trans. Med. Imaging **20**, 1228–1241 (2001)
87. Ji, S.-Y., Smith, R., Huynh, T., Najarian, K.: A comparative analysis of multi-level computer-assisted decision making systems for traumatic injuries. BMC Med. Inform. Decis. Mak. **9**, 2 (2009)
88. Polat, K., Akdemir, B., Güneş, S.: Computer aided diagnosis of ECG data on the least square support vector machine. Digit. Signal Process. **18**, 25–32 (2008)
89. Watrous, R.L., Thompson, W.R., Ackerman, S.J.: The impact of computer-assisted auscultation on physician referrals of asymptomatic patients with heart murmurs. Clin. Cardiol. **31**, 79–83 (2008)
90. Lisboa, P.J., Taktak, A.F.G.: The use of artificial neural networks in decision support in cancer: a systematic review. Neural Netw. **19**, 408–415 (2006)
91. De Andrade, L., Lynch, C., Carvalho, E., Rodrigues, C.G., Vissoci, J.R.N., Passos, G.F., Pietrobon, R., Nihei, O.K., de Barros Carvalho, M.D.: System dynamics modeling in the evaluation of delays of care in ST-segment elevation myocardial infarction patients within a tiered health system. PLoS One **9**, e103577 (2014)
92. Zhou, Y., Yu, F., Duong, T.: Multiparametric MRI characterization and prediction in autism spectrum disorder using graph theory and machine learning. PLoS One **9**, e90405 (2014)
93. Cabezas, M., Oliver, A., Valverde, S., Beltran, B., Freixenet, J., Vilanova, J.C., Ramió-Torrentà, L., Rovira, A., Lladó, X.: BOOST: A supervised approach for multiple sclerosis lesion segmentation. J. Neurosci. Meth. **237**, 108–117 (2014)
94. Suk, H.-I., Lee, S.-W., Shen, D.: Subclass-based multi-task learning for Alzheimer's disease diagnosis. Front. Aging Neurosci. **6**, 168 (2014)
95. Li, Q., Rajagopalan, C., Clifford, G.D.: A machine learning approach to multi-level ECG signal quality classification. Comput. Meth. Programs Biomed. **117**, 435–447 (2014)
96. Mitchell, M.T.: Pattern Recognition and Machine Learning (1997)
97. Witten, I.H., Eibe, F., Hall, M.A.: Data Mining: Practical Machine Learning Tools and Techniques. Morgan Kaufmann, San Francisco (2011)
98. Duda, R.O., Hart, P.E., Stork, D.G.: Pattern Classification. Wiley-Interscience, Hoboken (2000)
99. Wang, Y., Wu, X., Mo, X.: A novel adaptive-weighted-average framework for blood glucose prediction. Diabetes Technol. Ther. **15**, 792–801 (2013)
100. Bremer, T., Gough, D.A.: Is blood glucose predictable from previous values? A solicitation for data. Diabetes **48**, 445–451 (1999)
101. Gani, A., Gribok, A.V., Rajaraman, S., Ward, W.K., Reifman, J.: Predicting subcutaneous glucose concentration in humans: data-driven glucose modeling. IEEE Trans. Biomed. Eng. **56**, 246–254 (2009)
102. Lu, Y., Rajaraman, S., Ward, W.K., Vigersky, R.A., Reifman, J.: Predicting human subcutaneous glucose concentration in real time: a universal data-driven approach. In: Conference on Proceedings of the IEEE Engineering in Medicine and Biology Society 2011, pp. 7945–7948 (2011)
103. Zanderigo, F., Sparacino, G., Kovatchev, B., Cobelli, C.: Glucose prediction algorithms from continuous monitoring data: assessment of accuracy via continuous glucose error-grid analysis. J. Diabetes Sci. Technol. **1**, 645–651 (2007)

104. Robertson, G., Lehmann, E.D., Sandham, W., Hamilton, D.: Blood glucose prediction using artificial neural networks trained with the AIDA diabetes simulator: a proof-of-concept pilot study. J. Electr. Comput. Eng. **2011**, 1–11 (2011)

105. Stahl, F.: Diabetes Mellitus Glucose Prediction by Linear and Bayesian Ensemble Modeling. control.lth.se. (2012)

106. Pappada, S.M., Cameron, B.D., Rosman, P.M.: Development of a neural network for prediction of glucose concentration in type 1 diabetes patients. J. Diabetes Sci. Technol. **2**, 792–801 (2008)

107. Zainuddin, Z., Pauline, O., Ardil, C.: A neural network approach in predicting the blood glucose level for diabetic patients. Int. J. Comput. Intell. **5**, 1–8 (2009)

108. Bondia, J., Tarin, C., Garcia-Gabin, W., Esteve, E., Fernandez-Real, J.M., Ricart, W., Vehi, J.: Using support vector machines to detect therapeutically incorrect measurements by the MiniMed CGMS(R). J. Diabetes Sci. Technol. **2**, 622–629 (2008)

109. Daskalaki, E., Prountzou, A., Diem, P., Mougiakakou, S.G.: Real-time adaptive models for the personalized prediction of glycemic profile in type 1 diabetes patients. Diabetes Technol. Ther. **14**, 168–174 (2012)

110. Pappada, S.M., Cameron, B.D., Rosman, P.M., Bourey, R.E., Papadimos, T.J., Olorunto, W., Borst, M.J.: Neural network-based real-time prediction of glucose in patients with insulin-dependent diabetes. Diabetes Technol. Ther. **13**, 135–141 (2011)

111. Heinemann, L., Franc, S., Phillip, M., Battelino, T., Ampudia-Blasco, F.J., Bolinder, J., Diem, P., Pickup, J., Hans Devries, J.: Reimbursement for continuous glucose monitoring: a European view. J. Diabetes Sci. Technol. **6**, 1498–1502 (2012)

112. Sudharsan, B., Peeples, M., Shomali, M.: Hypoglycemia prediction using machine learning models for patients with type 2 diabetes. J. Diabetes Sci. Technol. **9**, 86–90 (2015)

113. Bondia, J., Tarin, C., Garcia-Gabin, W., Esteve, E., Fernandez-Real, J.M., Ricart, W., Vehi, J.: Using support vector machines to detect therapeutically incorrect measurements by the MiniMed CGMS(R). J. Diabetes Sci. Technol. **2**, 622–629 (2008)

114. Qu, Y., Jacober, S.J., Zhang, Q., Wolka, L.L., DeVries, J.H.: Rate of hypoglycemia in insulin-treated patients with type 2 diabetes can be predicted from glycemic variability data. Diabetes Technol. Ther. **14**, 1008–1012 (2012)

115. Bastani, M.: Model-free intelligent diabetes management using machine learning (2014)

116. Zitar, R.A., Al-jabali, A.: Towards neural network model for insulin/glucose in diabetics-II. Informatica, **29**, 227–232 (2005)

117. Ruch, N., Joss, F., Jimmy, G., Melzer, K., Hänggi, J., Mäder, U.: Neural network versus activity-specific prediction equations for energy expenditure estimation in children. J. Appl. Physiol. **115**, 1229–1236 (2013)

118. Ellis, K., Kerr, J., Godbole, S., Lanckriet, G., Wing, D., Marshall, S.: A random forest classifier for the prediction of energy expenditure and type of physical activity from wrist and hip accelerometers. Physiol. Meas. **35**, 2191–2203 (2014)

119. Gärtner, A.: Patientendatamanagementsysteme als Softwaremedizinprodukt ? Eine regulatorische Betrachtung, Erkrath (2011)

120. Holzinger, A., Jurisica, I.: Knowledge discovery and data mining in biomedical informatics: the future is in integrative, interactive machine learning solutions. In: Holzinger, A., Jurisica, I. (eds.) Interactive Knowledge Discovery and Data Mining in Biomedical Informatics. LNCS, vol. 8401, pp. 1–18. Springer, Heidelberg (2014)

121. Holzinger, A.: Availability, Reliability, and Security in Information Systems and HCI. Springer, Heidelberg (2013)

State-of-the-Art and Future Challenges in the Integration of Biobank Catalogues

Heimo Müller[1]([✉]), Robert Reihs[1], Kurt Zatloukal[1], Fleur Jeanquartier[2],
Roxana Merino-Martinez[3], David van Enckevort[4], Morris A. Swertz[4],
and Andreas Holzinger[2]

[1] Institute of Pathology, BBMRI.at, Medical University Graz,
Neue Stiftingtalstraße 2/B61, 8036 Graz, Austria
heimo.mueller@medunigraz.at
[2] Institute for Medical Informatics, Statistics and Documentation Research Unit HCI-KDD,
Medical University Graz, Auenbruggerplatz 2/V, 8036 Graz, Austria
[3] Department of Medical Epidemiology and Biostatistics (MEB), Karolinska Institutet,
PO Box 281, 171 77 Stockholm, Sweden
[4] Genomics Coordination Center, University Medical Center Groningen,
PO Box 30.001, 9700 RB Groningen, The Netherlands

Abstract. Biobanks are essential for the realization of P4-medicine, hence indispensable for smart health. One of the grand challenges in biobank research is to close the research cycle in such a way that all the data generated by one research study can be consistently associated to the original samples, therefore data and knowledge can be reused in other studies. A catalogue must provide the information hub connecting all relevant information sources. The key knowledge embedded in a biobank catalogue is the availability and quality of proper samples to perform a research project. Depending on the study type, the samples can reflect a healthy reference population, a cross sectional representation of a certain group of people (healthy or with various diseases) or a certain disease type or stage. To overview and compare collections from different catalogues, we introduce visual analytics techniques, especially glyph based visualization techniques, which were successfully applied for knowledge discovery of single biobank catalogues. In this paper, we describe the state-of-the art in the integration of biobank catalogues addressing the challenge of combining heterogeneous data sources in a unified and meaningful way, consequently enabling the discovery and visualization of data from different sources. Finally we present open questions both in data integration and visualization of unified catalogues and propose future research in data integration with a linked data approach and the fusion of multi level glyph and network visualization.

Keywords: Biobank catalogue · Linked data · Minimum information about biobank data sharing (MIABIS) · Knowledge discovery · Visualization · Glyph

1 Introduction

Biobanking is a relatively new concept that has been evolving over the years to become an essential part of biomedical research. Thousands of biobanks worldwide have been

© Springer International Publishing Switzerland 2015
A. Holzinger et al. (Eds.): Smart Health, LNCS 8700, pp. 261–273, 2015.
DOI: 10.1007/978-3-319-16226-3_11

collecting *bio-specimens*, clinical and research data from millions of individuals in different stages of their lives, before, during and after disease. All this information is a great source of knowledge for fundamental biomedical research and has the potential to dramatically contribute to the development of better predictive, preventive, personalized and participatory (P4) healthcare.

The biobanking landscape is evolving from insulated local biospecimen repositories to robust organizations providing services that cover a large part of the biomedical research cycle, from the biobanking processes up to large scale molecular profiling. High-throughput technologies are more accessible to research-biobanking and the number of biobanks providing services that require large storage capability and parallel data analysis is increasing.

One of the major challenges in biobank research is to close the research cycle in such a way that all the data generated by one research study can be consistently associated to the original samples and hence data and knowledge can be reused in other studies.

Another challenge is to achieve a real informatics integration of biobanks. Even when the technical conditions are created to establish networks of biobanks where bio-resources can be visible to clinicians and researchers regardless of the geographical location, the harmonization process is still in a very early state, not only due to the heterogeneous representation of biobank data but also and most importantly, to the lack of standards for representing and implementing governing policies for ethics and regu-lation involving sharing of biobank human samples and data (Fig. 1).

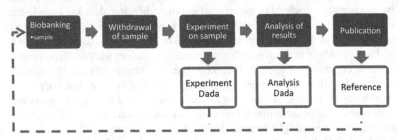

Fig. 1. Example of biomedical research cycle involving biobanking. Data generated in several steps of the research process should be associated to the original samples in the biobank for further reuse.

A high level of collaboration is necessary in the biobank community to gather suffi-cient resources to be pooled in order to reach statistical significance and hence derive consistent associations and meaningful knowledge. At the same time, data disclosure should be carried out in compliance with legal and regulatory issues at different levels: national, institutional, biobank, study participant, etc. Harmonization, standardization and regulations need to be in place in order to stimulate the development of infrastruc-tures for biobank interoperability in such a way that all these resources can be visible to the biomedical research community.

Several initiatives are on-going in that direction. For instance, MIABIS: Minimum Information About Biobank data Sharing [1] defines guidelines where several components represent different actors in the biomedical research process involving biobanking. Each component has a minimum list of attributes required to provide valuable information.

At the European level, an increasing number of countries and projects are implementing biobank catalogues aiming to make their bioresources visible and hence stimulate biobank data sharing. MIABIS is being implemented by several of these initiatives as part of their data models.

The *key question* when searching a biobank catalogue is where one can get the proper samples to perform a research project. Depending on the study type, the samples should reflect a healthy control population, a cross sectional representation of a certain group of people (healthy or with various diseases) or a certain disease type or stage. To support this first level of a query, harmonized disease and phenotype ontologies are needed. The typical next step of a query is which samples are available. Different study types require different types of samples (e.g., blood, serum plasma, tissue, urine, isolated biomolecules, such DNA, RNA, or proteins), and depending on the planned analytical challenge since currently there is no unique description of sample quality available. However the level of compliance with ISO and CEN standards as well as results from spot check quality testing will provide a common description of key quality-relevant parameters. Most research projects not only require access to samples but also access to detailed information on the sample and donor. To provide this information in an internationally standardized manner requires an enormous international collaborative effort addressing many as yet unsolved issues of health care informatics. The next level of information required to initiate a biobank-based research project refers to ethical and legal conformity and terms of access. All this above mentioned information should be provided in an aggregated manner to avoid privacy issues. However, the level of detail should be appropriate in order to allow the definition of a research project and to obtain approval by a research ethics committee or to pass scientific review. Finally, after successful approval of a research project by the respective bodies and after signature of a material transfer agreement, coded data related to individual samples and donors should be made available to users. All these different steps should be efficiently supported by an integrated biobank catalogue, thereby minimizing the time period from the first query to a biobank catalogue to the actual release of samples and data to start the research project. This time period is the most important performance indicator for biobanks.

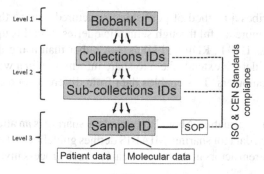

Fig. 2. Different levels of a biobanking catalogue. These levels correspond to the steps of user access needs.

To overview and compare collections from different catalogues and to search for new hypotheses, we must find unexpected patterns and interpret evidence in ways that frame new questions and suggest further explorations. Multilevel glyphs and visual analytics methods will help us to (1) overview collections within a catalogue as the human visual sense is optimized for parallel processing, (2) connect the global view with detail information, (3) provide different contextual views depending on users' needs and experience levels and (4) deal with heterogeneous data sets and different levels of data quality.

Current research highlights the need for interactive data visualization of biobank catalogues, while first approaches of visualization are already emerging [2, 3]. To further address this need it is essential to combine results of knowledge discovery in biobank catalogues and make use of visualization to benefit from the high visual data analysis capacities of humans in order to achieve new fundamental findings for predictive analytics in the medical domain.

2   Glossary and Key Terms

BBMRI-ERIC: is a pan-European distributed research infrastructure of biobanks and biomolecular resources. BBMRI-ERIC facilitates the access to biological resources as well as biomedical facilities and support high-quality biomolecular and medical research.

Biobank: is a collection of biological samples (e.g. tissues, blood, body fluids, cells, DNA etc.) in combination with their associated data. Here this term is mostly used for collections of samples of human origin.

BioSampleDB: The BioSamples database of the EMBL-EBI aggregates sample information for reference samples (e.g. Coriell Cell lines) and samples for which data exist in one of the EBI's assay databases such as ArrayExpress, the European Nucleotide Archive or PRoteomics IDentificates DatabasE.

Glyph: In the context of data visualization, a glyph is the visual representation of a piece of data where the attributes of a graphical entity are dictated by one or more attributes of a data record [4].

Linked Data: describes a method of publishing structured data so that it can be interlinked and become more useful through semantic queries. It builds upon standard Web technologies such as HTTP, RDF and URIs, but rather than using them to serve web pages for human readers, it extends them to share information in a way that can be read automatically by computers. This enables data from different sources to be connected and queried.

MIABIS: Minimum Information About Biobank data Sharing is an attempt to harmonize biobank and research data for sharing. MIABIS defines guidelines where several components represent different actors in the biomedical research process involving biobanking.

P4 Medicine: Preventive, Participatory, Pre-emptive, Personalized, Predictive, *Pervasive (= available to anybody, anytime, anywhere).*

TNM staging: The TNM Classification of Malignant Tumours (TNM) is a cancer staging notation system that gives codes to describe the stage of a person's cancer, when this originates with a solid tumor: T describes the size of the original (primary) tumor and whether it has invaded nearby tissue: N describes nearby (regional) lymph nodes that are involved: M describes distant metastasis.

Sample Collection: A collection of biological specimens (tissue, blood, blood components, cell lines, biopsies, etc.) having at least one common characteristic.

3   State-of-the-Art

3.1   Tools and Data Structure for Catalogue Harmonizations

3.1.1   State of the Art Publications

Data integration is about combining heterogeneous data sources in a unified and meaningful way, enabling the discovery and monitoring of data from different sources. Data integration is synonymous with sharing. When it comes to biomedical data, complexity, diversity and sensitivity are major factors driving the modelling of the integration process. An additional factor is the need to comply with the ethics and regulations for sharing clinical data or research data involving human samples.

The DataSHaPER (Data Schema and Harmonization Platform for Epidemiological Research) is both a scientific approach and a suite of practical tools. Its primary aims are to facilitate the prospective harmonization of emerging biobanks, provide a template for retrospective synthesis and support the development of questionnaires and information-collection devices, even when pooling of data with other biobanks is not foreseen. [5].

The integration of biomedical data is preceded by harmonization and standardization processes. The *BioSHaRE* project [6] demonstrated how retrospective harmonization could make it possible to perform complex statistical analysis on distributed data without compromising personal data protection when using DataSHIELD method [7]. Another interesting sharing tool is eagle-i [8] that allows bio-resources discovery among research institutions. Eagle-i uses the ontology approach to model research resources as instruments, platforms, protocols, bio-specimens, etc. in a distributed environment.

MIABIS is the BBMRI-ERIC's approach to harmonize biobank data for sharing. MIABIS 1.0 standardized high-level biobank data. The main components were "Biobank" and "Sample Collection" [1] (level 1 and level 2 as in Fig. 2). MIABIS paved the way for the creation of the first ontology for biobanking: omiabis [9]. These two steps in the biobank harmonization process have raised interest from the biobank community. Projects such as BiobankCloud (http://www.biobankcloud.com/), BioMed-Bridges (http://www.biomedbridges.eu/) and RD-Connect (http://rd-connect.eu/) are implementing MIABIS in their data models. Several catalogue initiatives from BBMRI-ERIC member states and BCNet (http://bcnet.iarc.fr/) are also implementing MIABIS. MIABIS 2.0 is currently being designed and a widespread adoption of this standard in Europe is expected.

In the biomedical research domain, integration and interoperability strongly depend on good methods and open source tools that facilitate the adoption of standards and hence stimulate the sharing culture. Harmonization is frustrating hard work that requires significant human intervention. Biomedical informatics systems are not easily modifiable or adaptable to new standards. We need best practice guidelines for semantics and data formats which at the same time, allow biobanks and researchers to continue using their own idiosyncratic semantics. Biobank management systems should be queried to discover what data they can offer and they should return references to data in the form of URIs (Uniform Resource Identifiers). In that way, biobanks and researchers will use their own semantic annotations rather than imposed specific labels and attributes. At some point the biomedical research domain will need to embrace the Internet of Thing (IoT) concept which is perfectly adaptable when it comes to cataloguing biobank and research bioresources.

Started in the BBMRI Netherlands, the MOLGENIS/catalogue tool was developed as a unified framework to create and federate local and national biobank catalogues. The result is an open source software that is now collaboratively developed between BBMRI, CTMM/TraIT, LifeLines, BioMedBridges and RD-Connect to name a few. The catalogue can host four levels of information: (1) biobank/study descriptions using custom or MIABIS standard format; (2) data schema/data dictionary of data elements; (3) aggregate data/sample availability counts and (4) the individual level data ready for analysis. Increasingly bigger datasets are required for epidemiological and genetic analysis and hence it is important to enable pooling of data from multiple biobanks.

The MOLGENIS/catalogue is building on the open source MOLGENIS platform [10]. This platform was chosen because its data structure can be completely configured using a meta-data definition in the Excel file. It offers pre-build components that allow users to (i) upload data (ii) visualize the data in aggregated or tabular form (iii) securely share the data through a comprehensive security model (iv) integrate data from different domains. In addition there are programmatic interfaces in R for statisticians and in javascript for systems integrators, which also allows data federation of multiple MOLGENIS/catalogues as demonstrated in the BioMedBridges project.

In collaboration with BioSHaRE, Biobank Standardisation and Harmonisation for Research Excellence in the European Union, MOLGENIS also addresses the challenge of data harmonization and integration via the BiobankConnect [11] toolbox aids, designed to assist with this arduous task.

3.1.2   Advantages and Disadvantages of Data Exchange Scenarios

With the growing possibilities of biobank data sharing, (associative) studies can achieve the power necessary to unveil biologically relevant associations for complex traits or diseases. However, sharing phenotypic and genotypic information opens up a complex world of regulatory compliance and privacy concerns. When this information is shared and can be linked back, re-identification of the subject becomes a real concern. Minimal information models help to reduce the risk of re-identification by reducing the available parameters. Study subject selection for most associative studies can be performed on coarser information that aggregates subjects in larger cohorts of similar patients and therefore protects their privacy.

Standardisation of the data items in the models improves the ability to find and reuse biobank data, but simplification of complex phenotypic information in coarse data vocabularies can lead to a loss of precision. Data vocabularies and ontologies need to be extensive and up to date with the current insights into the biology of diseases. A linked data model provides the ability to maintain the precision of rich ontologies by using linkage instead of tying a data model to a specific ontology.

3.2 Visual Analytics for Biobank Catalogues

3.2.1 State of the Art Publications

When dealing with the integration of biological data for analysis, visualization plays a major role in the process of understanding and sense-making [12, 13]. An overview about the state of the art in the visualization of multivariate data is given by Peng and Laramee [14] as well as Bürger and Hauser, where they discuss how different techniques take effect at specific stages of the visualization pipeline and how they apply to multivariate data sets being composed of scalars, vectors, and tensors. Moreover they provide a categorization of these techniques with the aim of a better overview of related approaches [15], with an update published 2009 [16].

Visual data exploration methods on large data sets were described by several authors, and particularly Keim [17], Hege et al. [18], Fayyad, Wierse and Grinstein [19], Fekete and Plaisant [20], and Santos and Brodlie [21] provide a good introduction to this topic. A recent state-of-the-art report on glyph based visualization and a good overview on theoretic frameworks, e.g. on the semiotic system of Bertin, was given by Borgo et al. [22].

Krzywinski et al., [23] introduce a network structure called hive plots, a graph visualization with nodes as glyphs in the context of systems biology. The layout and format of their glyphs is extensible and editable. Genes that connect cancer subsystems to other systems are represented differently. Another interesting application of glyphs for a visual analytics is an approach for understanding biclustering results from microarray data that has been presented by Santamaria, Theron and Quintales [24] and another one by Gehlenborg and Brazma [25] and Helt et al. [26] and a recent work by Konwar et al. [27]. The closest work to using glyphs with an adaptive layout is the work of Legg et al. [28] in the application domain of sport analysis. Here the data space is event based, and the adaptive layout strategy is focused on overlapping events with so called "macro glyphs", which combine several glyphs into one. In the "macro glyph" approach only scaling and no level of detail suitable for different screen spaces are applied. Maguire describes a taxonomy based glyph design with an application of biological workflow analysis [29, 30]. Last but not least Müller et al. [2] also show the usage of data glyphs in a visual analytics application and provide an outlook to a biomedical web visualization scenario, the combination of focus and context principle and different level of details are shown in Fig. 3.

A glyph visualizes the mortal state, disease free survival time and the T-Staging of a diagnosis, related to a sample, see Fig. 4.

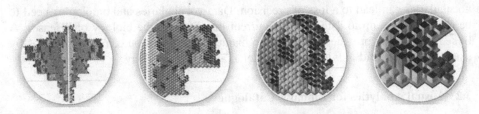

Fig. 3. Visualization of a collection of approx. 10.000 colon cancer samples, shown in 4 zoom levels [2]

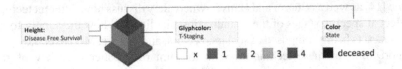

Fig. 4. Mapping of sample attributes to a 3D glyph

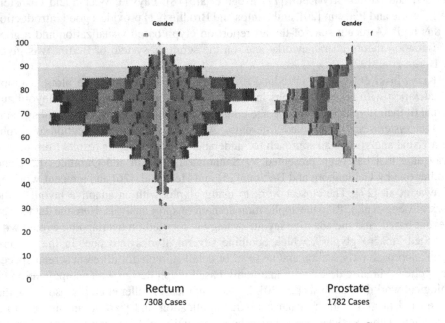

Fig. 5. Comparison of two sample collections of the Biobank Graz

In Fig. 5 the comparison of two sample collections of the Biobank Graz, each covering the same time range of 25 years is shown. The spatial arrangement of the glyphs is done in an age pyramid. All male cancer patients are on the left side and female patients on the right side. The vertical position of a glyph is determined by the patients' age and the horizontal position by the T-staging. We can clearly see the differences in the overall number of rectum and prostate cancer cases as well as the different distributions of T-Staging. Beside of the overview and comparison of two medium size groups, outliers and data errors can be identified easily, e.g. patients with age of 0 years and female prostate cancer cases.

3.2.2   Advantages and Disadvantages of Glyph Visualization

Glyph visualization is a natural way to map information about a sample to a visual symbol (glyph). However, the data density in this application area is very high, therefore we propose higher dimensional (2,5D and 3D) visualization methods. There are certain advantages and disadvantages when using 2D, 2.5D and 3D glyph visualizations, including different possibilities for placement strategies, linking and brushing, mapping low- to high-dimensional data, projection and interaction, up to benefitting from depth perception while dealing with issues such as occlusion and overlapping glyphs. A comprehensive comparison of 2D, 2.5D and 3D glyphs are still a matter to be researched: Systematically comparing visual complexity levels of 2D, 2.5D and 3D glyph visualization and methods for smooth transitions between different levels of graphical complexity are therefore fundamental research questions yet to be solved [2, 22].

Nonetheless, glyph based visualization is less abstract for effectively conveying information compared to other (visual) representations. By combining glyphs with graphs, certain visualization issues can be solved. For instance, by presenting complex glyphs as nodes in a network, the network itself shrinks and glyph visualization benefits from the graph's spatial arrangement.

Compare also Sect. 4 regarding Challenges and Sect. 5 regarding the fusion of Glyph and Network visualization.

4   Open Problems

Challenge 1: Harmonization of data is a huge challenge in the interchange of biobank data. Minimal data models such as MIABIS are a first attempt to harmonize the field, however, cannot solve the problem of harmonizing the data between different institutes. There is a **difference in the definition of data items.**

Challenge 2: tightly connected with challenge 1 there is also a **difference in the manner in which data is encoded.** Data is often encoded in non-standardized text (often called: "free text") and in the respective national language and there is a plethora of incompatible or only partially compatible ontologies and thesauri, often with merely a national scope.

Challenge 3: **Legal and ethical requirements** in the protection of patient privacy and concerns about losing control of research data lead to hurdles for sharing of data. Even though technical solutions exist to pseudonymize data, manual code lists are often used, which leads to **risk of privacy breaches.**

Challenge 4: At the same time sharing and linking data can **lead to re-identification through combination of data from different sources.**

Challenge 5: When the data elements are (well) structured and connected to ontologies we can analyse and compare collections in a catalogue. For this purpose glyph visualization techniques can be applied, i.e. for visual comparison, hypothesis generation and quality control. Here an appropriate glyph design is important, the development of glyph assessments algorithms and a **comparison of visual complexity levels of 2D, 2½ D and 3D glyph visualization** has to be done.

Challenge 6: Additionally to challenge 5, we have to find methods for **smooth transitions between different levels of graphical complexity.** The main research question here is, on how a high-density design (along with the challenges of the realization of such aspects, e.g. occlusion, depth perception and visual cluttering), indeed influence the user perception and recognition rate in glyph visualization. In particular it is necessary to look at the composition and interferences of visual variables and to carry out a systematic evaluation of shape/placement methods. There are a lot of studies comparing 2D versus 3D visualization techniques in the visualization of spatial related data, e.g. medical renderings or geographic data. However, for abstract information no inherent mapping of the data either to the 3D shape of a glyph nor the spatial position is given, which would be a natural model for visualization. In current solutions the glyph rendering method is changed due to the glyph size in the screen space. Future work should focus on methods for automatic glyph transitions (fusion of semantic and graphical zoom) and evaluate the results in a study.

Challenge 7: After the open problems of dimensionality and transitions of level of details are solved, algorithms for the **optimization of the sample/catalogue attribute mapping to visual variables** and methods for the **spatial arrangement of glyphs derived from network structures** have to be developed.

Challenge 8: In the fusion of glyph and network visualization a central research question is, **how a network topology can be mapped to glyph attributes** (e.g. relations of a sample to several studies) and/or to spatial positioning (e.g. temporal relation of a sample within a disease trajectory).

5 Future Outlook

A major task in the integration and harmonization of biobank catalogues is the provision of a terminology mapping service to overcome the non comparability of data from different sources. This results from the circumstance that institutions usually define their own best fitting data schema for sole use. As a consequence, they often omit to describe the exact meaning of their data, because they don't take into account, that it could be useful for future research performed by others. However, for the correct interpretation of data, especially for third parties, this is essential. Another problem is the fact that the partnering scientists have to consent on a common data schema, which is time-consuming and assumes willingness for compromises.

Within a terminology-mapping service attributes of structured data sets are described in a detailed both formal as well as descriptive manner. This should, in an ideal world, be done by data creators, who usually know their domain well. Future research will develop methods to support this process as well as motivating the users in doing it. This can e.g. be done with a visual analytics application, which indicates possible matches between attributes from different data schemas already during the data creation process and supports the description of data schema by presenting possible existing metadata sets matching as a starting point.

In the terminology mapping data elements are described by a set of overlapping ontologies, which can are modelled as Linked Data objects and stored together with sample attributes in a (federated) triple store. A toolbox for the curation of a triple store is essential to describe and improve data quality and completeness of a biobank catalogue. For the visualization part of such a toolbox glyphs together with focus and context techniques can be applied. To overcome certain issues with spatial placement of glyphs and benefitting from the fact that common graphs are easy to read, glyph visualization together with network visualization of Linked Data and enrichments on linked data graphs should be combined. In addition, nesting graphs by putting related biobank data into a formal graph structure may enable further exploration. With the emerging standards in biobank data sharing, this approach can be applied to visualise unified biobank catalogues and consequently, unveil and make sense of biologically relevant associations.

Acknowledgements. The work was performed and supported in the context of BBMRI.at the Austrian national node of BBMRI-ERIC. Our thanks are due to all partners for their contributions and various discussions and to Ms Penelope Kungl for proofreading.

References

1. Norlin, L., Fransson, M.N., Eriksson, M., Merino-Martinez, R., Anderberg, M., Kurtovic, S., Litton, J.-E.: A minimum data set for sharing biobank samples, information, and data: MIABIS. Biopreservation Biobanking **10**(4), 343–348 (2012). doi:10.1089/bio.2012.0003
2. Müller, H., Reihs, R., Zatloukal, K., Holzinger, A.: Analysis of biomedical data with multilevel glyphs. BMC Bioinform. **15**(Suppl 6), S5 (2014). doi:10.1186/1471-2105-15-S6-S5
3. Huppertz, B., Holzinger, A.: Biobanks – A source of large biological data sets: open problems and future challenges. In: Holzinger, A., Jurisica, I. (eds.) Knowledge Discovery and Data Mining. LNCS, vol. 8401, pp. 317–330. Springer, Heidelberg (2014)
4. Ward, M.O.: Multivariate data glyphs: Principles and practice. In: Handbook of Data Visualization, pp. 179–198. Springer, Berlin (2008). doi:10.1007/978-3-540-33037-0_8
5. Fortier, I., Doiron, D., Little, J., et al.: Is rigorous retrospective harmonization possible? Application of the DataSHaPER approach across 53 large studies. Int. J. Epidemiol. **40**, 1314–1328 (2011). doi:10.1093/ije/dyr106
6. Doiron, D., Burton, P., Marcon, Y., Gaye, A., Wolffenbuttel, B.H.R., Perola, M., Stolk, R.P., Minelli, F.L., Waldenberger, M., Holle, R., Kvaløy, K., Hillege, H.L., Tassé, A.M., Ferretti, V., Fortier, I.: Data harmonization and federated analysis of population-based studies: the BioSHaRE project. Emerg. Themes Epidemiol. **10**(1), 12 (2013). doi:10.1186/1742-7622-10-12

7. Wolfson, M., Wallace, S.E., Masca, N., Rowe, G., Sheehan, N.A., Ferretti, V., LaFlamme, P., Tobin, M.D., Macleod, J., Little, J., Fortier, I., Knoppers, B.M., Burton, P.R.: DataSHIELD: resolving a conflict in contemporary bioscience–performing a pooled analysis of individual-level data without sharing the data. Int. J. Epidemiol. **39**(5), 1372–1382 (2010). doi:10.1093/ije/dyq111

8. Vasilevsky, N., Johnson, T., Corday, K., Torniai, C., Brush, M., Segerdell, E., Wilson, M., Shaffer, C., Robinson, D., Haendel, M.: Research resources: curating the new eagle-i discovery system. Database (Oxford). 2012 Mar 20;2012:bar067. doi:10.1093/database/bar067

9. Brochhausen, M., Fransson, M.N., Kanaskar, N.V., Eriksson, M., Merino-Martinez, R., Hall, R.A., Litton, J.-E.: Developing a semantically rich ontology for the biobank-administration domain. J. Biomed. Semant. **4**(1), 23 (2013). doi:10.1186/2041-1480-4-23

10. Swertz, M.A., Dijkstra, M., Adamusiak, T., van der Velde, J.K., Kanterakis, A., Roos, E.T., Lops, J., Thorisson, G.A., Arends, D., Byelas, G., Muilu, J., Brookes, A.J., de Brock, E., Jansen, R.C., Parkinson, H.: The MOLGENIS toolkit: rapid prototyping of biosoftware at the push of a button. BMC Bioinform. **11**(Suppl 1), S12 (2010). doi:10.1186/1471-2105-11-S12-S12

11. Pang, C., Hendriksen, D., Dijkstra, M., van der Velde, K.J., Kuiper, J., Hillege, H., Swertz, M.: BiobankConnect: software to rapidly connect data elements for pooled analysis across biobanks using ontological and lexical indexing. J. Am. Med. Inform. Assoc. 2014 Oct 31. doi:10.1136/amiajnl-2013-002577. [Epub ahead of print] PubMed PMID: 25361575

12. O'Donoghue, S.I., Gavin, A.-C., Gehlenborg, N., Goodsell, D.S., Hériché, J.-K., Nielsen, C.B., Olson, A.J., Procter, J.B., Shattuck, D.W., Walter, T., Wong, B.: Visualizing biological data-now and in the future. Nat. Methods **7**(3 Suppl), S2–S4 (2010). doi:10.1038/nmeth.f.301

13. Turkay, C., Jeanquartier, F., Holzinger, A., Hauser, H.: On computationally-enhanced visual analysis of heterogeneous data and its application in biomedical informatics. In: Holzinger, A., Jurisica, I. (eds.) Knowledge Discovery and Data Mining. LNCS, vol. 8401, pp. 117–140. Springer, Heidelberg (2014)

14. Peng, Z., Laramee, R.S.: Higher dimensional vector field visualization: A survey. In: Tang, W., Collomosse, J. (eds.) Theory and Practice of Computer Graphics, pp. 149–163. The Eurographics Association (2009). doi:10.2312/LocalChapterEvents/TPCG/TPCG09/149-163

15. Bürger, R., Hauser, H.: Visualization of multi variate scientific data. In: Proceedings of EuroGraphics, pp. 117–134 (2007)

16. Fuchs, R., Hauser, H.: Visualization of multi-variate scientific data. Comput. Graph. Forum **28**(6), 1670–1690 (2009). doi:10.1111/j.1467-8659.2009.01429.x

17. Keim, D.A.: Visual exploration of large data sets. Commun. ACM **44**(8), 38–44 (2001). doi:10.1145/381641.381656

18. Hege, H.-C., Hutanu, A., Kähler, R., Merzky, A., Radke, T., Seidel, E., Ullmer, B.: Progressive retrieval and hierarchical visualization of large remote data. Scalable Comput. Pract. Exp. **6**(3), 60–72 (2001)

19. Fayyad, U., Grinstein, G.G., Wierse, A.: Information Visualization in Data Mining and Knowledge Discovery. Morgan Kaufmann, San Francisco (2002)

20. Fekete, J.-D., Plaisant, C.: Interactive information visualization of a million items. In: IEEE Symposium on Information Visualization, INFOVIS 2002, pp. 117–124. IEEE Computer Society (2002). doi:10.1109/INFVIS.2002.117315

21. Dos Santos, S., Brodlie, K.: Gaining understanding of multivariate and multidimensional data through visualization. Comput. Graph. **28**(3), 311–325 (2004). doi:10.1016/j.cag. 2004.03.013
22. Borgo, R., Kehrer, J., Chung, D.H.S., Laramee, R.S., Hauser, H., Ward, M., Chen, M.: Glyph-based visualization: Foundations, design guidelines, techniques and applications. In: Eurographics 2013-State of the Art Report, pp. 39–63. The Eurographics Association (2012)
23. Krzywinski, M., Birol, I., Jones, S.J.M., Marra, M.A.: Hive plots–rational approach to visualizing networks. Briefings Bioinform. **13**(5), 627–644 (2012). doi:10.1093/bib/bbr069
24. Santamaría, R., Therón, R., Quintales, L.: A visual analytics approach for understanding biclustering results from microarray data. BMC Bioinform. **9**, 247 (2008). doi: 10.1186/1471-2105-9-247
25. Gehlenborg, N., Brazma, A.: Visualization of large microarray experiments with space maps. BMC Bioinformatics **10**(Suppl 13), O7 (2009). doi:10.1186/1471-2105-10-S13-O7
26. Helt, G.A., Nicol, J.W., Erwin, E., Blossom, E., Blanchard, S.G., Chervitz, S.A., Harmon, C., Loraine, A.E.: Genoviz Software Development Kit: Java tool kit for building genomics visualization applications. BMC Bioinform. **10**, 266 (2009). doi:10.1186/1471-2105-10-266
27. Konwar, K.M., Hanson, N.W., Pagé, A.P., Hallam, S.J.: MetaPathways: A modular pipeline for constructing pathway/genome databases from environmental sequence information. BMC Bioinform. **14**, 202 (2013). doi:10.1186/1471-2105-14-202
28. Legg, P.A., Chung, D.H.S., Parry, M.L., Jones, M.W., Long, R., Griffiths, I.W., Chen, M.: MatchPad: Interactive glyph-based visualization for real-time sports performance analysis. Comput. Graph. Forum **31**(3pt4), 1255–1264 (2012). doi:10.1111/j.1467-8659.2012.03118.x
29. Maguire, E., Rocca-Serra, P., Sansone, S.A., Davies, J., Chen, M.: Taxonomy-based glyph design – with a case study on visualizing workflows of biological experiments. IEEE Trans. Vis. Comput. Graph. **18**(12), 2603–2612 (2012)
30. Maguire, E., Rocca-Serra, P., Sansone, S.A., Davies, J., Chen, M.: Visual compression of workflow visualizations with automated detection of macro motifs. IEEE Trans. Vis. Comput. Graph. **19**(12), 2576–2585 (2013)

Author Index

Printed in the United States
By Bookmasters